Human Blood Group Systems and Haemoglobinopathies

Edited by Osaro Erhabor and Anjana Munshi

Published in London, United Kingdom

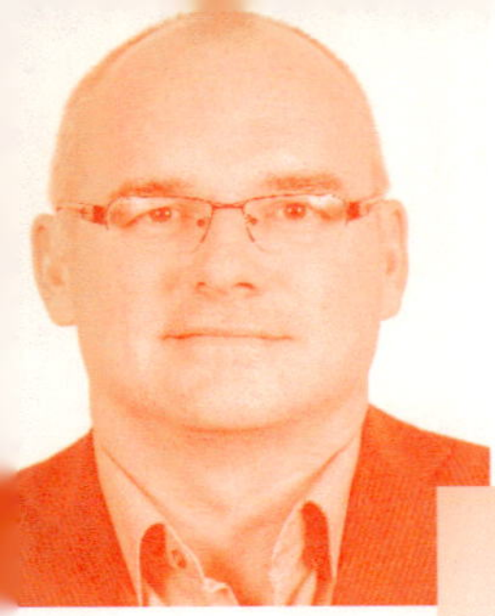
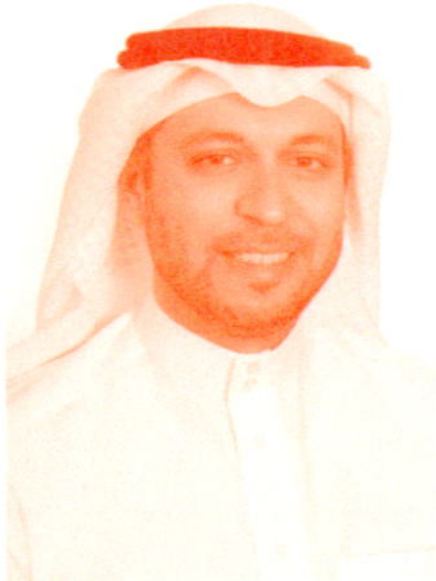
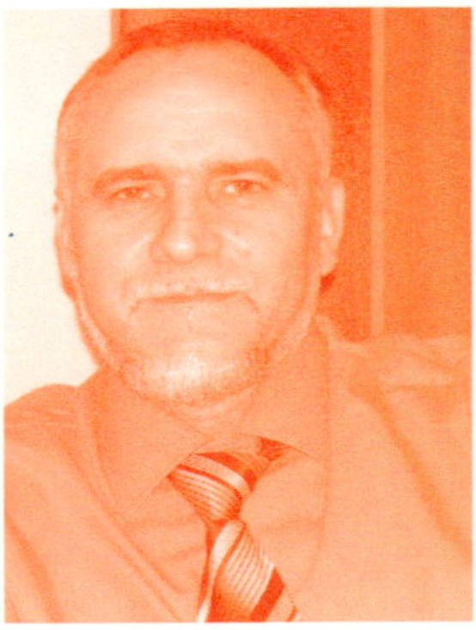
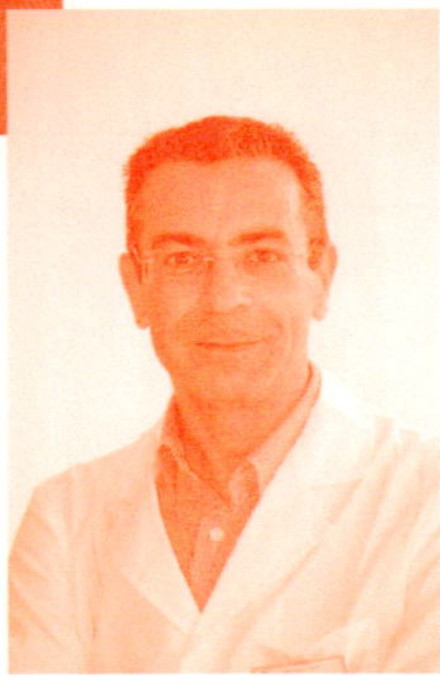
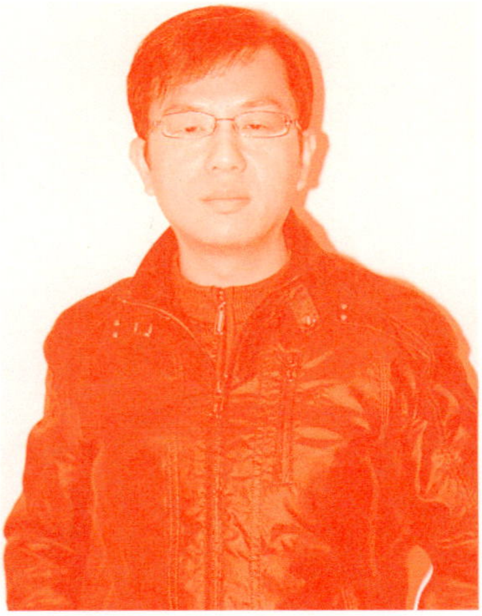
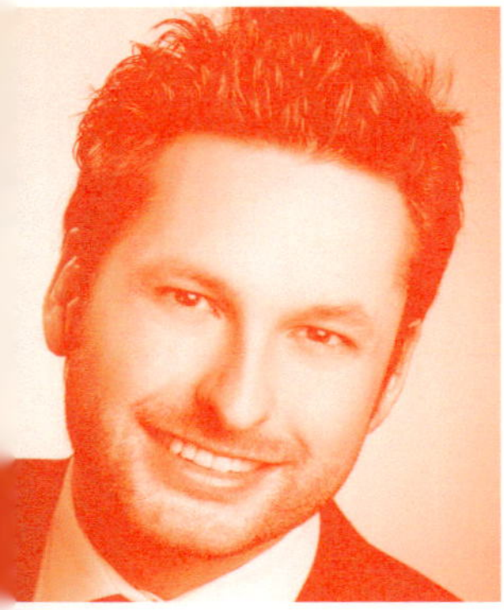
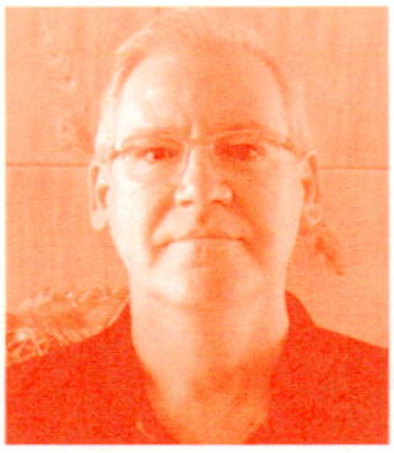

IntechOpen

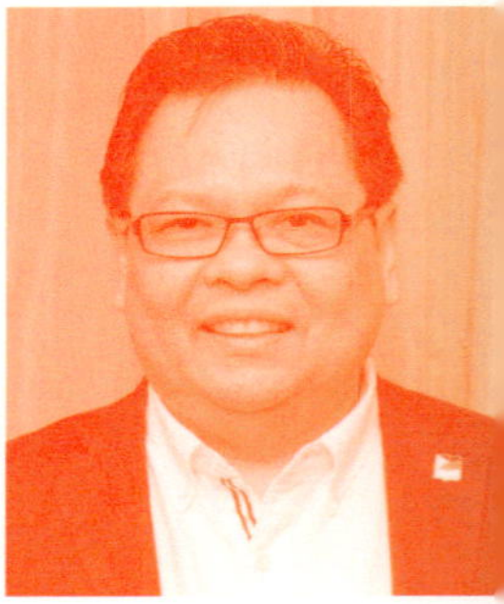
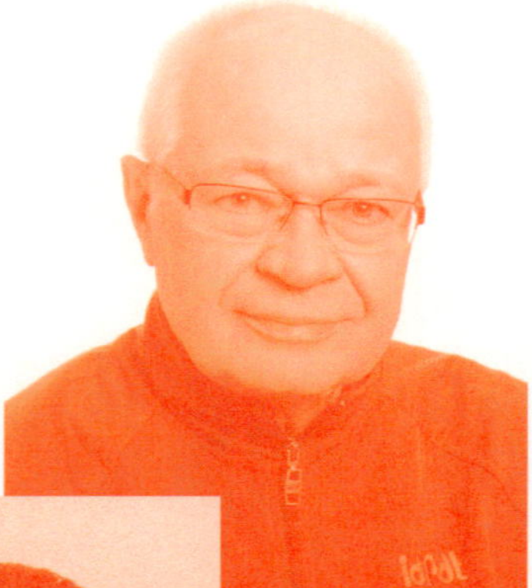
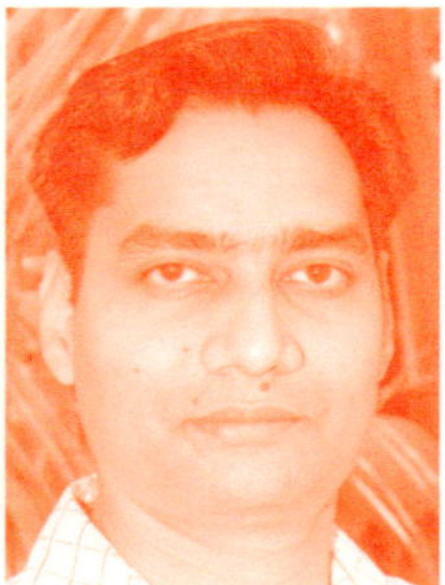
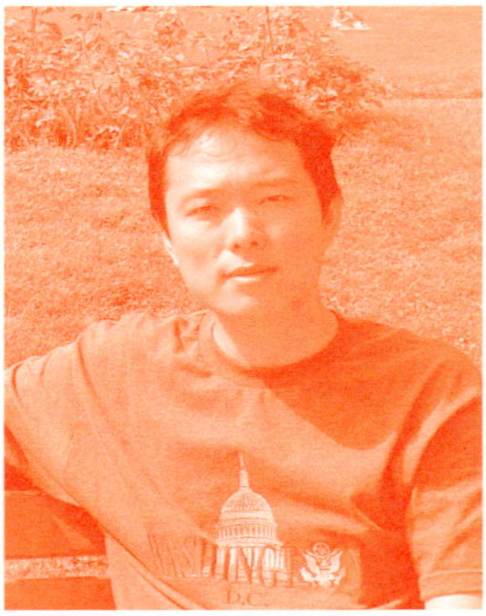
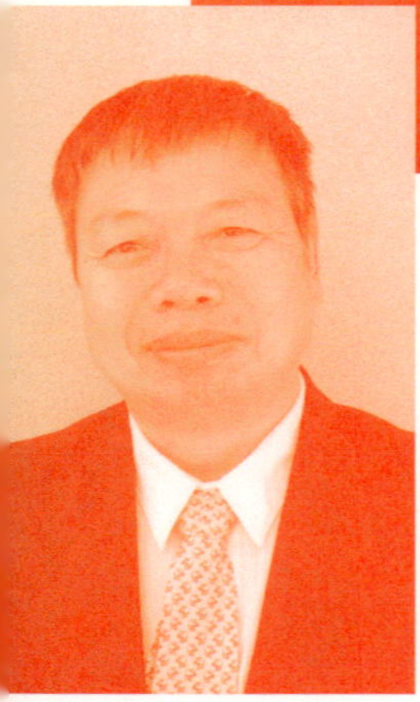
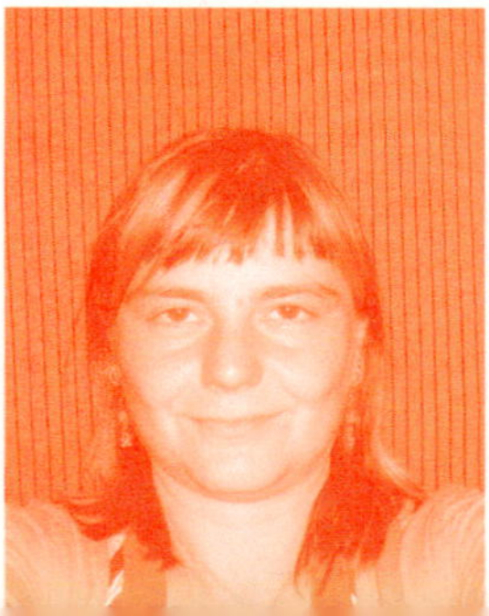

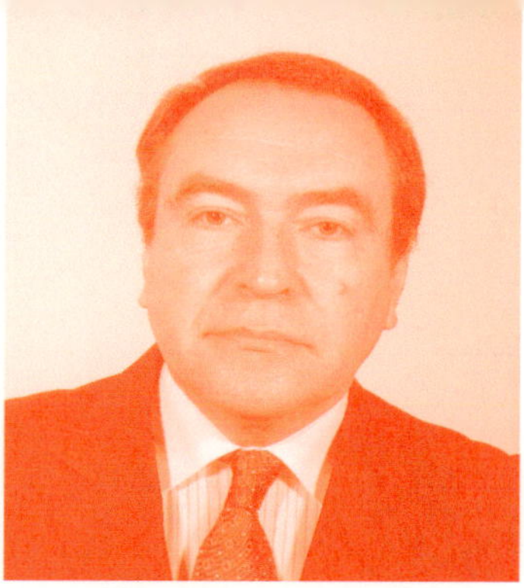

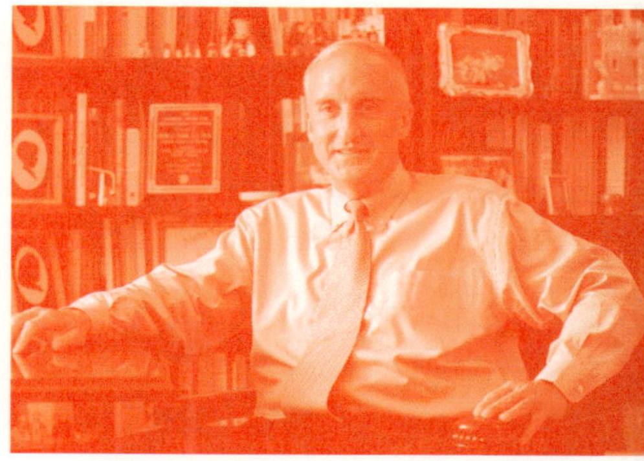

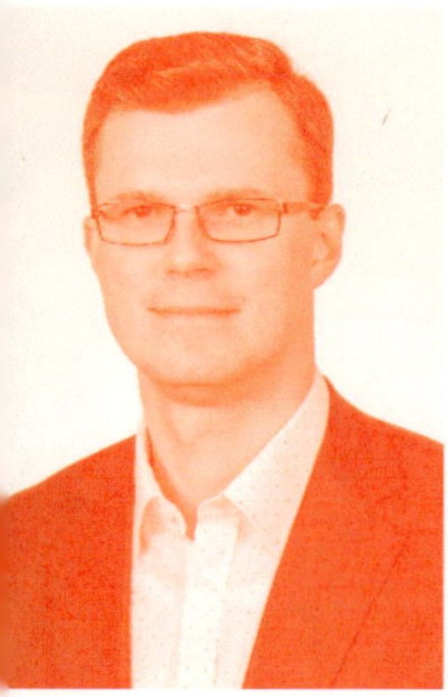

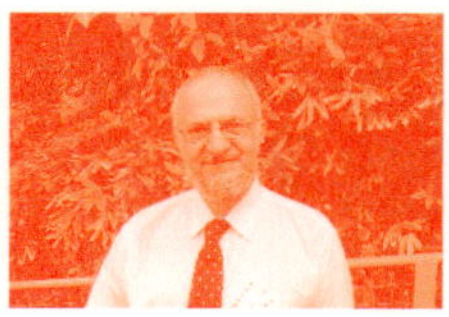

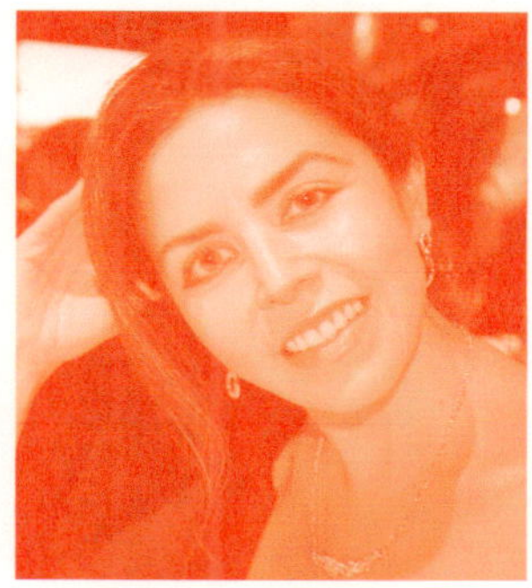

Supporting open minds since 2005

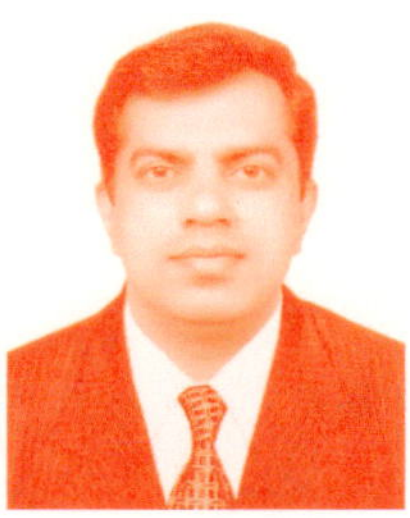

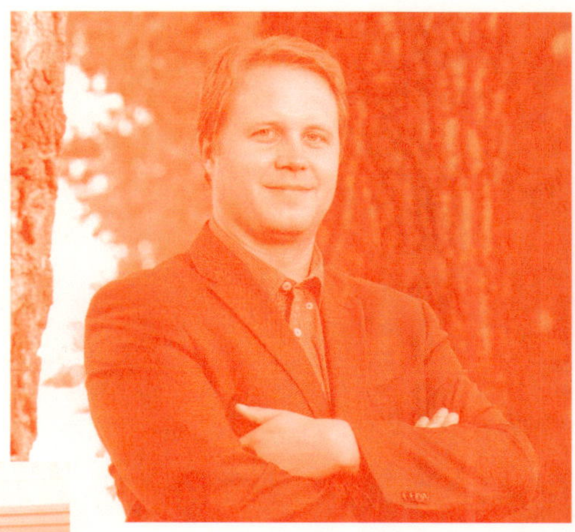

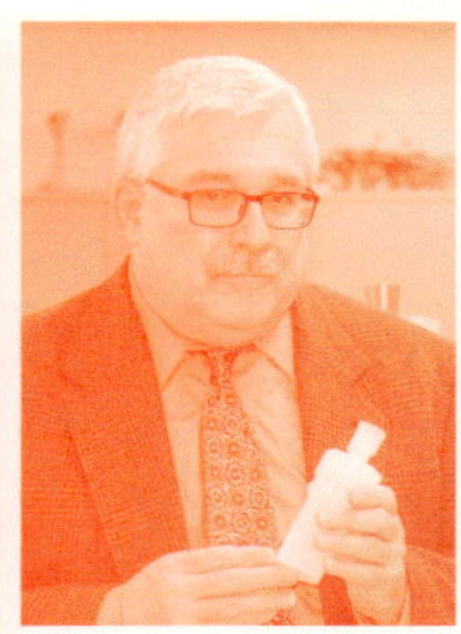

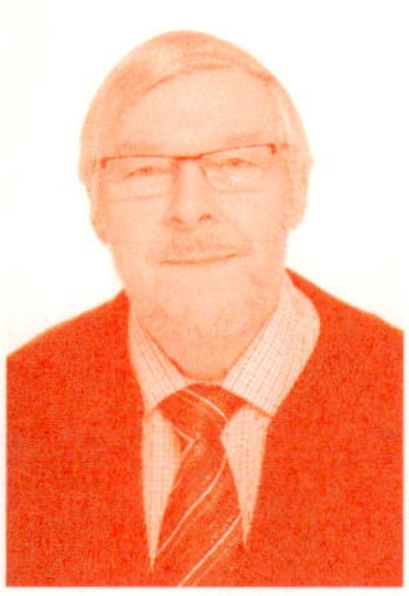

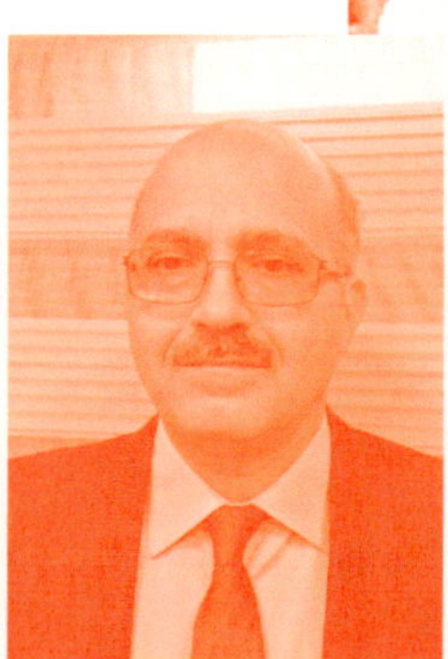

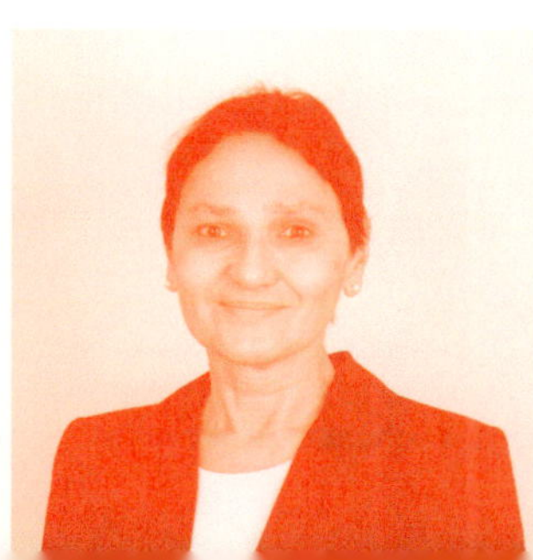

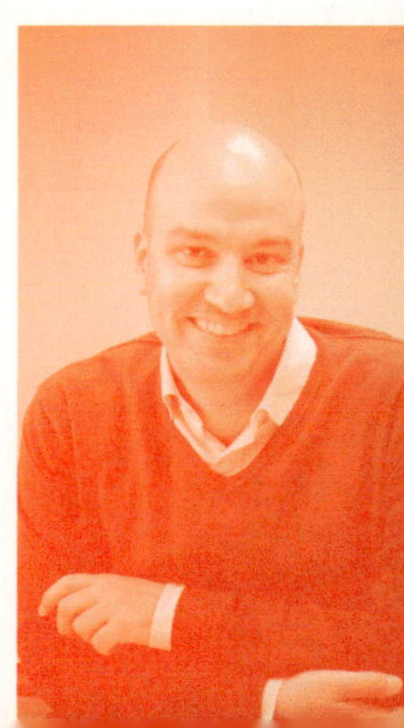

Human Blood Group Systems and Haemoglobinopathies
http://dx.doi.org/10.5772/intechopen.82992
Edited by Osaro Erhabor and Anjana Munshi

Contributors
Bruna Policiquio, Vivian Gonzaga, Cristiane Wenceslau, Irina Kerkis, Fatima A. Aldarweesh, Jolanta Korsak, Anna Piotrowska, Osaro Erhabor, Teddy Charles Adias, Tosan Erhabor, Iwueke Ikechukwu, Maria Rios, Emilia Sippert, Evgeniya Volkova, Rocio Aguilar-Quesada, Veronica Valdivieso-Gomez, Javier Garrancho-Pérez, Inés Aroca-Siendones, Hassan Njifon Nsangou, Régine Scelles, Vincent Kabwe Mulunda-A-Mulunda, Pierre Kouam, Taty Oke Ingwen, Parijat De, Jessica Siew Hua Lee, Kinda Al-Hourani, Edith Christiane Christianne Bougouma, Sodiomon Bienvenu Sirima

First published in London, United Kingdom, 2021 by IntechOpen
IntechOpen is the global imprint of INTECHOPEN LIMITED, registered in England and Wales, registration number: 11086078, 5 Princes Gate Court, London, SW7 2QJ, United Kingdom
Printed in Croatia

British Library Cataloguing-in-Publication Data
A catalogue record for this book is available from the British Library

Additional hard and PDF copies can be obtained from orders@intechopen.com

Human Blood Group Systems and Haemoglobinopathies
Edited by Osaro Erhabor and Anjana Munshi
p. cm.
Print ISBN 978-1-83880-313-1
Online ISBN 978-1-83880-314-8
eBook (PDF) ISBN 978-1-83881-969-9

For EU product safety concerns:
IN TECH d.o.o., Prolaz Marije Krucifikse Kozulić 3, 51000 Rijeka, Croatia, info@intechopen.com or visit our website at intechopen.com.

Meet the editors

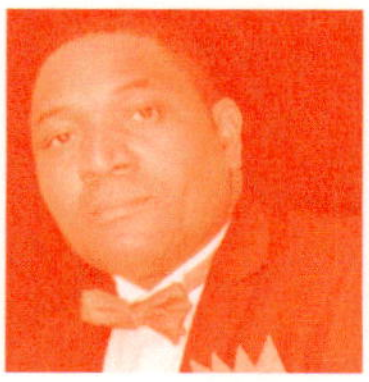

Professor Erhabor Osaro is a Chartered Scientist and fellow of the Institute of Biomedical Science of London. He holds a Ph.D. in Immunohematology from the Rivers State University of Science and Technology, Nigeria. He completed the University of Greenwich, UK Specialist Training in Blood Transfusion and Laboratory Quality Management System. He holds a Specialist Certificate in Transfusion Science Practice from the British Blood Transfusion Society (BBTS). He is also an alumnus of Francis Tuttle College of Technology in Oklahoma, USA. His teaching experience spans both the African continent and Europe. Dr. Osaro is the chair of the equality and diversity working group of the BBTS and recipient of the Margaret Kenwright Scientist award from the same organization. He is a registered portfolio verifier/examiner for the Institute of Biomedical Science of London. He has authored five scientific books and five book chapters. A well-published contributor with more than 160 published articles in the fields of infectious diseases, occupational health, immunohematology, and transfusion medicine, Dr. Osaro is also an editorial board member and reviewer for several international scientific journals.

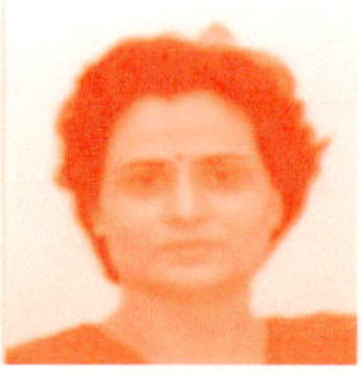

Professor Anjana Munshi, M.Sc, M.Phil, Ph.D., is head of the Department of Human Genetics and Molecular Medicine at the Central University of Punjab, Bathinda, Punjab, India. She is also Dean for the School of Health Sciences and Dean of Research at the Central University of Punjab. Her expertise includes stroke genetics, hemoglobinopathies, pharmacogenetics, molecular cancer biology, epilepsy and bioinformatics. She has published 125 papers in international peer reviewed journals and contributed to 20 book chapters in books published by reputed international publishing houses. She is a reviewer for several international research journals of global reputation.

Contents

Preface

Blood transfusion and hematology are associated with significant advances in science and technology. This book provides a comprehensive overview of some clinically significant blood group systems, hemolytic blood transfusion reactions, and hemoglobinopathies. The aim of this book is to empower biomedical, clinical, and allied medical professionals with the tools required for evidenced-based best practice in the field of blood transfusion and management of hemoglobinopathies.

Osaro Erhabor,
Professor,
Usmanu Danfodiyo University Sokoto,
Nigeria

Anjana Munshi
Central University of Punjab,
India

Section 1

Disorders

Chapter 1

Inherited Disorders of Hemoglobin and *Plasmodium falciparum* Malaria

Edith Christiane Bougouma and Sodiomon Bienvenu Sirima

Abstract

An estimated 300,000 babies are born each year with severe Inherited Disorders of Hemoglobin (IDH). Despite major advances in the understanding of the molecular pathology, control, and management of the IDH thousands of infants and children with these diseases are dying due to the accessibility to appropriate medical care. In addition, as malaria has been the principal cause of early mortality in several parts of the world for much of the last 5000 years, as a result, it is the strongest force for selective pressure on the human genome. That is why, in the world, there is an overlap of malaria endemicity and IDH. Over the past twenty years several studies have shown that IDH such us hemoglobin and/or red cell membrane abnormalities confer resistance to malaria reducing hence the mortality during the first years of life. This has led to the selection of populations with IDH in malaria-endemic areas. This may explain the overlap between these two pathologies. This chapter aims to present the relationship between IDH and malaria susceptibility, make an overview of the current state of knowledge and the burden of IDH, and highlight steps that require to be taken urgently to improve the situation.

Keywords: Hemoglobin, Inherited Disorders, malaria, host genetics

1. Introduction

Despite health better care and new strategies of disease control of, mortality remains high in many countries and worldwide [1]. Malaria is the biggest cause of childhood mortality in Africa.

In 2018, malaria was the cause of about 405 000 deaths, More than 90% of these deaths occurred in sub-Saharan Africa [2].

Malaria parasites enter red blood cells during key stages of their life cycle so that there is no surprise that a change of red blood structures or make-up could affect malaria infection. Some changes of red blood cells make more resistant to malaria infection whereas others create the potential for a harmful reaction to certain antimalarial drugs [3].

Falciparum malaria has had a profound effect on human evolution, evidenced by the high frequencies of malaria protective mutations observed in populations from historically malarious regions. This big pressure has resulted in the selection of many genetic variants that confer protection against severe malaria and reducing death due to malaria in some populations [4–6].

Gene (chromosome)		Mutation		Protein	Function	Reported Genetic Associations with Malaria	Mechanistic hypotheses Proposed protective mechanism	Distribution	High Frequency
		Change	Number						
G6PD (Xq28)		Asn126Asp A376	1	G6PD	Enzyme That protects against oxidative tress	G6PD deficiency protect against severe malaria and uncomplicated malaria	Increased phagocytosis of ring-parasitised variant RBCs due to enhanced oxidative stress [94, 103]. Increased vulnerability of the G6PD deficient erythrocyte to oxidant stress causes its protection against parasitization and Reduced parasite replication in G6PD-deficient erythrocytes [94, 103].	Africa	0.4
		Val68Met G202A	1					Africa	2.5
HBA (16p13.3)	α - thalassemia (α-thal)	α + or α one gene deleted	Many	α-Globin	Component of hemoglobin	Thalassemia protects against severe malaria and severe malaria aneamia but appears to enhance mild malaria episodes in some environments	Specific protection against malaria-induced anemia [94, 103]. Reduced pathogenicity through reduced cytoadherence or resetting [86, 87]. Immunological priming through cross-species immunity between *P.vivax and P.falciparum* [74]. Increased phagocytosis of infected variant RBCs by monocytes and enhanced antibody binding and subsequent clearance of infected variant RBCs [88, 89]. Reduced resetting. Increased micro-erythrocyte count in homozygotes reduces the amount of Hb lost for given parasite density, thus protecting against SMA [43, 82, 88, 90].	Mediterranean area, South / East Asia, Pacific	0.8
		α 0 or - - both genes deleted	Many						0.03
HBB (11p15.5)	β-thalassemia (β-thal)	Many	Many	β-Globin	Component of hemoglobin	Thalassemia protects against severe malaria	Enhanced removal of parasite-infected red blood cells [96]. Reduced invasion and growth of *P. falciparum* parasites [97, 98]. Reduced pathogenicity through reduced cytoadherence or resetting [99].	sub-Saharan Africa	0.1

Gene (chromosome)	Mutation		Protein	Function	Reported Genetic Associations with Malaria	Mechanistic hypotheses Proposed protective mechanism	Distribution	High Frequency
	Change	Number						
						Enhanced antibody binding and subsequent clearance of infected variant RBCs [88]. Increased phagocytosis of ring-parasitised variant RBCs [80, 96, 100].		
S (HbS)	Glu6Val GAG/GTG	2–5	β-Globin	Component of hemoglobin	HbS alleles protect againstuncomplicated malaria and severe malaria. Reduced parasitaemia	Impairment of *P. falciparum* red cell invasion and growth under conditions of low oxygen tension [31, 43]. Enhanced removal of parasite-infected HbAS red blood cell [31, 44]. Reduced pathogenicity of *P. falciparum* infected red blood cells because of reduced expression of PfEMP1 [33, 41]. Improved acquisition of malaria-specific immunity [33, 46, 48]. Selective sickling of infected sickle trait erythrocytes leading to enhanced clearance by the spleen [49]. Reduced erythrocyte invasion, early phagocytosis, and inhibited parasite growth under oxygen stress in venous micro vessels. [49]. Enhancement of innate and acquired immunity [41]. Increased clearance of sickled infected RBCs by the spleen Acquired host immunity and increased phagocytosis of ring-parasitised variant RBCs [44]. Reduced cytoadherence and rosetting Impaired trafficking of parasite proteins to RBC surface [49]. And Inhibition of	Africa	0.2

Gene (chromosome)	Mutation		Protein	Function	Reported Genetic Associations with Malaria	Mechanistic hypotheses Proposed protective mechanism	Distribution	High Frequency
	Change	Number						
						parasite growth due to oxygen-dependent polymerization of HbS [30].		
C (HbC)	Glu6Lys GAG/AAG	2			HbC alleles protect against uncomplicated malaria and severe malaria.	Increased immune clearance of infected erythrocytes [29, 35] Impairment of *P. falciparum* red cell invasion and growth under conditions of low oxygen tension [31, 43, 47] Improved acquisition of malaria-specific immunity [33, 47, 58] Reduced pathogenicity of P. falciparum infected red blood cells because of reduced expression of PfEMP1 [33, 64, 65] and Reduced cyto-adherence of infected erythrocyte [23] increased immune clearance of infected erythrocytes [22, 29]	West Africa	0.5
E (HbE)	Glu26Lys GAG to AAG	1–3			HbE allele reduces parasite invasion and protects against severe malaria.	Impairment of *P. falciparum* red cell invasion and growth [75]. AE heterozygotes appear to have protection from invasion into erythrocytes by *P. falciparum* malaria [53, 73]. Reduced erythrocyte invasion by merozoites, lower intra-erythrocytic parasite growth, and enhanced phagocytosis of infected erythrocytes [22, 75].	Southeast Asia	0.7

Note: The variants at the β- and α-globin loci that confer resistance to malaria and information about them, including their chromosomal location, the mutations, the protein, function and also the reported Genetic Associations with Malaria, Mechanistic hypotheses and finally their distribution.

Table 1.
Common erythrocyte variants that affect susceptibility and resistance to P. falciparum *malaria.*

The high mortality and widespread impact of malaria have resulted in this disease being the strongest evolutionary selective force in recent human history, and genes that confer resistance to malaria [7].

The history of genetics and the study of malaria are much linked. Indeed Burden of disease due to malaria across much of the world has selected for a series of traits, including the alleles of genes encoding hemoglobin, red cell enzymes, and membrane proteins.

Each year more than 7000000 babies born with either a congenital abnormality and/or a genetic disease, mainly (up to 90%) in low or middle-income countries [8].

About 25% of these births consist of five disorders, two of which, the inherited disorders of hemoglobin and glucose-6-phosphate dehydrogenase (G6PD) deficiency, are monogenic diseases [8].

In recent years there has been a major revival in scientific studies interest in the study of interactions between the inherited hemoglobin disorders and *P. falciparum* malaria, work that has been the subject of several extensive reviews [5, 9, 10].

This chapter focuses on IDH that are common enough to be of public health concern particularly those significantly associated with malaria as summarized in **Table 1**.

By presenting the relationship between IDH and malaria susceptibility, making an overview of the current state of knowledge and the burden of IDH, this chapter outline some of the more important protective genetic variants that have been identified as far as summarized in the **Table 1**. The knowledge of our understanding of the interaction between hemoglobin variants and malaria could give point to novel preventive and/or therapeutic approaches.

2. Inherited disorders of hemoglobin (IDH) and *Plasmodium falciparum (P. falciparum)* malaria

2.1 Brief review of malaria infection

Malaria is a severe infectious disease caused by parasites of the genus *Plasmodium. Plasmodium* is one of the longest-known parasites, which are transmitted to humans by a bite of an infected female mosquito of the species Anopheles.

Indeed, after inoculation into a human by a mosquito, the *P. falciparum* parasites enter the erythrocytic stage of their life cycle after a brief silent incubation in life (**Figure 2**). It is during this time that parasites sequentially invade and egress from their host RBCs and cause the signs and symptoms of malaria. Hemoglobin is the oxygen - carrying component and major protein of the RBC [11]. Indeed, the RBC is essential for the spread of malaria parasites, as summarized in **Figures 2** and **3**.

Despite progress towards its control of malaria, it is still the most important parasitic disease and then, one of the world's worst health problems. In 2018, about 228 million cases of malaria occurred worldwide. Most of these cases (93%) occurred in African Africa region In the same year malaria was responsible for 405 000 deaths made up to 67% (272000) of children under 5 years recognized as the most vulnerable group [12]. However, early diagnosis and fast-acting treatment prevent unwanted outcomes. Until recently it was thought that only four species of malarial parasite (Plasmodium) especially *Plasmodium. falciparum (P. falciparum), Plasmodium.vivax (P.vivax), Plasmodium. malariae (P.malariae), and Plasmoduim. ovale (P.ovale)*, have humans as their natural hosts. But, it has been found that many cases of malaria that were previously diagnosed as being due to P. malariae infection are in fact due to a fifth parasite, *Plasmodium. knowlesi (P. knowlesi)* mostly in Malaysia [13].

It has long been thought that *P. falciparum* was the only cause of severe malaria cases and deaths, until the equally destructive, if not worse, the role of *P. vivax* is gradually highlighted and established especially in South East Asia and in Latin America [2, 14–16].

Regarding the relationship between the severity of malaria and host genetics, it appears that *P. falciparum* malaria is one of the deadly forms of malaria with a life cycle including alternatives hosts: a sexual cycle in the insect vector, an Anopheles mosquito, and a human cycle in a liver stage and an erythrocyte stage. However, the resistance mechanisms have been described in the sporozoite entry to liver cells and in the erythrocyte invasion by merozoites (**Figures 1** and **3**) [17, 18]. Genetically based resistance is involved in either altering erythrocyte invasion by merozoites, in lowering parasite growth or in impairing merozoite viability after being released from schizonts [17, 19]. The genetic resistance in the blood stage step has been extensively documented [12].

There are multiple points in the parasite lifecycle that have impacted host genetic variation, but the majority of the malaria-protective variants described so far have various important impacts on the structure and function of the RBC [2].

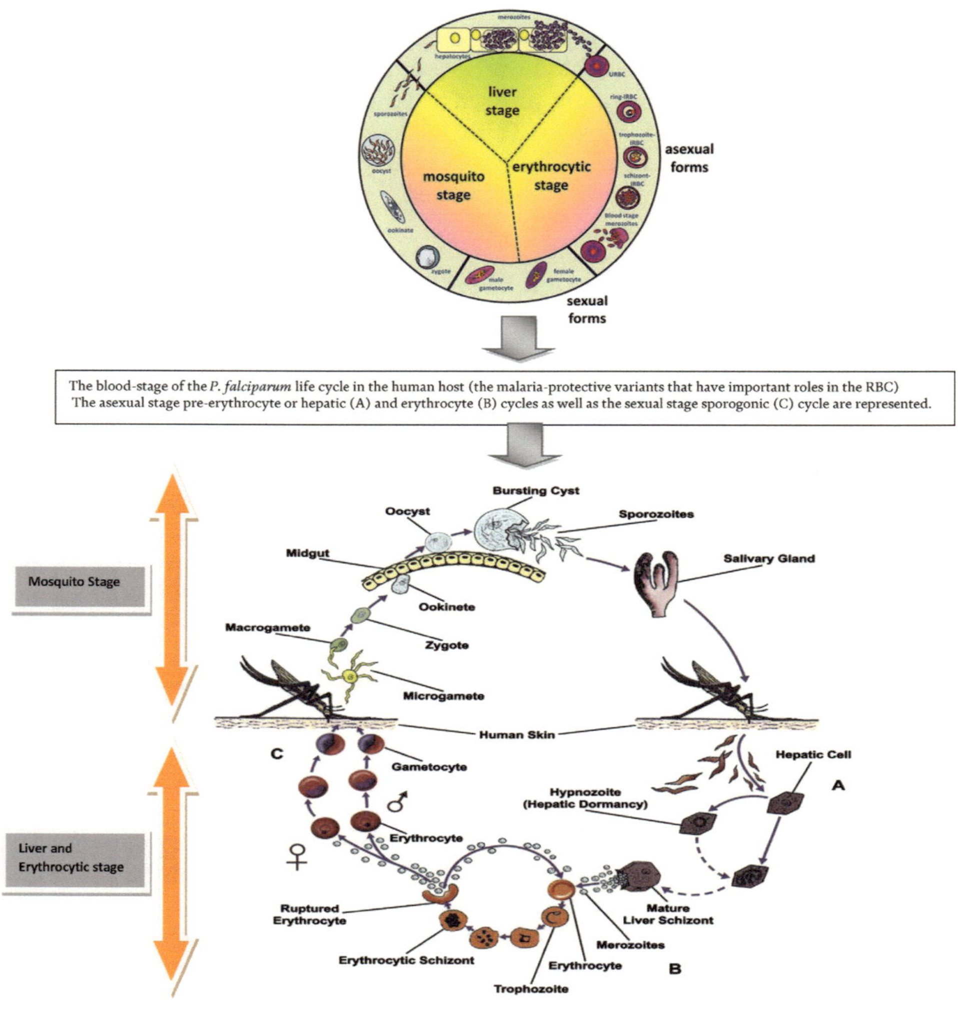

Figure 1.
The life cycle of the malaria parasite (schematic diagram illustrating life cycles of P. falciparum, *involving Anopheles mosquito and human hosts). Adapted from: Figure from Lopez et al. (2010). [Lopez C, Saravia C, Gomez A, Hoebeke J, Patarroyo MA: Mechanisms of genetically-based resistance to malaria. Gene 2010, 467:1–12.] and lee et al.(2019) [Wenn-Chyau lee, Bruce Russell, Laurent Rénia sticking for a cause: The falciparum Malaria parasites Cytoadherence paradigm immu.2019.01444].*

P. falciparum malaria is a major cause of mortality and morbidity, particularly in endemic areas of sub-Saharan Africa [2, 20]. Indeed the disease etiology is variable and is attributable to environmental factors, parasite virulence and mostly host genetics [21]. Variations in the severity of *P. falciparum* infections considered as different phenotypes include parasitaemia (hyperactive or asymptomatic), severe malaria anemia and cerebral malaria. Host genetic factors contribute to the variability of malaria phenotypes [22] and thus, should help to determine some of the mechanisms involved in susceptibility to *P. falciparum* infection. Some authors have summarized common mechanisms by which hemoglobinopathies may attenuate the pathogenesis of *P. falciparum* malaria (**Figure 2**) [11].

The knowledge gained with several studies has produced undisputed evidence about polymorphisms associated with malaria resistance. Indeed, several gene mutations and polymorphisms in the human hosts confer survival advantage and have increased in frequency through natural selection over generations. These include the classical polymorphisms that cause Sickle Cell Disorders (SCD) and haemoglobinopathies such as α-thalassaemias and G6PD deficiency and the major RCB group variants [23]. However, with news technology and experimental design, other polymorphisms have been identified that include the Dantu blood group variant, polymorphisms in the red cell membrane protein ATP2B4, and some variants related to the immune response (**Figure 3**) [10].

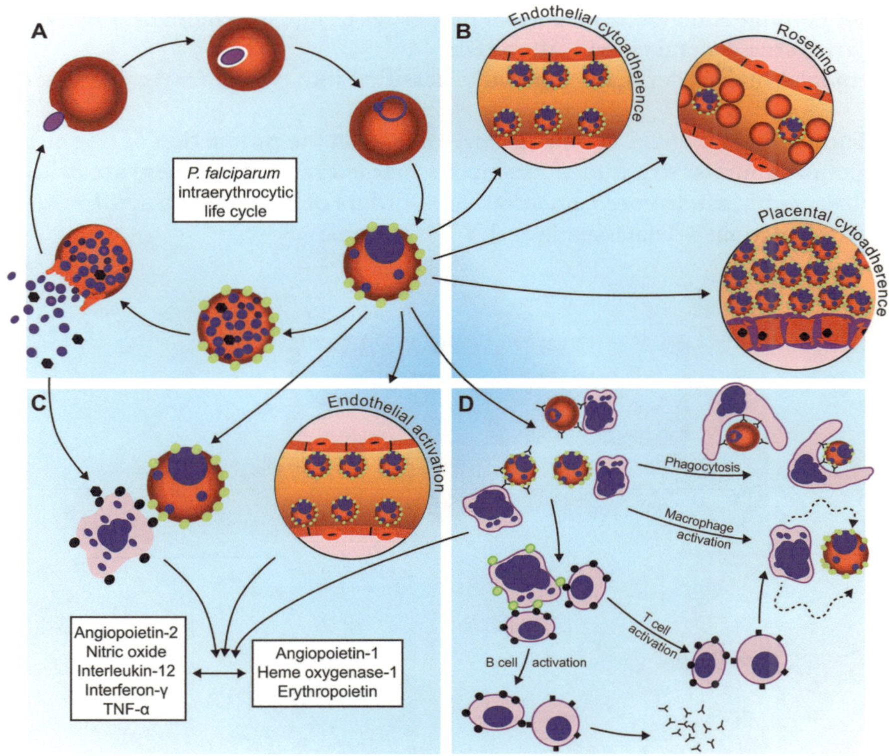

Figure 2.
Common mechanisms by which hemoglobinopathies may attenuate the pathogenesis of P. falciparum *malaria. (A) Restriction of RBC invasion or intraerythrocytic growth, thereby suppressing parasite densities in Vivo; (B) Interference with parasite-derived mediators of pathogenesis, including those involved in the binding of parasite-infected RBCs to extracellular host receptors; (C) Modulation of innate host defenses to favor protective, anti-inflammatory responses over those that drive pathogenic, pro-inflammatory responses; (D) Enhancement of adaptive cell-mediated and humoral immune responses that clear iRBCs from the blood. Source: Taylor SM, Cerami C, Fairhurst RM (2013) Hemoglobinopathies: Slicing the Gordian Knot of Plasmodium falciparum Malaria Pathogenesis. PLOS Pathogens 9(5): e1003327. https://doi.org/10.1371/journal.ppat.1003327. https://journals.plos.org/plospathogens/article?id=10.1371/journal.ppat.1003327.*

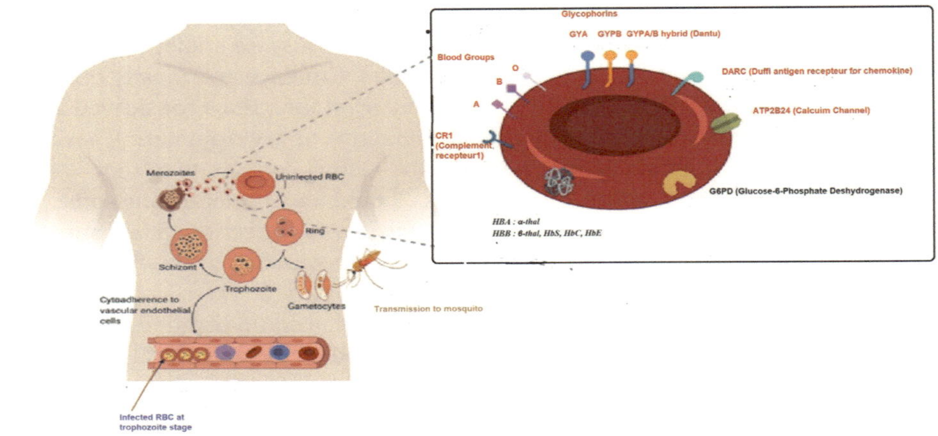

Figure 3.
Representation of the blood-stage of P. falciparum *life cycle in the human host and the malaria-protective variants that have important roles in the red blood cell (RBC). Image adapted from [1].*

2.2 Overview of inherited hemoglobin disorders

Inherited hemoglobin disorders include all disorders that are passed down through families and affect the normal properties of blood in humans. **Figure 4** summarizes the general classification IDH.

Hemoglobin disorders can be broadly classified into two general categories [24].

1. Those in which there is a quantitative defect in the production of one of the globin subunits, either total absence or marked reduction. These are called the thalassemia syndromes (quantitative disorders of globin chain synthesis/accumulation: β-Thalassemia and α-Thalassemia

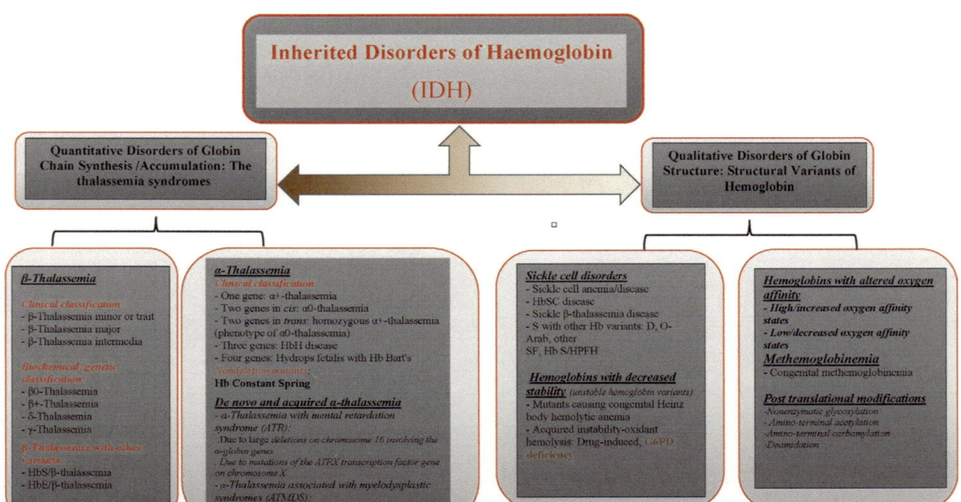

Figure 4.
Flow chart of general classification inherited disorders of Hemoglobin. Note: In this chapter we are interested in inherited hemoglobin disorders that are common enough to be of public health significance and particularly in those with a link to malaria (G6PD, α –thal, β-thal, HbS, HbC, HbE). Adapted from table of classification of hemoglobin disorders from Forget al. (2013). [Forget BG, Bunn HF: Classification of the disorders of hemoglobin. Cold Spring Harb Perspect Med 2013, 3:a011684].

2. Those in which there is a qualitative disorders of globin structure defect in one of the globin subunits: Structural variant of hemoglobin

    - Sickle cell disorders: Sickle Cell trait, Sickle cell anemia disease, SC disease, sickle β-thalassemia disease

    - Hemoglobin with decreased stability (unstable hemoglobin variants): G6PD deficiency

Hemoglobin includes four globin chains:

- fetal hemoglobin (HbF), the main hemoglobin in the fetal period which has two alpha (α) and two gamma (γ) chains (a2γ2),

- adult hemoglobin (HbA), which increases after birth up to more than 96% of total hemoglobin, has two α and two β chains (α2β2).

Human Hemoglobin genes are located in the α-globin and β-globin gene clusters in chromosomes 16 and 11. Due to spontaneous mutation, hemoglobin gene variants are present at low prevalence in all sizeable populations [5].

They fall into two broad groups structural variants that change the amino acid sequence and produce an unusual hemoglobin, [8] and thalassaemias that lower or abolish production of globin chains [12].

Morbidity and mortality rates from SCD and β-thalassemia are still very high and represent an important challenge. Increased understanding of pathophysiological aspects has lead to significant improvements in the treatment and prevention of these diseases [25]. However most hemoglobin gene variants are rare and many are harmless, but some are common because carriers are less likely than others to die from *falciparum* malaria.

We are interested in inherited hemoglobin disorders that are common enough to be of public health significance and particularly in those with a link to malaria.

2.2.1 Sickle cell disorders

SCD is a group of inherited RBC disorders; it is by far the most common IDH worldwide. SCD is caused by a variation in the gene that codes for hemoglobin, the protein in our red blood cells that helps carry oxygen to all parts of the body. The altered protein found in people with SCD is called hemoglobin S and occurs in people who have inherited the hemoglobin S (HbS), the red blood cells become hard and sticky [12].

Hemoglobin S results from an amino acid substitution at the sixth residue of the β-globin subunit: β6-Glu → Val. RBCs of persons with HbAS typically have 40% HbS and 56–58% HbA [24]. The frequency of allele S is up to 0.2 in some parts of sub-Saharan Africa [26–28]. In equatorial Africa, where malaria is endemic, the prevalence of HbAS is much higher and can reach over 30% in some populations because of the survival advantage of HbAS heterozygotes from complications of *P. falciparum* malaria. Individuals with HbAS are typically asymptomatic; severe hypoxia is required for them to experience manifestations of SCD, called sickling.

Persons who have inherited the HbS gene from only one parent are Heterozygote for the Sickle gene (AS). They carry the gene certainly, but they usually do not have the disease and are more tolerant of malaria infection, making them more likely to survive the disease [12, 29].

SCD is most common in Africa where limited resources and these resources carefully targeted are often directed towards sectors other than health. However, it should be noted that the symptoms of SCD are often serious, substantially reducing life expectancy and often requiring intensive treatment throughout the patient's life.

Hemoglobin C results from a variation in the gene that codes for hemoglobin (β6-Glu → Lys), the protein in our RBC that helps carry oxygen around the body, It causes hemolytic anemia, splenomegaly in homozygous state and provides a degree of protection against malaria infection [12, 26]. Persons with hemoglobin C trait (Hb AC) are phenotypically normal, with no clinical evident limitations or symptoms. However, their heterozygous status, gives them a degree of protection against developing severe malaria HbC is common in malarious areas of West Africa, especially in Burkina Faso, the prevalence of HbAC is much higher and can reach over 21% [26, 28, 30, 31].

HbS and HbC caused by point mutations in the beta-globin gene, offer both substantial malaria protection. Despite the fact that the blood disorder caused by homozygosity for HbC is much less severe than that caused by homozygosity for HbS [9, 12, 26, 32], it is the sickle mutation which has come to dominate many old-world malarious regions, whilst HbC is highly restricted in its geographical distribution [33]. It is probable that this discrepancy (blood disorder between HbC and HbS) may be due to sickle cell heterozygotes enjoying a higher level of malaria protection than heterozygotes for HbC. A probable higher fitness of HbS heterozygotes relative to HbC heterozygotes could certainly have allowed the sickle cell allele to spread more rapidly. However, observations that carrying either HbC or HbS enhances an individual's capacity to transmit malaria parasites to mosquitoes could also shed light on this hypothesis [32].

Hemoglobin E results from a glutamate to lysine substitution in codon 26 (β26 Glu-Lys and GAG-AAG). Besides being a structural variant, the E variant also causes the production of an abnormal mRNA with less b-globin being synthesized. It is synthesized at a slightly reduced rate and has a homozygous phenotype similar to heterozygous β thalassemia [34].

HbE is the second commonest abnormal hemoglobin after sickle cell hemoglobin (HbS). HbE is common in South-East Asia, where its prevalence can reach 30–40% in some parts of Thailand, Cambodia and in Laos [35].

2.2.2 Thalassemia syndromes

The thalassemia syndromes are inherited disorders characterized by absence or markedly decreased accumulation of one of the globin subunits of hemoglobin. Individuals with thalassemia disease are not able to make enough hemoglobin, which causes severe anemia [24].

There is two primary types of thalassemia disease: alpha (α) thalassemias and beta (β) thalassemia disease. In the α-thalassemias, there is absent or decreased production of α-globin subunits, whereas, in the β-thalassemias, there is absent or reduced production of β-globin subunits. Thalassemias affecting the production of delta (δ)- or gamma (γ)-globin subunits are also been described but are rare and not clinically significant disorder

2.2.2.1 α-thalassemia

The α-thalassemia syndromes are usually caused by the deletion of one or more α-globin genes and are sub classified according to the number of α-globin genes that are deleted or mutated [24].

There is two primary types of α-thalassemia:

- α+ - thalassemia, in which one pair of the genes is deleted or inactivated by a point mutation,

- α 0-thalassemia, in which both pairs of genes are deleted or inactivated.

The frequency of a α thalassemia is generally 41% in regions where malaria is prevalent and in some populations, such as in Nepal, parts of India, and Papua New Guinea, it is over 80% [36]. However, in sub-Saharan African populations, a α-thalassemia frequencies do not exceed 50% despite intense malaria selection and some authors [37] suggested that this might occur because of negative epistasis with the S allele.

2.2.2.2 β-thalassemia

The β-thalassemias are characterized by a quantitative deficiency of β-globin chains, can be sub classified into those in which there is a total absence of normal b-globin subunit synthesis or accumulation. The β^{-}thalassemias are divided into two main varieties (β0-thalassemia, there is no β-chain production and β^{+}thalassemia, there is a partial deficiency of β-chain production) [24]. The molecular basis of the β-thalassemias is very heterogeneous, with over 200 different mutations having been described [38]. In general, the mutations causing β-thalassemia are point mutations affecting a single nucleotide, or a small number of nucleotides, in the b-globin gene. The frequency of carriers of β-thalassemia variants is from 5 to 20% in some areas, although not as high as the frequency of α-thalassemia variants [39].

2.2.3 Glucose-6-phosphate dehydrogenase deficiency and P. falciparum *malaria*

Glucose-6-phosphate dehydrogenase (G6PD) deficiency is a genetic disorder that results in impaired enzyme activity.

This X-linked genetic condition is characterized by reduced G6PD enzyme activity, which can remain asymptomatic. Red blood cells obtain reduced glutathione (GSH) solely from the G6PD/reduced nicotinamide adenine dinucleotide phosphate (NADH) pathway [7, 12, 30, 40, 41].

The deficiency makes red cells more susceptible to oxidative haemolysis, this disease that can cause jaundice in newborn babies and haemolytic anemia (when red blood cells break up) throughout life. This is, usually caused by an infection or exposure to certain foods or chemicals [41, 42]. One of the chemicals that can trigger severe symptoms in people with G6PD deficiency is Primaquine, the only drug currently available to clear the relapsing life stages of the *Plasmodium vivax* parasite from the liver.

G6PD and a number of other human genetic traits including sickle cell anemia and related haemoglobinopathies are predominantly found in populations living in malaria endemic countries and have been suggested to provide the host protection from severe forms of malaria [30, 43–45] and asymptomatic malaria [27].

G6PD deficiency can be common in populations with high levels of malaria infection, indeed the prevalence is even higher (8%) in malaria-endemic countries [8]. Malaria control programs need to know this to inform their policies on using Primaquine as a treatment and as a malaria control measure.

2.3 Epidemiology of inherited hemoglobin disorders and *P. falciparum* malaria

For a very long time, human beings have interacted with malaria parasites and thus the parasite has had largely time to adapt and evolve with the human host [40]. Immune processes and genetic traits have contributed to reducing the profligacy of the malaria parasite and a wide range of genetic polymorphisms has been developed to modify the individual response to this disease. Gene mutations involved in susceptibility and resistance to *P. falciparum* malaria. It has been shown that the severity of several malaria infections (such as asymptomatic, CM and SMA) varies significantly between individuals and between populations [5]. Many of the protective variants identified thus far affect erythrocytes, where the malaria parasite spends a crucial stage of its life cycle. Several of the best studied mutations affect the globin genes encoding hemoglobin [46]. Haemoglobinopathies and G6PD deficiency are among the most common single-gene disorders, which affect RBC stability and integrity [47].

More than 700 abnormal hemoglobin have been described worldwide and more than 200 million people worldwide have RBC enzyme abnormality [48].

These genetic mutations are major causes of morbidity and mortality around the world [49]. Sickle hemoglobin and G6PD deficiency are genetically independent, their loci is located on chromosome 11 for sickle and chromosome X for G6PD deficiency genes.

Table 1 summarizes the Common Erythrocyte variant that affects malaria infection particularly *P. falciparum* malaria.

2.3.1 Sickle hemoglobin (HbS), hemoglobin C (HbC) and P. falciparum *malaria*

Sickle hemoglobin (HbS) and hemoglobin C (HbC) are both caused by point mutations in the beta globin gene, and both offer substantial malaria protection.

2.3.1.1 HbS and P. falciparum *malaria*

Heterozygosity for the sickle mutation (genotype AS) offers considerable protection against all forms of severe malaria, as well as protection against uncomplicated malaria [26, 32, 33] and parasitaemia [26, 32, 50, 51]. The different potential protective mechanisms that have been proposed and supported for sickle cell include, the growth of malarial parasites is suppressed in sickle cells [52], the abnormal display of PfEMP-1 [53], and the acceleration of acquired immunity [54]. It has also been shown that the growth rate of *P. falciparum* is retarded in HbS containing erythrocytes under conditions of low oxygen tension in vitro [55]; inhibition parasite growth by [44], miRNAs found more commonly in sickle cell trait cells than in normal cells inhibit parasite growth [56, 57].

The mechanism of the most strongly protective variant (HbS) against *P. falciparum* [1], is very complex. However studies have been shown here are two plausible mechanisms, which are not mutually exclusive, in suppression of parasite growing in red cells [55] and enhanced splenic clearance of parasitized erythrocytes [58]. Furthermore, a study summarized other possible protective effects of HbC. Indeed effects may result from [59]:

- Impairment of *P. falciparum* red cell invasion and growth under conditions of low oxygen tension [39, 55, 59]

- Enhanced removal of parasite-infected red blood cell [39, 58, 59]

- Reduced pathogenicity of *P. falciparum* infected RBC because of reduced expression of PfEMP1 [53, 60, 61]

- Improved acquisition of malaria-specific immunity [60, 62–64]

- Inhibition of parasite growth due to oxygen-dependent polymerization [37]

- Selective sickling of infected sickle trait erythrocytes leading to enhanced clearance by the spleen. Reduced erythrocyte invasion, early phagocytosis, and inhibited parasite growth under oxygen stress in venous micro vessels [65].

- Enhancement of innate and acquired immunity [53]

- oxygen-dependent polymerization of HbS is responsible for *P. falciparum* growth inhibition [66]

A study with children (between the ages of 2 and 10 years) found that the protective effect of HbAS against malaria increased from 20% to 56%, which implies that it enhances or acts in synergy with the acquired immune response [54, 67].

The compromise between risks and benefits allows us to maintain the HbS polymorphism at allele frequencies of environ 10% in many parts of Africa, despite the lethal consequences for homozygotes, which provides the most striking known example of heterozygote advantage in human genetics [9].

- Severe *P. falciparum* malaria

Some case–control and prospective cohort studies [10, 33, 54, 68–71] indicate that HbAS is consistently associated with large reductions in the risk of severe malaria.

- Uncomplicated *P. falciparum* malaria

A comparative studies [33, 44, 71–73] and several prospective studies [5, 26, 37, 74] have shown the reduction of risk in malaria attributable to HbS. In fact, the HbAS genotype protects against uncomplicated *P. falciparum* malaria by about 30% [33, 71]. In addition, this has been further confirmed by some genome-wide association studies [70, 71].

- *P. falciparum* parasitaemia

Cross-sectional studies have reported conflicting data on the prevalence of *P. falciparum* parasitemia in asymptomatic HbAS children compared with HbAA children.

A lower prevalence of parasitaemia in HbAS children was reported in some studies, [6, 26, 75], when others studies found contrary results of similar prevalence [72, 76, 77] or of higher prevalence [78, 79].

In these surveys, parasite densities were reported in HbAS children as lower [6, 62, 76, 79, 80] or similar [27, 78, 81, 82] to those in HbAA children. We can conclude that HbAS does not consistently protect from *P. falciparum* parasitaemia.

2.3.1.2 HbC and P. falciparum *malaria*

A recent meta-analysis concluded that homozygotes for βC (Hb CC) were strongly protected against severe malaria, and heterozygotes (HbAC) were mildly protected [10, 33]. It has also been found that both both heterozygotes and homozygotes of HbC are protected against severe malaria [26, 30, 31, 44, 83] but the protective effect appears to be substantially greater in homozygotes [44].

Although a cohort study in Mali reports an increase in the incidence of clinical malaria in AC individuals relative to AA [84].

HbC genotypes are not fully elucidated [56], but several mechanisms have been proposed to explain the malaria protection offered by HbC [32], including abnormal intra-erythrocytic development of the parasite leading to lower *P. falciparum* replication rates in subsets of CC erythrocytes [65]; *abnormal P. falciparum* erythrocyte membrane protein 1 (PfEMP-1) display, leading to reduced cytoadherence and possibly reduced parasite sequestration [85], and accelerated acquisition of immunity against malaria [63]. In addition, the protective effect of HbC may result from:

- Increased immune clearance of infected erythrocytes [36, 46].
- Impairment of *P. falciparum* red cell invasion and growth under conditions of low oxygen tension [39, 55, 63]
- Improved acquisition of malaria-specific immunity [60, 63, 78]
- Reduced pathogenicity of *P. falciparum* infected red blood cells because of reduced expression of PfEMP1 [60, 85, 86] and Reduced cyto-adherence of infected erythrocyte [30]
- increased immune clearance of infected erythrocytes [28, 36]
- Besides, on observations of reduced parasite cytoadherence abnormal PfEMP1 expression, clustering of erythrocyte band3 protein, and altered surface topography of the erythrocyte membrane in the presence of HbC, it would appear that the protective effect of HbC works by increasing the immune clearance of infected erythrocytes [85, 87, 88].

2.3.1.3 Severe P. falciparum *malaria*

Compared to healthy children, HbC appears to protect against severe malaria to a lesser degree than HbS and in proportion to allele frequency [31, 33, 44, 73, 89]. Protection from specific severe malaria syndromes has not been fully investigated in HbCC; in one study [90] HbAC showed mild protection from cerebral malaria (CM) and severe malarial anemia (SMA). When compared to children with uncomplicated malaria, protection from severe malaria is inconsistent: non-significant protection is reported from severe malaria in some studies [30, 33, 44, 69] of HbCC and HbAC, and from SMA in other studies [30, 33, 69] that combined homozygotes and heterozygotes. Significant protection from CM was reported in one study of Malian children that combined homo- and heterozygotes [30, 33] Prospective studies have not reported the incidence of severe syndromes in HbC children. Thus, convincing evidence for protection from severe malaria owing to HbC derives largely from few case–control studies. Also, a further strong evidence for overall protection comes from a recent GWAS, which concluded that for each copy of the HbC allele, the risk for severe *P. falciparum* malaria was reduced by 29% [56, 70].

- Uncomplicated *P. falciparum* malaria

Few studies have reported the risk of uncomplicated malaria associated with HbC. However some comparative studies [44, 72] and prospective studies have yielded conflicting results [26, 33, 74, 91]. Further studies are still needed to show the evidence of protection from uncomplicated malaria afforded by HbCC and HbAC.

- *P. falciparum* parasitaemia

In most studies cross-sectional surveys with adults and children, HbC has not been associated with a reduced prevalence of *P. falciparum* parasitaemia

[76, 78, 80, 92, 93] or *P. falciparum* density [76, 78, 80, 94]. The incidence of asymptomatic parasitaemia did not differ between HbAC and HbAA children in Mali study [26, 74]. However, in Burkina Study HbAC genotype was associated with a lower incidence of clinical malaria relative to AA among children. Thus, HbC does not appear to modify the risk of *P. falciparum* parasitaemia.

2.3.1.4 HbE and P. falciparum *malaria*

HbE is an extremely most common structural hemoglobin variant that occurs at high frequencies throughout Southeast Asia and has reached an allele frequency of up to 70% in some areas of northern Thailand and Cambodia [52]. It is a β-hemoglobin variant, which is produced at a slightly reduced rate and hence has the phenotype of a mild form of β thalassemia [95].

Generally, none of HbS or C variants are present in Southeast Asia and HbE is in general also absent from populations in which HbS and HbC are present [52].

HbE is an extremely most common structural hemoglobin variant that occurs at high frequencies throughout Southeast Asia and has reached an allele frequency of up to 70% in some areas of northern Thailand and Cambodia [34].

AE heterozygotes appear to have protection from invasion into erythrocytes by *P. falciparum* malaria [4, 65, 72, 96]. Moreover, the protective effect of HbE may result from impairment of *P. falciparum* red cell invasion and growth [96], lower intra-erythrocytic parasite growth, and enhanced phagocytosis of infected erythrocytes [28, 96].

When the frequency of HbE is high, some other red cell disorders, such as a-thalassemia, can be also in high frequency. Although extensive sequence analysis has not been carried out. [97]. However, the E allele found in China is on the same haplotype as that found in Thailand [98], suggesting that it does not have a different origin.

Few studies have been done to characterize the mechanisms of malaria protection. Three categories of effects are relevant: reduced parasite growth and development, altered adhesion of parasitized RBCs to endothelium, and impact on the immune system. In vitro studies of HbEE and HbAE RBCs have found reduced invasion and growth of HbE [96, 99]. Clearly, more work needs to be done to answer further questions about the protective impact of HbE.

- Severe *P. falciparum* malaria

Meta-analysis of few studies [21, 33, 100] that compared the prevalence of HbE in severe and uncomplicated malaria cases demonstrated no evidence of protection, though this should be interpreted cautiously given the significant.

Considering heterogeneity of the findings and the highly selected settings of the studies, more investigations are necessary to conclude on possible protection of HbE.

- Uncomplicated *P. falciparum* malaria

We have not identified studies that have quantified clearly susceptibility to malaria by HbE.

- *P. falciparum* parasitaemia

A cross-sectional study conducted in India reported a significantly lower prevalence of *P. falciparum* parasitaemia in patients with HbE (AE or EE) compared with patients with HbAA [101].

2.3.1.5 Hemoglobins S/C and malaria transmission

Some studies suggest that human genetic variation at the β-globin locus can influence the transmission of malaria. Indeed the same genetic variants that are protective against infection also showed an association with the intensity of malaria transmission. Hemoglobin variants C and S protect against severe malaria but their influence probably on parameters not directly linked to disease severity such as gametocyte carriage and infection chronicity. Moreover, some studies provided evidence that hemoglobin variants selected for the protection against malaria might also have a broader impact on local epidemiology by influencing the frequency of parasite, including the carriage of gametocytes [3, 32].

2.3.2 Thalassemia (α and β) and P. falciparum malaria

The thalassemias are the most common Mendelian diseases of humans and constitute a major global health problem [39]. This is a group of clinical disorders that result from defective production of α- or β-globin chains, which arise from deletions or other disruptions of the globin gene clusters on chromosomes 11 and 16 [9].

A study in Kenyan children found that both heterozygous and homozygous a1 thalassemia was protective against severe malaria [102], whereas a study in Ghanaian children found that heterozygotes were protected [103]. However, a study conducted in Papua New Guinea, founded the risk of severe malaria (other childhood infections) was reduced by 60% in children who were homozygous for α1 thalassemia and to a lesser degree in heterozygotes [104]. The protective mechanism of thalassemia is not well known. Flow-cytometry studies in vitro have shown that erythrocytes with the thalassemia phenotype show reduced parasite growth [105] and increased binding of antibodies from malaria-immune [106].

2.3.2.1 α - thalassemia

The distribution of both a and b thalassemia variants seems to correspond closely to the regions that have historically had high rates of malaria [23] and the local distribution of these variants also corresponds to endemic malaria [36, 107]. Several studies have shown protection from severe malaria for individuals with a α-thalassemia, compared with individuals without thalassemia [37, 103, 104]. In addition, some authors. In a case–control study have shown protection from severe malaria for a α heterozygotes and homozygotes compared to normal aa/aa genotype [7, 37]. Overall, it appears that.

many haplotypes that reduce the expression of α-globin provide a selective advantage in resistance to severe malaria. Indeed some mechanisms have been proposed to explain the malaria protection offered by α thalassemia:

- Specific protection against malaria-induced anemia [90, 104]
- Reduced pathogenicity through reduced cytoadherence or resetting [108, 109]
- Immunological priming through cross-species immunity between *P. vivax and P. falciparum* [94]
- increased phagocytosis of infected variant RBCs by monocytes and Enhanced antibody binding and subsequent clearance of infected variant RBCs [110, 111]

- Increased micro-erythrocyte count in homozygotes reduces the amount of Hb lost for given parasite density, thus protecting against SMA [55, 104, 110, 112]

- Severe *P. falciparum* malaria

Some studies [90, 102–104] investigated α-thalassaemia showed protection against severe malaria, malarial anemia and additionally, protection from cerebral malaria [94].

- Uncomplicated *P. falciparum* malaria

Several prospective studies have assessed the incidence of uncomplicated malaria in α-thalassaemic children, with conflicting results. Indeed some studies showed the incidence of falciparum malaria was higher in α-thalassemia homozygotes and heterozygotes [94]; in contrast, other studies, found a lower incidence [37, 113]. However, other studies have found no protection for both homozygotes and heterozygotes

- *P. falciparum* parasitaemia

In cross-sectional studies, α-thalassaemia was not associated with the prevalence of parasitaemia [79, 103, 112, 114, 115]. In prospective study of children conducted in Papua New Guinea, both α- thalassaemia homozygotes and heterozygotes had fewer episodes of PCR-detectable parasitaemia than those without α thalassaemia, [115, 116] though this outcome has not been investigated in other studies.

Finally, there is no evident data to confirm a protective effect of α-thalassaemia against asymptomatic parasitaemia [112, 114].

2.3.2.2 β–thalassemia

Haldane has explain the very high level of β-thalassemia in some Mediterranean populations by the 'malaria hypothesis' of Haldane [117].

There is ordinarily only one copy of the HBB gene and βþ and β0 thalassemia showing the reduction and loss, respectively, of the production of functional protein. Individuals with α-thalassemia major, have profound anemia while Heterozygotes typically have mild anemia, however, symptoms can vary greatly in severity from having severe anemia to being a symptomless carrier. [118]

Generally, β-thalassemia is more of a public health problem because of this higher morbidity than α-thalassemia.

Several mechanisms have been also proposed to explain specific protection against malaria-induced

- Enhanced removal of parasite-infected RBC [45]

- Reduced invasion and growth of *P. falciparum* parasites [119, 120]

- Reduced pathogenicity through reduced cytoadherence or resetting [121]

- Enhanced antibody binding and subsequent clearance of infected variant RBCs [110]

- Increased phagocytosis of ring-parasitised variant RBCs [45, 102, 122]

- Severe *P. falciparum* malaria

To our knowledge, no studies have investigated the risk of severe malaria in patients with β-thalassaemia.

- Uncomplicated *P. falciparum* malaria

A case–control study in Liberia, have showed a low prevalence of β-thalassaemia in participants with uncomplicated malaria compare to community controls [72].

- *P. falciparum* parasitaemia

A other study that was done in Northern Liberia, found no differences, although they did report lower parasite densities in those with β-thalassaemia [46].

2.3.3 Deficiency Glucose-6-phosphate dehydrogenase (G6PD) and P. falciparum *malaria*

G6PD deficiency is a common X-linked recessive genetic disorder inherited from parents. Although, in most cases, G6PD-deficient individuals appear normal, it can lead to life-threatening anemia in severely G6PD-deficient individuals during oxidative stress-induced by the consumption of certain foodstuff (fava beans), legumes, and taking such as particular antimalarial (primaquine and pamaquine), sulfonamide, sulfamethoxazole, and other drugs and chemicals [123] and also probably infection with microorganisms [124]. Additionally, some authors show that G6PD deficiency increases the risk of severe neonatal hyperbilirubinemia, which can lead to lifetime disability with kernicterus if inadequately treated [115, 125].

However, there is a big beneficial effect of G6PD deficiency. Some studies have reported that G6PD deficiency provides resistance against malaria as the malaria parasite cannot complete its life cycle in compromised G6PD deficient RBC which have a decrease in life span or because of early phagocytosis of deficient RBC [126, 127]. Deficient G6PD enzyme activity has been shown to correlate with protection against severe malaria [43, 89]. Reduced parasite replication in G6PD-deficient erythrocytes is thought to be the mechanism of protection [128], but the parasite appears to counter this by manufacturing G6PD itself [129].

The geographical distribution of G6PD deficiency is consistent with evolutionary selection by malaria [130], and a hypothesis of positive selection [131–133]. The results of studies examining the risk of malaria for various G6PD-deficient genotypes are not consistent. Some authors [43, 134] found in Gambia and Kenya that the reduction in risk of severe malaria in male hemizygotes was 58% and that the reduction in risk for heterozygous females was 46%. Other hand, other authors found that in two populations in Mali, the reduction in risk of severe malaria in male hemizygotes was also 58%, but no reduction in risk in the female heterozygotes [93]. Some authors [27, 133] found no protective effect for either male hemizygotes or female heterozygotes. However, a protective effect has been reported on for females that were found to be G6PD deficient. This finding appears to be based on the incomplete correlation of genotype and phenotype for G6PD deficiency in female heterozygotes due to variable inactivation of the two X chromosomes [127].

Several mechanisms have been proposed to explain the malaria protection offered by G6PD deficiency [45, 127].

- Increased phagocytosis of ring-parasitized variant RBCs due to enhanced oxidative

- Increased vulnerability of the G6PD deficient erythrocyte to oxidant stress causes its protection against parasitization

- Reduced parasite replication in G6PD-deficient erythrocytes

2.4 Global burden of the hemoglobin disorders

Hemoglobinopathies are a group of IDH initially described in the subtropical regions, they are now spread all around the world. Their high frequency and clinical severity make them a global health burden mostly in Africa where there is a huge lack of resources. The measure of the yardstick of under-5 mortality has been used to assess the broad effect of hemoglobin disorders on health because most affected children can die in early childhood and most survivors can have a chronic disease. Some authors show that the disease may be cause of at least 3.4% of deaths in children aged under 5 years [135]. However, it is very difficult to estimate the burden especially as inherited disorders affect families and then communities. Worldwide, over 1% of couples are at risk for IDH most have at least one affected child. Most affected children could die in early childhood although there are now better health facilities and medical care.

Although the West African death rate in children aged under 5 years is 18.4%, This rate is 16.5% for children born to couples, not at risk for sickle-cell disorders, and 40% for children born to couples who are at risk [135]. Clearly, methods to assess the health burden of inherited disorders must include also a family perspective [135].

The burden of disease due to malaria across worldwide vary according to selected visible traits of major medical importance, including the alleles of genes encoding hemoglobin. There are several reasons for the extremely high frequency and uneven distribution of inherited hemoglobin disorders. Natural selection is by far the most important, because of the frequency of the heterozygote and the protection against malaria afforded to the homozygotes of thalassemia and HbC, followed by consanguineous marriages [9, 136]. The epidemiological transition whereby, owing to improvements of health care services, nutrition, and health positive social and behavioral factors, babies who would have probably died from the more severe hemoglobin disorders survive nowadays [39]. Then, the migration from areas of high frequency of SCD into regions like Europe and the United States are also cited.

Currently, there are only limited data on the gene frequencies and the number of births of patients with common hemoglobin disorders, particularly in Africa. Micro mapping studies involving many different centers in these countries have recently found that there is remarkable diversity in the frequency of the hemoglobin disorders even over small geographical distances [137–139].

For the future more micro mapping data are then needed to provide an accurate picture global burden according selective factors distribution [60]. Hemoglobinopathies are so common that they provide a convenient model for working out a genetic approach to the control of chronic childhood diseases. At present, about 250 million people (4.5% of the world population) carry a potentially pathological haemoglobinopathy gene. Haemoglobinopathy control programs, based on WHO approaches and recommendations, have been established in different countries in all WHO Regions and have been successful in the management of the problem by reducing the burden of the Hemoglobin Disorders [108].

Nowadays effective prevention programs have been carried out successfully in many developed countries concerning medical care for hemoglobinopathies. The programs should be extended and followed to African regions where hemoglobin disorders are frequency very high. Indeed this frequency accounts for more than 70% of total hemoglobinopathies in the world [140]. Reducing the incidence of IDH, better prevention against IDH should remain the major priority of health services in order to reduce the burden of heamoglobinopathies.

2.5 Global burden of the Malaria

Despite the global awareness with the promulgation of malaria eradication goals, despite the colossal efforts deployed in many forms: international and bilateral cooperation, foundations and humanitarian agencies, philanthropic works. Malaria remains a crucial public health concern within the world in general and in tropical countries in particular. According to the latest Global Malaria Report, there were 228 million cases of malaria in 2018, of which there were 405,000 deaths. Almost all of the morbidity and associated lethality, respectively 93% and 94%, occur in Africa (WMR, 2019) more than 50% of the disease burden of malaria is borne by only 6 countries namely: Nigeria (25%), the Democratic Republic of Congo (12%), Uganda (5%) and Côte d'Ivoire, Mozambique and Niger (4% each). With 67% of malaria-related deaths, children under 5 remain the most vulnerable group [2]. These health consequences of malaria bring with them very important economic and social tragedies. In some cases, the resulting disruption of family structures has consequences for the family itself and for the whole community over several generations [141]. The incidence of malaria is inversely proportional to the level of development of the affected societies. The global distribution of gross domestic product per capita shows a strong correlation between malaria and poverty. Malaria generates direct costs (medical care) and indirect costs (loss of productivity linked to disabilities and deaths due to malaria) [141]. The relief of all this sharp and stifled pain requires strengthening malaria prevention programs and promoting multidisciplinary research on effective and safe antimalarial drugs and vaccines.

3. Discussion

This review confirms that the malaria parasite has co-evolved with its human host, each struggling for survival. The resulting stigmas appear as polymorphisms of the human genome. This process resulted in a symbiotic association, conferring to the host a relative protection against parasitic infection on one hand and allowing the parasite a greater longevity and proliferation due to host acquired resistance on other hand About polymorphisms of the proteins of red blood cells conferring an innate relative resistance to malaria, it is established that with an effect size >80%, the HbS variant confers the strongest protective effect against severe malaria, while the α- thalassemia confers a protective effect of about 40% in homozygotes [70, 71].

Other genes such as G6PD deficiency have also been shown to be present at high frequencies in endemic malaria populations [9, 10, 22, 142]. However, taking into account the limited mapping specific gene variants of early studies, recent studies have shown that the significant effects of known candidate genes would explain only a small fraction of the heritability of malaria [10, 22, 63, 143, 144]. This indicates that the genetic architecture of susceptibility to malaria is much more complex and that "missing heritability" could be explained by polygenetic or epigenetic effects or by gene–gene and gene–environment interactions [10, 145].

The MalariaGEN consortium has greatly contributed to understanding the correlation between the pathogenesis of malaria and polymorphisms in human RBC.

A better understanding of how changes in RBC physiology affects malaria pathogenesis may uncover new strategies to combat the disease. Understanding the

DOI: http://dx.doi.org/10.5772/intechopen.93807

molecular basis of these polymorphisms may shed additional light on the variation in human susceptibility to malaria and offer insight into mechanisms of malaria pathogenesis likewise, a better understanding of red cell membrane structure and function will offer opportunities for the discovery of new and urgently needed therapeutic targets for the treatment of malaria.

4. Conclusions

Hemoglobinopathies are among the most common monogenic diseases in populations. The complexity of their pathophysiological processes, the severity and diversity of their clinical manifestations reflect the relevance of their scientific interests. Genetic polymorphisms that affect the structure and production of the β- or α-chains of hemoglobin are variously associated with protection from a range of clinical manifestations of *P. falciparum* infection. The degree of protection conferred by hemoglobinopathies, in general, is greatest against severe malaria, moderate against uncomplicated malaria, and probably absent against asymptomatic *P. falciparum* parasitaemia. Therefore, there is a positive relationship between the frequency of either βC or βS and malaria selection intensity favors.

However, people with hemoglobin disorders could be high-risk groups. Indeed subjects admitted with malaria are twice more likely to die than those admitted for other pathologies. The screening and genetic counseling for hemoglobin disorders should be an intrinsic part of health care in most countries. Health facility's services should be designed to provide a foundation for more comprehensive community genetics services because hemoglobin disorders are commonly a point of entry for genetic approaches into health systems.

Although information about the precise world distribution and frequency of the inherited hemoglobin disorders is still limited, there is no doubt that they are going to pose an increasing burden on global health resources in the future. Increased knowledge of the biological basis of these diseases would offer significant advances in their therapeutic management and in the prevention of the occurrence of new cases. Indeed the high frequency of IDH because of natural selection associated due to consanguineous marriages in some countries could be reduced through public awareness campaigns. Improving health care conditions in general and those related to pathologies associated with IDH would enhance affected children's survival. Hemoglobin variants could shape the distribution of malaria parasites in human populations and their transmission potential. Therefore, the knowledge of our understanding of the interaction between hemoglobin variants and malaria parasites is still being incomplete even if it has improved these last years. Nonetheless, with the interest in malaria elimination, knowledge on how these prevalent genetic variants influence parasite distribution and probably cumulative host transmission potential would be particularly valuable and necessary.

The malaria parasite has co-evolved with its human host in a struggle for their survival. The scars of this war on the human genome are polymorphisms conferring an innate resistance to malaria. Regarding relationships between malaria and human genetic alterations of RBC proteins, it appears that the MalariaGEN studies have clearly opened new doors to understand the malaria burden on human RBC polymorphisms and thus malaria pathogenesis. These new pieces of knowledge will help to redefine or readjust malaria control strategies.

In fact, despite the complexity of these interactions, hemoglobin variants in general and hemoglobinopathies, in particular, show a good model and natural experiment identifying cellular and molecular mechanisms by which *P. falciparum* produces morbidity.

Vaccines are unquestionably the most cost-effective way for malaria control. The new generation of vaccine delivery systems is increasingly moving towards co-administration of certain immunostimulants and the use of more than one antigen in the same system. In any event, the best vaccine should be effective, safe, low cost, available, and easy to administer.

5. Perspectives

WHO has announced an ambitious goal of global malaria elimination by 2030. Malaria elimination is possible but will require adaptive and well-managed programs and the implementation of evidence-based surveillance strategies and strong national responses, with adequate funding and human resources.

Over the past 20 years, significant progress has been made in the fight against malaria worldwide, with impressive reductions in transmission in many endemic regions. However, the successful outcome of the global malaria eradication research program will depend on the development of new and more effective tools, including rapid diagnostic tests, drugs, vaccines, insecticides, and awareness raising. Nowadays, genetic and genomic knowledge of malaria parasites, vectors (mosquitoes), and human hosts are available. These bits of knowledge could and should be used for the development of the latest generation tools that are more efficient and secure. The situation is all the more urgent and worrying as there is the emergence of a resistance of *Plasmodium falciparum* to the first-line drug, namely artemisinin.

In any event, the development of an effective, safe and operational malaria vaccine remains the ultimate objective that we must achieve. In this perspective, we must watch and take into account the genetic variation of the parasite population, which threatens to undermine our efforts.

A big significant milestone in scientific advancements of the last twenty years was already the elucidation of the genomes, transcriptomes, and proteomes of many pathogens, including malaria parasites. These informations give a clearer and more detailed picture that provides the foundation for new approaches to refine existing targets as well as to identify new target antigens for the development of more efficient and effective vaccines, drugs and diagnostic tests. It is clear that further progress is needed for the development of a malaria vaccine, based on basic research, in order to identify new target antigens and better understand how different adjuvants will affect balance, sustainability, and the effectiveness of the responses. To hope for an effective vaccine, emphasis should be placed on mixtures of antigens combined with potent adjuvants, not only to induce the necessary effective responses, but also to increase the possibility of inducing at least partial cross-immunity by including a range of Plasmodium epitopes.

Innovative genome-based vaccination strategies have shown the potential of a number of pathogens, including malaria. A rational genome-based vaccine design, allowing the selection of the best possible targets by prioritizing antigens according to clinically relevant criteria (frequency and magnitude of the clinically relevant immune response and/or biological function), will overcome the problem of poor immunogenicity and poor vaccine protection that have undermined the development of malaria vaccines in the past 30 years.

The use of gene drive technology could revolutionize ecosystem management. These emerging technologies with potential global effects are being offered to researchers and now subject to public discussions regarding environmental and safety concerns. The relative protection against malaria that heamoglobinopathies would confer, justify justly that we are still investigating this correlation to determine all its nature and its power. Despite this relative advantage over the manifestations of malaria in subjects with sickle cell trait, gene therapy is a new approach to healing patients with hemoglobinopathies, which must be popularized. In this sense, clinical trials are underway with promising results. However, there are still frontiers to explore that could improve this approach: the stoichiometry between transgenic hemoglobin and endogenous hemoglobin in relation to the different genetic mutations of globins; the supply of donor cells, such as the use of induced pluripotent stem cells (iPSC); and the use of safer gene insertion methods to prevent oncogenesis.

The overall prospects for malaria elimination are clear, encouraging and the potential opportunities are endless. Technological discoveries and advances are happening at an incredibly fast pace. The context of discovery and use of new technologies makes the eradication of malaria within the reach of the test tube. However, regardless of the time it will take, we must increase our efforts; intensify networking, with the financial support and strong political will of our leaders, especially in Africa where the problem of malaria is the most important.

Acknowledgements

We would like to acknowledge all authors whose articles were cited in this chapter.

Conflicts of interest

The authors have declared no conflict of interest.

Authorship contributions

BEC wrote the manuscript. SBS read and approved the final manuscript and agree to be accountable for all aspects of the work.

Contributor information

Bougouma Edith Christiane, Email: eddy.cnrfp@gmail.com/e.bougouma@gras.bf. Sirima Bienvenu Sodiomon, Email: s.sirima@gras.bf/gras@fasonet.bf

Funding statement

The authors received no specific funding for this work.

Competing interests

The authors declare no competing financial interests.

Ethics approval

There is no ethical approval for this article.

Disclosures

None.

Acronyms and Abbreviations

Acronyms

INSP	Institut National de Sante Publique
GRAS	Groupe de Recherche Action en Santé

Abbreviations

INSP	Institut National Sante Publique
GRAS	Groupe de Recherche Action en Santé
IDH	Inherited Disorders of Hemoglobin
SCD	Sickle Cell Disorders
RBC	Red Blood Cells
P. falciparum	*Plasmodium falciparum*
P. malaria	Plasmodium. malariae
P. vivax	Plasmodium. vivax
P. ovale	Plasmoduim. ovale
P. knowlesi	Plasmodium. knowlesi
HbS	Sickle hemoglobin
HbC	hemoglobin C
HbE	hemoglobin E
HbAA	normal genotype (hemoglobin AA genotype)
HbCC	homozygotes for βC (hemoglobin CC genotype)
HbAC	heterozygotes for βC (hemoglobin AC genotype)
HbSS	homozygotes for βS (hemoglobin SS genotype)
HbAS	heterozygotes for βS (hemoglobin AS genotype)
HbSC	heterozygotes for βS and βC (hemoglobin AS genotype)
HbEE	homozygotes for βE (hemoglobin EE genotype)
HbAE	heterozygotes for βE (hemoglobin AE genotype)
G6PD	Deficiency Glucose-6-phosphate dehydrogenase
CM	cerebral malaria
SMA	severe malarial anemia
PfEMP-1	*P. falciparum* erythrocyte membrane protein 1
WHO	World Health Organization
RDTs	Rapid diagnostic Tests
ITNs	insecticide-treated nets
ACT	Artemisinin-based Combination Therapies
IRS	Indoor Residual insecticide Spray
GWA	genome-wide association study

Author details

Edith Christiane Bougouma[1] and Sodiomon Bienvenu Sirima[2]*

1 Institut National de Sante Publique (INSP), Ouagadougou, Burkina Faso

2 Groupe de Recherche Action en Santé (GRAS), Ouagadougou, Burkina Faso

*Address all correspondence to: s.sirima@gras.bf

References

[1] Kariuki SN, Williams TN. Human genetics and malaria resistance. Human Genetics. 2020

[2] WHO. World Malaria Report. https://wwwwhoint/malaria/publications/world-malaria-report-2019/en/2019.

[3] Goncalves BP, Sagara I, Coulibaly M, Wu Y, Assadou MH, Guindo A, et al. Hemoglobin variants shape the distribution of malaria parasites in human populations and their transmission potential. Scientific Reports. 2017;**7**:14267

[4] Roberts DJ, Williams TN. Haemoglobinopathies and resistance to malaria. Redox Report. 2003;**8**:304-310

[5] Weatherall DJ. Genetic variation and susceptibility to infection: The red cell and malaria. British Journal of Haematology. 2008;**141**:276-286

[6] Allison AC. Protection afforded by sickle-cell trait against subtertian malareal infection. British Medical Journal. 1954;**1**:290-294

[7] Hedrick PW. Population genetics of malaria resistance in humans. Heredity (Edinb). 2011;**107**:283-304

[8] Christianson AD, Howson CP, Modell B. Global report on birth defects. White Plains, New York: March of Dimes Birth Defects Foundation; 2006. p. 84

[9] Kwiatkowski DP. How malaria has affected the human genome and what human genetics can teach us about malaria. American Journal of Human Genetics. 2005;**77**:171-192

[10] Kariuki SN, Williams TN. Human genetics and malaria resistance. Human Genetics. 2020;**139**:801-811

[11] Taylor SM, Cerami C, Fairhurst RM. Hemoglobinopathies: Slicing the Gordian knot of plasmodium falciparum malaria pathogenesis. PLoS Pathogens. 2013;**9**:e1003327

[12] Howes R, Battle K, Gething P: Inherited Blood Disorders 2017. https://malariaatlasorg/research.

[13] Singh B, Kim Sung L, Matusop A, Radhakrishnan A, Shamsul SS, Cox-Singh J, et al. A large focus of naturally acquired plasmodium knowlesi infections in human beings. Lancet. 2004;**363**:1017-1024

[14] Mendis K, Sina BJ, Marchesini P, Carter R. The neglected burden of plasmodium vivax malaria. The American Journal of Tropical Medicine and Hygiene. 2001;**64**:97-106

[15] Rogerson SJ, Carter R. Severe vivax malaria: Newly recognised or rediscovered. PLoS Medicine. 2008;**5**:e136

[16] Martinsen ES, Blumberg BJ, Eisen RJ, Schall JJ. Avian hemosporidian parasites from northern California oak woodland and chaparral habitats. Journal of Wildlife Diseases. 2008;**44**:260-268

[17] Lopez C, Saravia C, Gomez A, Hoebeke J, Patarroyo MA. Mechanisms of genetically-based resistance to malaria. Gene. 2010;**467**:1-12

[18] Yuthavong Y, Wilairat P. Protection against malaria by thalassaemia and haemoglobin variants. Parasitology Today. 1993;**9**:241-245

[19] Smith TG, Ayi K, Serghides L, McAllister CD, Kain KC. Innate immunity to malaria caused by plasmodium falciparum. Clinical and Investigative Medicine. 2002;**25**:262-272

[20] Snow RW, Guerra CA, Noor AM, Myint HY, Hay SI. The global distribution of clinical episodes of

plasmodium falciparum malaria. Nature. 2005;**434**:214-217

[21] Hutagalung R, Wilairatana P, Looareesuwan S, Brittenham GM, Aikawa M, Gordeuk VR. Influence of hemoglobin E trait on the severity of falciparum malaria. The Journal of Infectious Diseases. 1999;**179**:283-286

[22] Mackinnon MJ, Mwangi TW, Snow RW, Marsh K, Williams TN. Heritability of malaria in Africa. PLoS Medicine. 2005;**2**:e340

[23] Weatherall DJ, Clegg JB. Genetic variability in response to infection: Malaria and after. Genes and Immunity. 2002;**3**:331-337

[24] Forget BG, Bunn HF. Classification of the disorders of hemoglobin. Cold Spring Harbor Perspectives in Medicine. 2013;**3**:a011684

[25] Sonati Mde F, Costa FF. The genetics of blood disorders: Hereditary hemoglobinopathies. Jornal de Pediatria. 2008;**84**:S40-S51

[26] Bougouma EC, Tiono AB, Ouedraogo A, Soulama I, Diarra A, Yaro JB, et al. Haemoglobin variants and plasmodium falciparum malaria in children under five years of age living in a high and seasonal malaria transmission area of Burkina Faso. Malaria Journal. 2012;**11**:154

[27] Badoum ES, Sermé SS, Yaro JB, Coulibaly SA, Kargougou D, Diarra A, et al. Abnormalities of hemoglobin and Glucose-6-Phosphate-Dehydrogenase deficiency in children with uncomplicated malaria and living in Banfora and Saponé, two different malaria setting of Burkina Faso. International Journal of Tropical Disease & Health. 2019;**37**

[28] Modiano D, Bancone G, Ciminelli BM, Pompei F, Blot I, Simpore J, et al. Haemoglobin S and haemoglobin C: 'quick but costly' versus 'slow but gratis' genetic adaptations to plasmodium falciparum malaria. Human Molecular Genetics. 2008;**17**: 789-799

[29] Luzzatto L. Sickle cell anaemia and malaria. Mediterr J Hematol Infect Dis. 2012;**4**:e2012065

[30] Agarwal A, Guindo A, Cissoko Y, Taylor JG, Coulibaly D, Kone A, et al. Hemoglobin C associated with protection from severe malaria in the Dogon of Mali, a west African population with a low prevalence of hemoglobin S. Blood. 2000;**96**: 2358-2363

[31] Mockenhaupt FP, Ehrhardt S, Cramer JP, Otchwemah RN, Anemana SD, Goltz K, et al. Hemoglobin C and resistance to severe malaria in Ghanaian children. The Journal of Infectious Diseases. 2004; **190**:1006-1009

[32] Goncalves BP, Gupta S, Penman BS. Sickle haemoglobin, haemoglobin C and malaria mortality feedbacks. Malaria Journal. 2016;**15**:26

[33] Taylor SM, Parobek CM, Fairhurst RM. Haemoglobinopathies and the clinical epidemiology of malaria: A systematic review and meta-analysis. The Lancet Infectious Diseases. 2012;**12**: 457-468

[34] Rees DC, Clegg JB, Weatherall DJ. Is hemoglobin instability important in the interaction between hemoglobin E and beta thalassemia? Blood. 1998;**92**: 2141-2146

[35] Bachir D, Galacteros F. Hemoglobin E disease. In: Orphanet Encyclopedia. 2004

[36] Flint J, Harding RM, Boyce AJ, Clegg JB. The population genetics of the haemoglobinopathies. Baillière's Clinical Haematology. 1998;**11**:1-51

[37] Williams TN, Mwangi TW, Wambua S, Peto TE, Weatherall DJ, Gupta S, et al. Negative epistasis between the malaria-protective effects of alpha+−thalassemia and the sickle cell trait. Nature Genetics. 2005;**37**: 1253-1257

[38] Thein SL. The molecular basis of beta-thalassemia. Cold Spring Harbor Perspectives in Medicine. 2013;**3**: a011700

[39] Weatherall DJ, Clegg JB. Inherited haemoglobin disorders: An increasing global health problem. Bulletin of the World Health Organization. 2001;**79**: 704-712

[40] Troye-Blomberg M, Perlmann P, Mincheva Nilsson L, Perlmann H. Immune regulation of protection and pathogenesis in plasmodium falciparum malaria. Parassitologia. 1999;**41**:131-138

[41] Amoah LE, Opong A, Ayanful-Torgby R, Abankwa J, Acquah FK. Prevalence of G6PD deficiency and plasmodium falciparum parasites in asymptomatic school children living in southern Ghana. Malaria Journal. 2016; **15**:388

[42] Beutler E. G6PD: Population genetics and clinical manifestations. Blood Reviews. 1996;**10**:45-52

[43] Ruwende C, Khoo SC, Snow RW, Yates SN, Kwiatkowski D, Gupta S, et al. Natural selection of hemi- and heterozygotes for G6PD deficiency in Africa by resistance to severe malaria. Nature. 1995;**376**:246-249

[44] Modiano D, Luoni G, Sirima BS, Simpore J, Verra F, Konate A, et al. Haemoglobin C protects against clinical Plasmodium falciparum malaria. Nature. 2001;**414**:305-308

[45] Ayi K, Turrini F, Piga A, Arese P. Enhanced phagocytosis of ring-parasitized mutant erythrocytes: A common mechanism that may explain protection against falciparum malaria in sickle trait and beta-thalassemia trait. Blood. 2004;**104**:3364-3371

[46] Williams TN. Human red blood cell polymorphisms and malaria. Current Opinion in Microbiology. 2006;**9**: 388-394

[47] Kar BC, Agrawal KC, Panda A. Sickle haemoglobin, G-6PD deficiency and malaria in western Orissa. The Journal of the Association of Physicians of India. 1990;**38**:555-557

[48] Arya R, Layton DM, Bellingham AJ. Hereditary red cell enzymopathies. Blood Reviews. 1995;**9**:165-175

[49] Angastiniotis M, Modell B. Global epidemiology of hemoglobin disorders. Annals of the New York Academy of Sciences. 1998;**850**:251-269

[50] Mangano VD, Kabore Y, Bougouma EC, Verra F, Sepulveda N, Bisseye C, et al. Novel insights into the protective role of Hemoglobin S and C against plasmodium falciparum Parasitemia. The Journal of Infectious Diseases. 2015;**212**:626-634

[51] Billo MA, Johnson ES, Doumbia SO, Poudiougou B, Sagara I, Diawara SI, et al. Sickle cell trait protects against plasmodium falciparum infection. American Journal of Epidemiology. 2012;**176**(Suppl 7):S175-S185

[52] Weatherall DJ. Recent insights into the population genetics and dynamics of the inherited disorders of hemoglobin. Mediterr J Hematol Infect Dis. 2009;**1**: e200922

[53] Cholera R, Brittain NJ, Gillrie MR, Lopera-Mesa TM, Diakite SA, Arie T, et al. Impaired cytoadherence of plasmodium falciparum-infected erythrocytes containing sickle hemoglobin. Proceedings of the National Academy of Sciences of the

United States of America. 2008;**105**: 991-996

[54] Williams TN, Mwangi TW, Roberts DJ, Alexander ND, Weatherall DJ, Wambua S, et al. An immune basis for malaria protection by the sickle cell trait. PLoS Medicine. 2005;**2**:e128

[55] Pasvol G, Weatherall DJ, Wilson RJ. Cellular mechanism for the protective effect of haemoglobin S against P. falciparum malaria. Nature. 1978;**274**: 701-703

[56] Goheen MM, Wegmuller R, Bah A, Darboe B, Danso E, Affara M, et al. Anemia offers stronger protection than sickle cell trait against the Erythrocytic stage of falciparum Malaria and this protection is reversed by iron supplementation. eBioMedicine. 2016; **14**:123-130

[57] LaMonte G, Philip N, Reardon J, Lacsina JR, Majoros W, Chapman L, et al. Translocation of sickle cell erythrocyte microRNAs into plasmodium falciparum inhibits parasite translation and contributes to malaria resistance. Cell Host & Microbe. 2012; **12**:187-199

[58] Shear HL, Roth EF Jr, Fabry ME, Costantini FD, Pachnis A, Hood A, et al. Transgenic mice expressing human sickle hemoglobin are partially resistant to rodent malaria. Blood. 1993;**81**:222-226

[59] Lelliott PM, McMorran BJ, Foote SJ, Burgio G. The influence of host genetics on erythrocytes and malaria infection: Is there therapeutic potential? Malaria Journal. 2015;**14**:289

[60] Weatherall DJ. The inherited diseases of hemoglobin are an emerging global health burden. Blood. 2010;**115**: 4331-4336

[61] Kilian N, Srismith S, Dittmer M, Ouermi D, Bisseye C, Simpore J, et al. Hemoglobin S and C affect protein export in plasmodium falciparum-infected erythrocytes. Biol Open. 2015; **4**:400-410

[62] Guggenmoos-Holzmann I, Bienzle U, Luzzatto L. Plasmodium falciparum malaria and human red cells. II. Red cell genetic traits and resistance against malaria. International Journal of Epidemiology. 1981;**10**:16-22

[63] Verra F, Simpore J, Warimwe GM, Tetteh KK, Howard T, Osier FH, et al. Haemoglobin C and S role in acquired immunity against plasmodium falciparum malaria. PLoS One. 2007;**2**:e978

[64] Marsh K, Otoo L, Hayes RJ, Carson DC, Greenwood BM. Antibodies to blood stage antigens of plasmodium falciparum in rural Gambians and their relation to protection against infection. Transactions of the Royal Society of Tropical Medicine and Hygiene. 1989; **83**:293-303

[65] Fairhurst RM, Fujioka H, Hayton K, Collins KF, Wellems TE. Aberrant development of plasmodium falciparum in hemoglobin CC red cells: Implications for the malaria protective effect of the homozygous state. Blood. 2003;**101**: 3309-3315

[66] Archer NM, Petersen N, Clark MA, Buckee CO, Childs LM, Duraisingh MT. Resistance to plasmodium falciparum in sickle cell trait erythrocytes is driven by oxygen-dependent growth inhibition. Proceedings of the National Academy of Sciences of the United States of America. 2018;**115**:7350-7355

[67] Gong L, Maiteki-Sebuguzi C, Rosenthal PJ, Hubbard AE, Drakeley CJ, Dorsey G, et al. Evidence for both innate and acquired mechanisms of protection from plasmodium falciparum in children with sickle cell trait. Blood. 2012;**119**:3808-3814

[68] Aidoo M, Terlouw DJ, Kolczak MS, McElroy PD, ter Kuile FO, Kariuki S,

et al. Protective effects of the sickle cell gene against malaria morbidity and mortality. Lancet. 2002;**359**:1311-1312

[69] Guinet F, Diallo DA, Minta D, Dicko A, Sissoko MS, Keita MM, et al. A comparison of the incidence of severe malaria in Malian children with normal and C-trait hemoglobin profiles. Acta Tropica. 1997;**68**:175-182

[70] Malaria Genomic Epidemiology N, Malaria Genomic Epidemiology N. Reappraisal of known malaria resistance loci in a large multicenter study. Nature Genetics. 2014;**46**:1197-1204

[71] Goheen MM, Campino S, Cerami C. The role of the red blood cell in host defence against falciparum malaria: An expanding repertoire of evolutionary alterations. British Journal of Haematology. 2017;**179**:543-556

[72] Willcox M, Bjorkman A, Brohult J, Pehrson PO, Rombo L, Bengtsson E. A case-control study in northern Liberia of plasmodium falciparum malaria in haemoglobin S and beta-thalassaemia traits. Annals of Tropical Medicine and Parasitology. 1983;**77**:239-246

[73] Ackerman H, Usen S, Jallow M, Sisay-Joof F, Pinder M, Kwiatkowski DP. A comparison of case-control and family-based association methods: The example of sickle-cell and malaria. Annals of Human Genetics. 2005;**69**:559-565

[74] Kreuels B, Kreuzberg C, Kobbe R, Ayim-Akonor M, Apiah-Thompson P, Thompson B, et al. Differing effects of HbS and HbC traits on uncomplicated falciparum malaria, anemia, and child growth. Blood. 2010; **115**:4551-4558

[75] Ntoumi F, Mercereau-Puijalon O, Ossari S, Luty A, Reltien J, Georges A, et al. Plasmodium falciparum: Sickle-cell trait is associated with higher prevalence of multiple infections in Gabonese children with asymptomatic infections. Experimental Parasitology. 1997;**87**:39-46

[76] Danquah I, Ziniel P, Eggelte TA, Ehrhardt S, Mockenhaupt FP. Influence of haemoglobins S and C on predominantly asymptomatic plasmodium infections in northern Ghana. Transactions of the Royal Society of Tropical Medicine and Hygiene. 2010;**104**:713-719

[77] Aluoch JR. Higher resistance to plasmodium falciparum infection in patients with homozygous sickle cell disease in western Kenya. Tropical Medicine & International Health. 1997; **2**:568-571

[78] Ringelhann B, Hathorn MK, Jilly P, Grant F, Parniczky G. A new look at the protection of hemoglobin AS and AC genotypes against plasmodium falciparum infection: A census tract approach. American Journal of Human Genetics. 1976;**28**:270-279

[79] Allen SJ, Bennett S, Riley EM, Rowe PA, Jakobsen PH, O'Donnell A, et al. Morbidity from malaria and immune responses to defined plasmodium falciparum antigens in children with sickle cell trait in the Gambia. Transactions of the Royal Society of Tropical Medicine and Hygiene. 1992;**86**:494-498

[80] Thompson GR. Significance of haemoglobins S and C in Ghana. British Medical Journal. 1962;**1**:682-685

[81] Bernstein SC, Bowman JE, Kaptue Noche L. Population studies in Cameroon: Hemoglobin S, glucose-6-phosphate dehydrogenase deficiency and falciparum malaria. Human Heredity. 1980;**30**:251-258

[82] Motulsky AG, Vandepitte J, Fraser GR. Population genetic studies in the Congo. I. Glucose-6-phosphate dehydrogenase deficiency, hemoglobin

S, and malaria. American Journal of Human Genetics. 1966;**18**:514-537

[83] Rihet P, Flori L, Tall F, Traore AS, Fumoux F. Hemoglobin C is associated with reduced plasmodium falciparum parasitemia and low risk of mild malaria attack. Human Molecular Genetics. 2004;**13**:1-6

[84] Lopera-Mesa TM, Doumbia S, Konate D, Anderson JM, Doumbouya M, Keita AS, et al. Effect of red blood cell variants on childhood malaria in Mali: A prospective cohort study. Lancet Haematol. 2015;**2**:e140-e149

[85] Fairhurst RM, Baruch DI, Brittain NJ, Ostera GR, Wallach JS, Hoang HL, et al. Abnormal display of PfEMP-1 on erythrocytes carrying haemoglobin C may protect against malaria. Nature. 2005;**435**:1117-1121

[86] Cyrklaff M, Sanchez CP, Kilian N, Bisseye C, Simpore J, Frischknecht F, et al. Hemoglobins S and C interfere with actin remodeling in plasmodium falciparum-infected erythrocytes. Science. 2011;**334**:1283-1286

[87] Arie T, Fairhurst RM, Brittain NJ, Wellems TE, Dvorak JA. Hemoglobin C modulates the surface topography of plasmodium falciparum-infected erythrocytes. Journal of Structural Biology. 2005;**150**:163-169

[88] Tokumasu F, Fairhurst RM, Ostera GR, Brittain NJ, Hwang J, Wellems TE, et al. Band 3 modifications in plasmodium falciparum-infected AA and CC erythrocytes assayed by autocorrelation analysis using quantum dots. Journal of Cell Science. 2005;**118**: 1091-1098

[89] Gilles HM, Fletcher KA, Hendrickse RG, Lindner R, Reddy S, Allan N. Glucose-6-phosphate-dehydrogenase deficiency, sickling, and malaria in African children in South Western Nigeria. Lancet. 1967;**1**:138-140

[90] May J, Evans JA, Timmann C, Ehmen C, Busch W, Thye T, et al. Hemoglobin variants and disease manifestations in severe falciparum malaria. JAMA. 2007;**297**:2220-2226

[91] Crompton PD, Traore B, Kayentao K, Doumbo S, Ongoiba A, Diakite SA, et al. Sickle cell trait is associated with a delayed onset of malaria: Implications for time-to-event analysis in clinical studies of malaria. The Journal of Infectious Diseases. 2008;**198**:1265-1275

[92] Labie D, Richin C, Pagnier J, Gentilini M, Nagel RL. Hemoglobins S and C in upper Volta. Human Genetics. 1984;**65**:300-302

[93] Storey J, Fleming AF, Cornille-Brogger R, Molineaux L, Matsushima T, Kagan I. Abnormal haemoglobins in the Sudan savanna of Nigeria. IV. Malaria, immunoglobulins and antimalarial antibodies in haemoglobin AC individuals. Annals of Tropical Medicine and Parasitology. 1979;**73**:311-315

[94] Williams TN, Maitland K, Bennett S, Ganczakowski M, Peto TE, Newbold CI, et al. High incidence of malaria in alpha-thalassaemic children. Nature. 1996;**383**:522-525

[95] Fucharoen S, Weatherall DJ. The hemoglobin E thalassemias. Cold Spring Harbor Perspectives in Medicine. 2012;**2**

[96] Chotivanich K, Udomsangpetch R, Pattanapanyasat K, Chierakul W, Simpson J, Looareesuwan S, et al. Hemoglobin E: A balanced polymorphism protective against high parasitemias and thus severe P falciparum malaria. Blood. 2002;**100**: 1172-1176

[97] Fucharoen G, Fucharoen S, Sanchaisuriya K, Sae-Ung N, Suyasunanond U, Sriwilai P, et al. Frequency distribution and Haplotypic heterogeneity of beta(E)-globin gene

among eight minority groups of Northeast Thailand. Human Heredity. 2002;**53**:18-22

[98] Ohashi J, Naka I, Patarapotikul J, Hananantachai H, Brittenham G, Looareesuwan S, et al. Strong linkage disequilibrium of a HbE variant with the (AT)9(T)5 repeat in the BP1 binding site upstream of the beta-globin gene in the Thai population. Journal of Human Genetics. 2005;**50**:7-11

[99] Bunyaratvej A, Butthep P, Sae-Ung N, Fucharoen S, Yuthavong Y. Reduced deformability of thalassemic erythrocytes and erythrocytes with abnormal hemoglobins and relation with susceptibility to plasmodium falciparum invasion. Blood. 1992;**79**: 2460-2463

[100] Oo M, Tin S, Marlar T, O'Sullivan WJ. Genetic red cell disorders and severity of falciparum malaria in Myanmar. Bulletin of the World Health Organization. 1995;**73**:659-665

[101] Kar S, Seth S, Seth PK. Prevalence of malaria in Ao Nagas and its association with G6PD and HbE. Human Biology. 1992;**64**:187-197

[102] Williams TN, Wambua S, Uyoga S, Macharia A, Mwacharo JK, Newton CR, et al. Both heterozygous and homozygous alpha+ thalassemias protect against severe and fatal plasmodium falciparum malaria on the coast of Kenya. Blood. 2005;**106**:368-371

[103] Mockenhaupt FP, Ehrhardt S, Gellert S, Otchwemah RN, Dietz E, Anemana SD, et al. Alpha(+)-thalassemia protects African children from severe malaria. Blood. 2004;**104**: 2003-2006

[104] Allen SJ, O'Donnell A, Alexander ND, Alpers MP, Peto TE, Clegg JB. Weatherall DJ: Alpha+-thalassemia protects children against disease caused by other infections as well as malaria. Proceedings of the National Academy of Sciences of the United States of America. 1997;**94**:14736-14741

[105] Pattanapanyasat K, Yongvanitchit K, Tongtawe P, Tachavanich K, Wanachiwanawin W, Fucharoen S, et al. Impairment of plasmodium falciparum growth in thalassemic red blood cells: Further evidence by using biotin labeling and flow cytometry. Blood. 1999;**93**: 3116-3119

[106] Williams TN, Weatherall DJ, Newbold CI. The membrane characteristics of plasmodium falciparum-infected and -uninfected heterozygous alpha(0)thalassaemic erythrocytes. British Journal of Haematology. 2002;**118**:663-670

[107] Hill AV, Bowden DK, O'Shaughnessy DF, Weatherall DJ, Clegg JB. Beta thalassemia in Melanesia: Association with malaria and characterization of a common variant (IVS-1 nt 5 G——C). Blood. 1988;**72**:9-14

[108] Colbourne MJ, Edington GM. Sickling and malaria in the Gold Coast. British Medical Journal. 1956;**1**:784-786

[109] Cockburn IA, Mackinnon MJ, O'Donnell A, Allen SJ, Moulds JM, Baisor M, et al. A human complement receptor 1 polymorphism that reduces plasmodium falciparum rosetting confers protection against severe malaria. Proceedings of the National Academy of Sciences of the United States of America. 2004;**101**:272-277

[110] Luzzi GA, Merry AH, Newbold CI, Marsh K, Pasvol G. Protection by alpha-thalassaemia against plasmodium falciparum malaria: Modified surface antigen expression rather than impaired growth or cytoadherence. Immunology Letters. 1991;**30**:233-240

[111] Yuthavong Y, Bunyaratvej A, Kamchonwongpaisan S. Increased

susceptibility of malaria-infected variant erythrocytes to the mononuclear phagocyte system. Blood Cells. 1990;**16**: 591-597

[112] Fowkes FJ, Michon P, Pilling L, Ripley RM, Tavul L, Imrie HJ, et al. Host erythrocyte polymorphisms and exposure to plasmodium falciparum in Papua New Guinea. Malaria Journal. 2008;**7**:1

[113] Enevold A, Lusingu JP, Mmbando B, Alifrangis M, Lemnge MM, Bygbjerg IC, et al. Reduced risk of uncomplicated malaria episodes in children with alpha+−thalassemia in northeastern Tanzania. The American Journal of Tropical Medicine and Hygiene. 2008;**78**:714-720

[114] Wambua S, Mwangi TW, Kortok M, Uyoga SM, Macharia AW, Mwacharo JK, et al. The effect of alpha+−thalassaemia on the incidence of malaria and other diseases in children living on the coast of Kenya. PLoS Medicine. 2006;**3**:e158

[115] Veenemans J, Andang'o PE, Mbugi EV, Kraaijenhagen RJ, Mwaniki DL, Mockenhaupt FP, et al. Alpha+ −thalassemia protects against anemia associated with asymptomatic malaria: Evidence from community-based surveys in Tanzania and Kenya. The Journal of Infectious Diseases. 2008;**198**:401-408

[116] Lin E, Tavul L, Michon P, Richards JS, Dabod E, Beeson JG, et al. Minimal association of common red blood cell polymorphisms with plasmodium falciparum infection and uncomplicated malaria in Papua new Guinean school children. The American Journal of Tropical Medicine and Hygiene. 2010;**83**:828-833

[117] Haldane JB. A test for homogeneity of records of familial abnormalities. Annals of Eugenics. 1949;**14**:339-341

[118] Thein SL. Genetic association studies in beta-hemoglobinopathies. Hematology. American Society of Hematology. Education Program. 2013; **2013**:354-361

[119] Kaminsky R, Kruger N, Hempelmann E, Bommer W. Reduced development of plasmodium falciparum in beta-thalassaemic erythrocytes. Zeitschrift für Parasitenkunde. 1986;**72**: 553-556

[120] Senok AC, Li K, Nelson EA, Yu LM, Tian LP, Oppenheimer SJ. Invasion and growth of plasmodium falciparum is inhibited in fractionated thalassaemic erythrocytes. Transactions of the Royal Society of Tropical Medicine and Hygiene. 1997;**91**:138-143

[121] Carlson J, Nash GB. Gabutti V, al-Yaman F, Wahlgren M: Natural protection against severe plasmodium falciparum malaria due to impaired rosette formation. Blood. 1994;**84**: 3909-3914

[122] Penman BS, Pybus OG, Weatherall DJ, Gupta S. Epistatic interactions between genetic disorders of hemoglobin can explain why the sickle-cell gene is uncommon in the Mediterranean. Proceedings of the National Academy of Sciences of the United States of America. 2009;**106**: 21242-21246

[123] Beutler E. The hemolytic effect of primaquine and related compounds: A review. Blood. 1959;**14**:103-139

[124] Beutler E. Glucose-6-phosphate dehydrogenase deficiency: a historical perspective. Blood. 2008;**111**:16-24

[125] Nair PA, Al Khusaiby SM. Kernicterus and G6PD deficiency–a case series from Oman. Journal of Tropical Pediatrics. 2003;**49**:74-77

[126] Ginsburg H, Atamna H, Shalmiev G, Kanaani J, Krugliak M.

Resistance of glucose-6-phosphate dehydrogenase deficiency to malaria: Effects of fava bean hydroxypyrimidine glucosides on plasmodium falciparum growth in culture and on the phagocytosis of infected cells. Parasitology. 1996;**113**(Pt 1):7-18

[127] Cappadoro M, Giribaldi G, O'Brien E, Turrini F, Mannu F, Ulliers D, et al. Early phagocytosis of glucose-6-phosphate dehydrogenase (G6PD)-deficient erythrocytes parasitized by plasmodium falciparum may explain malaria protection in G6PD deficiency. Blood. 1998;**92**:2527-2534

[128] Luzzatto L, Usanga FA, Reddy S. Glucose-6-phosphate dehydrogenase deficient red cells: Resistance to infection by malarial parasites. Science. 1969;**164**:839-842

[129] Usanga EA, Luzzatto L. Adaptation of plasmodium falciparum to glucose 6-phosphate dehydrogenase-deficient host red cells by production of parasite-encoded enzyme. Nature. 1985;**313**: 793-795

[130] Ganczakowski M, Bowden DK, Maitland K, Williams TN, O'Shaughnessy D, Viji J, et al. Thalassaemia in Vanuatu, south-West Pacific: Frequency and haematological phenotypes of young children. British Journal of Haematology. 1995;**89**: 485-495

[131] Tishkoff SA, Varkonyi R, Cahinhinan N, Abbes S, Argyropoulos G, Destro-Bisol G, et al. Haplotype diversity and linkage disequilibrium at human G6PD: Recent origin of alleles that confer malarial resistance. Science. 2001;**293**: 455-462

[132] Sabeti PC, Reich DE, Higgins JM, Levine HZ, Richter DJ, Schaffner SF, et al. Detecting recent positive selection in the human genome from haplotype structure. Nature. 2002;**419**:832-837

[133] Johnson MK, Clark TD, Njama-Meya D, Rosenthal PJ, Parikh S. Impact of the method of G6PD deficiency assessment on genetic association studies of malaria susceptibility. PLoS One. 2009;**4**:e7246

[134] Guindo A, Fairhurst RM, Doumbo OK, Wellems TE, Diallo DA. X-linked G6PD deficiency protects hemizygous males but not heterozygous females against severe malaria. PLoS Medicine. 2007;**4**:e66

[135] Modell B, Darlison M. Global epidemiology of haemoglobin disorders and derived service indicators. Bulletin of the World Health Organization. 2008;**86**:480-487

[136] Weatherall D, Greenwood B, Chee HL, Wasi P: Science and Technology for Disease Control: Past, Present, and Future. In Disease Control Priorities in Developing Countries. Edited by nd, Jamison DT, Breman JG, Measham AR, Alleyne G, Claeson M, Evans DB, Jha P, Mills A, Musgrove P. Washington, DC 2006

[137] Colah R, Gorakshakar A, Phanasgaonkar S, D'Souza E, Nadkarni A, Surve R, et al. Epidemiology of beta-thalassaemia in Western India: Mapping the frequencies and mutations in sub-regions of Maharashtra and Gujarat. British Journal of Haematology. 2010;**149**: 739-747

[138] de Silva S, Fisher CA, Premawardhena A, Lamabadusuriya SP, Peto TE, Perera G, et al. Thalassaemia in Sri Lanka: Implications for the future health burden of Asian populations. Sri Lanka Thalassaemia Study Group. Lancet. 2000;**355**:786-791

[139] O'Riordan S, Hien TT, Miles K, Allen A, Quyen NN, Hung NQ, et al. Large scale screening for haemoglobin disorders in southern Vietnam: Implications for avoidance and

management. British Journal of Haematology. 2010;**150**:359-364

[140] Fattoum S. Evolution of hemoglobinopathy prevention in Africa: Results, problems and prospect. Mediterr J Hematol Infect Dis. 2009;**1**: e2009005

[141] Sachs J, Malaney P. The economic and social burden of malaria. Nature. 2002;**415**:680-685

[142] Opi DH, Swann O, Macharia A, Uyoga S, Band G, Ndila CM, et al. Two complement receptor one alleles have opposing associations with cerebral malaria and interact with alpha(+) thalassaemia. eLife. 2018;**7**

[143] Mangano VD, Clark TG, Auburn S, Campino S, Diakite M, Fry AE, et al. Lack of association of interferon regulatory factor 1 with severe malaria in affected child-parental trio studies across three African populations. PLoS One. 2009;**4**:e4206

[144] Damena D, Denis A, Golassa L, Chimusa ER. Genome-wide association studies of severe P. falciparum malaria susceptibility: Progress, pitfalls and prospects. BMC Medical Genomics. 2019;**12**:120

[145] Manolio TA. Cohort studies and the genetics of complex disease. Nature Genetics. 2009;**41**:5-6

Chapter 2

Sickle Cell Anemia, Representations and Care: Experience of a Brother of a Sick Child in Cameroon

Hassan Njifon Nsangou and Régine Scelles

Abstract

In Africa, families often with more than one child consult with both modern and traditional African medicine to treat their child with sickle cell anemia. This research aimed to understand how a child experiences both the medical and traditional care of his sister. We collected data from an interview and family drawing of a young boy growing up with an affected sister in Cameroon. Results showed this child persisted to feel as though his sister had fallen victim to a sorcerer and that he was at risk of the same fate even after the two of them received traditional treatment. He also felt neglected about his suffering because of his sister's disease by hospital professionals that were caring for her. It is therefore necessary to establish a support system for affected children and their family by providing a safe space in hospitals where they can express and contain their experiences with the disease.

Keywords: sickle cell anemia, care, tradition, modernity, siblings, Cameroon

1. Introduction

Sickle cell anemia is a genetic disease that confronts families with iterative, intense and unpredictable crises associated with the physical manifestation on the sick child [1] to his death thought to be imminent and inevitable. It is a taboo in most sub-Saharan African families [2] where it is difficult to meet unique children. Few psychological studies have focused on what happens to children who grow up with a sibling with sickle cell disease which is characterized by severe pain, frequent hospitalization and early death not to mention the high cost of treatment (traditional and medical) for families. However, it is unclear how families live the traditional and medical care of the disease.

This article includes an interview and drawing analysis done with a brother of a sick child in the context of research whose framework and method will be briefly presented. It highlights the way in which a child perceives the healthcare of his sister, both by Western medicine professionals and traditional healers—two types of care specialists with virtually different processes and goals. It is therefore a question of understanding the psychological impact of the concurrent consultation of medical and traditional care of a sick child on his brother. The article illuminates and questions the simultaneous existence of two sickle cell care systems within a

Cameroonian family and tries to understand its effects on a brother of a sick child. It shows the complexity of the experiences of children growing up with a sick sibling and its close interweaving with the family experiences as they care for the child. The objective is to build on this knowledge to open up the design of care devices that better take into account the specificity of the experiences of siblings of children with sickle cell anemia.

2. Theoretical consideration

2.1 The sickle cell anemia, a serious and deadly genetic disease

Sickle cell anemia is the most prevalent genetic disease in the world, with approximately 500 million individuals with sickle cell traits and 50 million individuals with the disorder itself worldwide [3]. Originally spread across malaria-endemic areas such as sub-Saharan African countries, historical migrations linked to the slave trade and the recent acceleration of migration flows have gradually changed its distribution worldwide [4]. It is found in almost all countries with large populations from Africa and regions around the Mediterranean. In France, for example, it is a rare disease, but nonetheless the most common genetic disease with a prevalence of one child per 1900 births [5].

With a prevalence rate of at least 2% in the general population and an estimated mortality rate of more than 70% among children under the age of 5 [6], the African continent is most affected by sickle cell anemia. Cameroon is one of the most affected countries, with a prevalence of 8.34% in the general population [7]. In sub-Saharan Africa, the unavailability of bone marrow transplantation—the only effective treatment for seizures—increases the risk of death in children under 5 years old [8].

The disease is an autosomal recessive pathology transmitted to the child by both parents. The presence of abnormal hemoglobin in the blood causes a deficiency in the supply of oxygen to various organs in the body by the red blood cells that have reduced life cycles. This leads to anemia and chronic, unpredictable pain [4, 9] that the patient identifies [1], resulting in multiple expensive hospitalizations and care organized by their parents [10] both in the hospital and among traditional healers.

2.2 The sickle cell anemia, a persecution figure of the family group

In the sub-Saharan African cultural context, sickle cell anemia is thought of as an "evil" that can attack any member of the family, even after the death of the patient [11]. The sick child is immersed in a society structured by traditional taboos, rituals and attitudes of which women are custodians [12]. The illness or handicap of the child is inscribed in this cultural structure, which gives it meaning and produces effects.

Sickle cell anemia is thought to be a manifestation of the possession of the sick child and his family by an evil spirit or bewitchment by a wizard [13]. It can also be perceived as a request of the ancestors to repair a transgression of an ancestral norm, addressed to the patient's family [14]. Generally, the mother is designated as responsible for this transgression and the overprotection of the sick child, by her and by the family members, constitutes a defense allowing them to feel guilt-free and to put the child in the family's history [14] alongside his brothers and sisters.

2.3 The specificities of the medical care of sickle cell anemia in Cameroon

The hospital is a place regularly frequented by sick children and their families. Described as the disease of hospitals in several African countries [15], sickle cell anemia makes hospital services a second home for the patient and their families around them. The frequency of hospitalizations in Cameroon is estimated to be between three and four hospitalizations per month in children under five, between five and seven hospitalizations per month in adolescents and two hospitalizations per month in adults [16]. The reasons for these hospitalizations are sometimes varied in one subject and identical in others. In general, sick children are regularly hospitalized for pain attacks, severe anemia and/or chronic complications (stroke and heart attacks). Stroke is also a cause of hospitalization for sickle cell patients. For the latter, the probabilities of having a stroke before the ages of 20, 30 and 45 are, respectively, 11, 15 and 24% [17]. In Cameroon, the prevalence of stroke is 6–7% in patients aged 7 months–35 years [18].

The medical management of patients has undergone an important evolution within the past 20 years due to the intensification of available treatments for children at risk of severe complications [19]. These treatments consist mainly of yoglycurea, transfusion programs and family transplants. Indeed, yoglycan significantly reduces the frequency of onset of occlusive seizures, acute thoracic syndrome and the degree of hemolysis. The establishment of transfusion programs for children detected as at risk of stroke by transcranial Doppler has significantly reduced this risk from 11 to 2% [19].

Allogeneic transplantation is currently the only treatment that can cure approximately 95% of children with sickle cell anemia [8, 20]. This treatment involves grafting from a brother or sister of the patient, based on their genetic compatibility with hematopoietic stem cells located in the bone marrow of the patient.

Sickle cell anemia is essentially a disease of the south whose treatment is in the north. This caricature seems more appropriate to address the lethal nature of this pathology in sub-Saharan African countries, including Cameroon, where it remains a chronic and orphan disease [21] because of the absence of hematopoietic stem cell allograft and the gene editing systems, the only treatments available against this disease [8, 9, 22]. Therefore, the therapeutic approach of the disease remains curative and focuses on the nature of the crises. The patient is supported in relation to the type of crisis he manifests. The primary purpose of medicine, in this case, is to alleviate the suffering of the patient by managing the symptoms. Crisis treatment incorporates several therapeutic products and postures. Severe attacks (mild pain, modeled fever) are often treated at home in collaboration with a doctor or by self-medication. The patient is advised to rest, drink abundantly and is given an analgesic treatment including acetylsalicylic acid, paracetamol or Di-Antalvic. In case of severe attacks involving localized or generalized pain, rest and rehydration are recommended. If these measures do not calm the crisis, a transfusion is performed.

The management of anemia, meanwhile, requires a transfusion of phenotyped erythrocyte concentrates, leukocyte depleted and filtered. The intervention in cases of severe pain attacks is based on the transfusion and/or hydroxyurea of the patient. Hydroxycarbamide is the only current attenuator therapy used in the management of vaso-occlusive seizures and severe anemias. The price of these products, combined with that of many hospitalizations, is relatively high for most Cameroonian families who generally do not have social security [16].

2.4 Balancing between traditional care and medical care

Parents of sick children, supported by the members of their extended families, are frequently searching for ways to relieve their suffering. With the advent of globalization, they resort to several therapies. The therapeutic route is, in this sense, a sort of mosaic between traditional therapies and imported Western and messianic therapies. In this way, the traditional therapist, the doctor and the Imam, pastor or priest are consulted at the same time. This system of "round care" [23] is one that perfectly summarizes the therapeutic path of most African families in sub-Saharan Africa. At each source, they seek the healing of a specific aspect of the child's suffering. The quests for meaning of the child's illness, ancestral protection and reconciliation with the ancestors lead parents to traditional healers. With the priest, the pastor or the Imam, families seek the divine therapy to ensure protection from God. They usually do this because they yearn for the healing of the child under the mercy of God. With the medical doctor, they seek the somatic healing of the child. These families are part of a permanent search for identity reconstruction [24, 25]. The identities of Africans remain very complex as they continually attempt to find their identities, following the effects of globalization [14, 26].

The traditional treatment of sickle cell anemia is based on cultural representations of this disease that people have. It does not aim to repair physiological disorders. It focuses on restoring social order by reconciling the patient and their groups with their social and supernatural environments [14]. This therapy considers the sick child as a messenger, a person who talks about the transgressions of ancestral norms by a member of his family or the persecution of his family by a wizard. This is the reason why parents, uncles, aunts, brothers, sisters and cousins of the patient are all also patients of the traditional therapists.

2.5 Cameroonian families oscillating between modernity and tradition

African families have retained certain intrinsic cultural values such as polygamy and the maintenance of family life through the births of several children. They have also opened up to modernity by gradually applying family planning practices.

In Cameroonian families, the cultural tradition is neither past nor "outdated" [14]. The behaviors of the subjects are always marked by identifiable traditional elements. These families have neither resisted nor surrendered to modernity. These are simultaneously modern and traditional families, not necessarily modern or traditional. In Cameroon, there are several types of families; nuclear families, extended families, polygamous families, monogamous families, etc. [27]. These categories reflect the diversity and complexity of family dynamics in Cameroon, and potentially the lives of children confronted by a sick sibling.

2.6 The experiences of the brothers and sisters of sick children

A child's illness has repercussions on their siblings who experience ambivalent feelings towards them. These relate specifically to shame, guilt, love, hatred, complicity, rivalry, anguish and the desire for the death of the sick child [28]. In order not to aggravate the suffering of their parents and that of the patient, brothers and sisters often attempt to prevent them from suffering [29].

Studies on sickle cell anemia patients indicate the psychological suffering of sick children and their parents [9, 14, 30]. The experiences of their siblings are often studied from the parents' stories. Overprotection of the child causes parents to progressively neglect caring for their other children [31]. The latter experience emotional breakdowns resulting in feelings of rejection, marginalization and exclusion on the part of parents and the extended family [32, 33]. They express jealousy towards the patient that they designate as the main person responsible for crises that destabilize the family financially and emotionally [34]. They feel guilty for having negative thoughts such as jealousy towards the patient; they consider themselves "bad siblings" [35]. They experience, at the same time, the desire for the death of the patient and the fear of this death [36]. Their experiences are usually influenced by parental intrusions in their relationships with the sick child because they are often parented by parents [36]. In the absence of the parents, they are the ones who supervise the sick child. Supervision ranges from daily monitoring of treatment and observation of medical instructions by the patient [2] to the bodily care of the patient and their assistance during hospitalization [37]. This has great implications on the sisters of sick children, particularly on girls' education. In many sub-Saharan African societies, the main objective is to bring up girls to be good mothers, thus making them the person most likely to take care of children [21].

3. Material and method

3.1 Specificities of the method

The methodology of this research is similar to that presented in a previous research [36]. In sub-Saharan African cultures, children who talk to professionals about themselves or anything else are supposed to have been given permission by their families to do so [38]. It is usually parents who talk to professionals about their children, who on their part are obliged to listen and to talk only when adults allow it [39]. Talking with children about sickle cell anemia is not easy and it requires the researcher to make an alliance with the family. This research, which took place in Cameroon worked to get parents to allow their children to talk with the researcher about the way they experience the care of their sick brother or sister. In fact, many children are not allowed to speak to strangers and to speak only to adults who are intimate with the family [40].

The parents signed consent forms concerning the participation of the family and children in the research and designated which of their children would participate. These children were allowed by their parents to speak with the researcher about their family, their sick brother or sister and his/her illness. Indeed they had a mission to talk to the researcher who informed them about their freedom to participate in this research. The method includes an individual interview with each child and a drawing, preceded and followed by a group time. Before the interview, the mother, in front of the whole family, talks about the relations between her sick child and his siblings; the children listen and keep quiet. After the interview and the drawing, the adults question the researcher and the participating child about the content of their meeting. It is therefore an individual meeting, but it takes place in a group setting allowing children to speak as freely as possible.

We report in this article the case of Jules. With Jules, we talked about the illness, his relationship with the sick child and the family. In Jules' interview, there is an important place for treatment and its effects on the sick child, on his siblings, on his mother and father and on extended family members. This interview was done in the absence of the other members of the family whom we asked to leave the family room to allow for confidentiality. The interview was followed by the drawing session after which the analysis of the drawing was done. The family drawing test followed the approach of [41], taking into account the cultural referent as advocated by [42]. We asked Jules to draw his family on a sheet. The drawing, complementary to the interview allows the child to project on the sheet what he thinks and experiences about his family, his sick brother and his place in the family.

3.2 Jules and his family

In accordance with the ethical requirements, we gave fictitious first names to the persons to guarantee the anonymity and the confidentiality of the meeting.

Aged eleven and a student in fifth grade, Jules is the third child out of five siblings and the older brother of Paulette, his sister with sickle cell anemia. After the death of his father, a nurse who had previously worked in his home village, Jules, accompanied by his sick sister and his mother emigrated from the village to settle in Yaoundé at his elder sister's home. This sister was a public school teacher. One of the reasons for this rural exordium is the medical follow-up of Paulette, eight, with sickle cell anemia. She is the second-to-last of the five siblings, three boys and two girls. The youngest of two siblings and three boys would probably have died, according to Jules's older sister, following sickle cell anemia crises. In Cameroon, sickle cell anemia is not well enough known by all public health professionals and some people still do not recognize nor know its symptoms.

Paulette's illness was diagnosed at the age of seven, when she was first hospitalized following an anemic crisis in a hospital in Yaoundé. The unavailability of prenatal diagnosis and the non-systematization of neonatal diagnosis of sickle cell anemia in Cameroon leads to children being diagnosed relatively late during one of their hospitalizations.

Paulette is usually hospitalized between one and two times a month following anemia attacks, the main symptom of her illness. Her mother, estimates the average duration of each of her hospitalizations to be between 2 and 3 days. During these hospitalizations, her older sister and her mother often assist her.

Jules lives with the eldest daughter in the family, his mother, his sick sister and his one-year-old niece. The eldest daughter of the siblings is separated from the father of her daughter and she is the only child who is a parent herself. Paulette is the only sick child and the mother of the family is unemployed. The eldest daughter and the second child of the siblings contribute to the financing of Paulette's care. Siblings are therefore a family resource in the financing of care. These first two siblings are employed and the last two are students.

4. Results

Paulette's fits give rise to many hospitalizations.

4.1 The financing of medical care

Jules does not know the cost of Paulette's medical care. He knows, however, that it is his older sister and his paternal uncle who finance this care. He exclaims "*Ah! I do not know the price. Mom and my older sister do not tell me the price. My older sister pays the hospital. There is also my uncle and my brother who also gives the money for the hospital.*"

He behaves as though he was forbidden and/or forbade himself from knowing or asking adults questions about the cost of his sister's medical care. However, he is grateful for the uncle's financial support to his mother and older sister. He does not mention the involvement of his brother who is a taxi driver in financing the care.

Her older sister and mother usually accompany Paulette to the hospital. This elder sister plays both the role of father and sister to Jules and Paulette. She finances the care and assists her mother at Paulette's bedside during hospitalizations. In the end, she plays the role of substitute for the deceased father and the mother for the sick sister. Her status as the eldest daughter of her siblings demands that she cares for her younger siblings, in keeping with the cultural norm that [40] makes the eldest son especially, and the eldest sister also, a parental figure for her brothers and sisters in African families. Jules specifies, "*My sister brings Paulette to the doctors of the foundation when the blood reduces.*" Therefore, he refers to this sister as a mother for both Paulette and himself.

Jules refers to the fact that the medical professionals at the hospital do not care about his family and his siblings. Their interest is in Paulette and the relief of her crises. Medical treatment is only given to the patient. Jules feels abandoned, forgotten and neglected by these professionals. He says, "*they do the remedies only to Paulette*" which signifies the sentiment of disregard of his own suffering at the hands of the professionals in the hospital.

4.2 The attendance at the hospital during crises

Jules refers to the fact that Paulette is usually brought to the hospital during her seizures. "*When her hands turn white or the eyes start to turn red, it's because the blood is already reducing. When the blood reduces, she becomes very tired and heats a lot. We bring her to the hospital.*"

The hospital is invested as having a curative function, given in urgency. All of this suggests that the family seeks hospital care only after failures of self-medication and preventive measures that it would have implemented to avoid or to relieve the crises. Obviously, this behavior of the family is an adaptation to the expensive nature of healthcare in a context where it is not reimbursed and where health insurance is non-existent [16]. This poses the problem of crisis prevention via the check-up of children with sickle cell anemia in sub-Saharan Africa, in general, and in Cameroon, in particular.

4.3 Recognition of non-effectiveness of crisis treatment in hospitals

Paulette's seizures are treated in the hospital via transfusions, which relieves seizures for a time without eliminating them. Jules evokes the infernal cycle of crises, hospitalizations and returns home. He says, "*in the hospital, she is given a lot of blood. When she takes the blood from the hospital, she comes home. It's always like that for Paulette.*" He recognizes the effectiveness of transfusion in relieving crises, but temporarily. What arouses him is an anguish of death concerning his sick sister "*When I see it like that, my body trembles.*"

Paulette's illness is thought of as "*a disease of the blood.*" Jules knows, therefore, that the "*affected*" blood must be removed from Paulette's body. "*In order for it to end, you have to empty all the blood from your body. Like that it will come out with the disease.*" In his view, this is not what hospital care professionals do because they put new blood in the sick child's body and do nothing about the "bad" blood.

Hospital care professionals are referred to as "responsible" for the chronicity of crises. Jules disqualifies them and thinks that they cannot permanently relieve these crises. "*The people in the hospital just put the blood into the bad blood. That is why the disease always comes back. When they put the good blood in their body, the bad blood eats up all the good blood, and the disease begins again.*" This recognition of the inefficiency of hospital care arouses his anger against these professionals whom he designates as ineffective against the worsening of his sister's state of health. It is possible that Jules, by this anger, projects on these professionals, his feeling of helplessness concerning the crises his sister goes through and the feeling of concomitant guilt. Medical professionals can also understand it as a cry for recognition and take into account his experience.

The hospital is designated as responsible for the death of the last daughter of the mother, who died from a sickle cell anemia crisis during her hospitalization. "*They put false blood in her body and she died. It was not necessary to put this blood in her body. When they put that blood, she died two days later. We were only called to be told that the child is dead, that we should take her body to the morgue.*" As a result, Jules shows distrust of the hospital, hospital professionals and the handling of crises by these professionals whom he designates as responsible for the death of his sister.

4.4 The traditional healer treats the patient and his family

The traditional healer cares for the sick child, her siblings, her parents and her extended family because the illness is considered an ailment of the patient and his family.

4.4.1 The care of the sick child

The traditional healer cares for the sick child's body. The body is thought to be possessed by an "evil spirit," an illness that manifests itself in the patient by chronic anemia and the seizures of pains in the back and feet. These symptoms inform the traditional healer about the extent of possession and persecution of the sick child's body by wizards. In response to this possession/persecution, the traditional healer provides bodily care to the patient.

Jules says that he was wounded on the body. The painful parts of the sick child's body are scarified to allow the therapist to act directly on the evil and to limit the destruction of the body by the wizards. He does this by administering a powder with magical powers, effective against sorcerers. Therefore, the care of the patient has a curative aim of "*freeing*" the patient from this possession and persecution by wizards. Thus, not only is the blood treated here, but also the body too.

4.4.2 Care of the brothers, sisters and the mother

Jules' mother and his paternal uncle accompanied Paulette to the traditional healer. The brothers and sisters, who were absent from the consultation, received through the uncle the treatment given by the traditional therapist. Jules refers to the fact that his paternal uncle administered on him and his other siblings scarifications and he applied the powder from the traditional healer. Because the father is deceased, the paternal uncle went accompanied his mother and the sick sister to the traditional practitioner. This shows the involvement of the extended family in traditional care and support for the mother in this process apart from acting as an intermediary between the traditional healer and the family. He is also responsible for monitoring the application of the traditional medication.

At the requestion of the traditional healer, his paternal uncle scarified Jules just as he did to his sister. The treatment was administered orally and via scarification of the back. "*Even my mother and my older sister ate the same medicine. After eating it, the remaining was put in the blood.*" Thus, Paulette's siblings and her mother who were considered at risk of becoming, and of being persecuted by witches were also subjected to the traditional treatment against sickle cell anemia. The goal of this treatment is to protect them against the ailment.

The traditional practitioner, through these treatments, sought to domesticate the harm represented by the disease. He did not seek to exclude this evil from the family, but to transform it into an entity likely to cohabit in harmony with family members. The "bad" blood of the sick child is thus transformed into "good" blood, into a blood that is no longer a threat to him or to the family members. This therapy does not aim at excluding the "evil" from the family, but to make the ailment an entity of the family and to bring the family members to accept it as such [43].

4.5 The experience of traditional treatment

With Jules, there is a before and an after of traditional treatment. An "unsecured" pre-treatment period where the threat of contamination by the disease looms, and a more "secure" post-treatment period when the threat is contained by receiving traditional treatment.

4.5.1 Treatment reduces feelings of insecurity

Jules thinks of the traditional treatment as a protection against its contamination by the disease. Taking this treatment is associated with a reduction of fear regarding the disease and possible contamination. He says, "*I'm not too scared. Before I was very scared. Now, with the remedy in my body, I'm not as afraid as I was before*." It is interesting to note that although the fear of his sister's death has diminished, it still lingers in his mind. He experiences his body as less vulnerable and more protected against the disease. This indicates that at this point, Jules feels safer with the disease and with the wizards.

The receiving of traditional treatment against sickle cell anemia thus helps Jules contain the fear and anguish that arises in him because of his sister's illness. It helps him to contain his feelings of persecution by the wizards and the fear of infection with the disease even if it does not totally eliminate this fear.

4.5.2 Treatment makes blood bad for wizards

For Jules, the blood of the patient is a dead blood, a blood possessed by the wizards. In this sense, "a bad blood" attacks the "good blood" transfused into the patient during hospitalizations. According to him, this gives meaning to the chronic anemia and the iterative crises of pain that his sick sister experiences.

The traditional treatment is thought by Jules to be effective against wizards. It makes the blood of the sick and the non-sick unassailable by wizards. His treatment reduces the feeling of persecution by wizards, even in the event that his sister dies. "*They will not look for me anymore*," he says. The traditional treatment is thus invested as a protection against the attacks of wizards, against the disease and, of course, against Paulette's and his own death.

Jules does not associate the death of a patient with the end of the disease as in the case of his mother's youngest daughter, which preceded that of their father. According to him, the disease survives and invests another child or family member. This leads Jules to think of himself as the next potential victim of the disease in the event of Paulette's death. "*If Paulette dies after her little sister, that means we're going to get another person to kill. If she dies, another person will die. That's what scares me*." Jules has a fear of death concerning his sister. He suffers more from this fear of death that he feels threatened by the disease, this "death". He thinks of his sister's imminent death and, therefore, his infection with the disease and his own death.

The administration of the traditional treatment leads Jules to say this about the wizards, "*it's over for them, everyone ate the cure, everyone is armored*," and specifically, "*when wizards enter the family they do not leave*." In connection with receiving traditional treatment, he says one thing and then contradicts it. He expresses ambivalent feelings of protection against and vulnerability to wizards. This suggests that the sense of security against witchcraft remains feeble, as the feelings of insecurity were never really eliminated.

4.6 The contribution of the drawing

The drawing was made, after the interview, on the dining table in the living room, lit by sunlight.

4.6.1 The complexity of the instructions

Following the instruction "*I would like you to draw your family*" Jules says he does not know how to draw human beings. Regarding his family, he thinks he is too tall to be represented on a sheet of paper and he asked for a second drawing sheet. He was told that for this drawing, it is recommended that he use a single sheet.

Jules persisted in his request by asking whether he could draw the other people on the back of the paper. To this question, the answer was negative. Following these requests for clarification of the instructions, he resigned himself to drawing according to the rules. This behavior is informative about the limits of family design in this context where the family is not limited to the father, the mother and the children. It is an extended family leading to the need to (re)think the handover, analysis and interpretation of this drawing in a sub-Saharan African context following [42].

4.6.2 The drawing of the extended family

The eldest daughter in the family ("grande soeur," on the drawing) is the first character drawn by Jules, followed by his father ("papa" on the drawing) the second character. This can signify in Jules that this sister is the most important person in the family because she provides a home near the hospital and money for medical bills. She took the role of the father. That can be why the father is then drawn second. Mother ("maman" on drawing), older brother ("grand frère Willie" on drawing), cousin ("grand frère Hugo" on drawing), maternal uncle and aunt, mother's aunt, paternal aunt, other maternal uncle, cousin mother ("grande soeur Manuella" on drawing), her maternal cousin ("petit frère" on the drawing) and her maternal grandmother were, respectively, drawn by Jules. All the characters in the drawing are real. There are no fictional characters. The drawing is invested as a projective support on which Jules illustrates what he lives and thinks about his family in connection with the illness of his sister.

That Jules's drawing includes his extended family reflects his sense of belonging to it and the support it brings to his immediate family in the face of his sister's illness and the successive deaths of his father and youngest sister. It is thus a drawing on which is projected the family solidarity surrounding his sister's illness (**Figure 1**).

The characters are not very invested by Jules, who drew them in a very minimalist way. It is possible that he wanted to draw all the members of the extended family, which would have led him to drawing his characters in a minimalist way on the sheet. It may also reflect an inhibition of affects in Jules concerning his family ties.

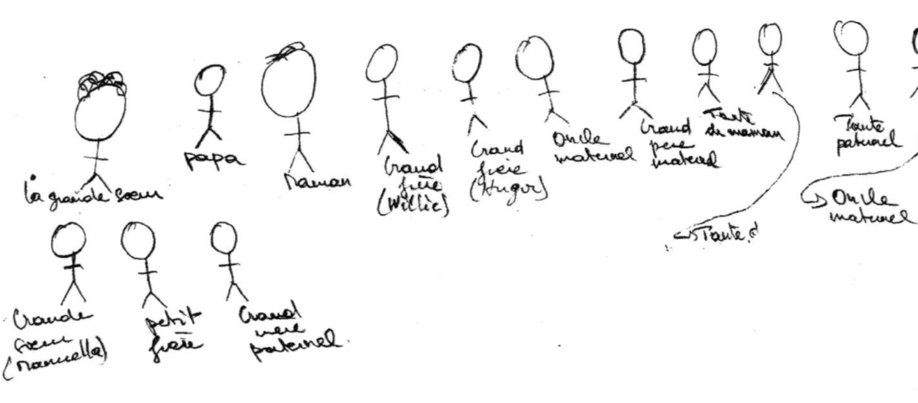

Figure 1.
Jules Family drawing.

Moreover, this is the first time that he drew human characters without drawing on a predefined model as he often does at school. However, a large part of the sheet is empty. The drawing is in the "upper central part" high center of the sheet, in a portrait orientation. The drawing location in the upper part of the document can signify the escape of the present, the escape towards the unreal and the distance from oneself according to [41]. It is therefore possible that this drawing signifies Jules' avoidance concerning his family, which is "inhabited" by death and disease. This may justify his lack of drawing.

No character is in contact with others as they do not touch each other. This can be interpreted as lack of family support and the isolation of family members according to [41]. This interpretation is questionable, however, in a cultural context where affection and support do not necessarily manifest themselves through physical contact [26] through touch, caress or hug, for example, thus reflecting the complexity of this child's life.

4.6.3 The elder sister, a father figure

Jules says he drew "*these people*" in his father's house, at his father's funeral in his village. Of all these characters, the elder sister ("la grande soeur" on the drawing) is designated as the happiest person. This is because, according to Jules, she bought the coffin for the burial of his father. The mother is referred to as the least happy person in the drawing because "*she was crying because she had lost her husband.*" The elder sister is invested psychologically and symbolically as the father of the family. She is the one who provided financial support for the funeral. She is designated as the nicest person in the drawing because she looks after her siblings. The fact that Jules first drew his older sister might reflect her emotional over-investment. She is invested as a mother emotionally and symbolically. The least kind person is the paternal aunt (paternal aunt, on the drawing). Jules justifies himself by declaring, "*It is they who caused the village to be fired. They are mean. They said that mom killed her husband.*"

When asked what role he would like to take within the family dynamic in the drawing, if he had the opportunity, Jules points to his mother saying, "*She is kind. As I go to school, she always buys me lunch.*" This reveals the mother's nurturing role in the family and invests her as an identification figure.

4.6.4 The absence of Jules on the drawing of a mourning scene

Jules said he had drawn his family members in his father's house during his father's funeral in his village. This tells us that he is still suffering grieving the death of his father. It is possible that Jules represents himself and associates his family with death, due to the past deaths of his father and his youngest sister, along with the imminent and distressing risk of the death of his sick sister. The family is therefore thought to be inhabited by death.

Jules's absence from the drawing may reflect his avoidance of the family, which he associates with disease and death. With this, he avoids living psychologically in this family dynamic, where he feels insecure about the circumstances. The sick child is also absent from the drawing. This can translate, for Jules, the anguish regarding the potential death of his sister. The sick sister is thus excluded from the family dynamic, thought of as not making/leaving her because of an illness that makes her a "dead" person. It could also be a way of distancing himself from this sister who reminds him of the suffering of the family. This absence contrasts with the presence of his later father.

The presence of the father in the drawing can explain in Jules the incomplete mourning process of this father who is still invested as alive. He remains present beyond his death; unlike the other daughter who died before him. While the dead father remains present (illustrated on the drawing), the sick sister' s absence from the drawing may signify Jules' avoidance of this sister and therefore, avoidance of the threat of death that accompanies her illness. On a psychological level, Jule's drawing may signify that, the living sister is dead, while the dead father remains alive. This complexity of Jules's experiences is illustrated within his drawing.

4.6.5 Friends and other supporters of Jules

Jules perceives the children in the neighborhood as helpers and supporters concerning his sister's illness. They are friends who support him by protecting his sister during games and other interactions with her. "*The children do not bother Paulette. They go to school and come back together. They do not cause any problems. Even when we play together, there are no provocations.*" Of course, these friends know that Jules is protective of his sick sister. They support him in this way by also protecting her and he is grateful for this.

Jules' friends are curiously absent from the drawing. He differentiates them from the members of the family. He does not make them part of his family; and hence their absence. In a cultural context where people with whom the subject has special relationships are considered to be members of their family [14], the absence of friends of the drawing is significant. This can tell you that Jules differentiates his friends from family members. Therefore, the support provided by the friends does not compensate for his feeling of abandonment by family members. They are considered outsiders and they may have no obligation over his situation. It could also exhibit his need for more support from within as the outside support could be a privilege.

4.6.6 The absence of care professionals

Healthcare professionals (hospital and traditional healers) are completely absent from the drawing. This absence can translate into their investment by Jules as outsiders to the family.

It is also possible that Jules did not draw them because their presence acts as that of the disease and, obviously, the risk of contamination and death. This absence can indicate a psychological effort to avoid anything that reminds him of the disease. In Jules, this absence can refer to the feeling that the traditional therapist does not protect him against the idea of possible contamination by the disease. It is possible that he did not draw the hospital professionals in order to protect himself against the feeling of abandonment by them.

4.6.7 The request for recognition of his experience

At the end of the drawing, Jules handed his drawing to me while smiling and he asked me to protect it well because it is very fragile. By a projection mechanism, he could be asking me to pay attention to his psychological suffering.

At the end of the meeting, with the agreement of Jules and following the requests of his elder sister, we presented the drawing to her and the mother. It is possible that Jules found by this means a way to make them understand his experience with Paulette's disease in a family context where talking about the disease remains taboo. Particularly moved by finding themselves in the drawing, the elder sister and the mother criticized the "non-human" nature of the characters he drew and the absence of the use of many colors on the drawing. The elder sister put this in relation to the pedagogical approaches used at school, which do not enable children to draw freely.

5. Discussion

With the exception of the sick child who is named by Jules during the interview, parents and siblings are referred to as parents or siblings. The eldest daughter is referred to as "*my big sister*," the brother who is a taxi driver as "*my older brother*," the sick sister as "*the last daughter of mother*," this is very important as she also died of sickle cell anemia. He does not refer to her as 'sister' maybe because he wants to distance himself from the condition which eventually led to her death, the things he fears most, and that have become a part of his family. This shows the specificity of his links to his sick sister. Jules refers to her niece as "*the daughter of my older sister*," thereby differentiating his brothers and sisters from his niece. He referred the father and mother as "*father*" and "*mother*."

Four people appear in Jules's drawing. Referred to in the interview as "*my older sister*," the eldest daughter is designated on the drawing as "*the big sister*." The brother who is a taxi driver is, however, named "*big brother Willie*" on the drawing while he is referred to as "*my big brother*" in the interview. The father and the mother are designated in the drawing by "*daddy*" and "*mother*." However, the father is absent from the interview. The absence of the father within Jules' speech is not synonymous with his absence in the psychological universe of the interviewee, as he is present on the drawing. This makes the drawing a mediator to speech and a complementary tool in the interview.

Not all the people mentioned in the interviews appear in the drawing, and those in the interviews are named differently in the interviews. This account for Jules' psychological dynamics concerning his links to family members and the complexity of these links.

The valorization of the traditional treatment (as financially expensive for the families as the medical treatment) contrasts with Jules persistence of the feeling of insecurity regarding wizards. It suggests that the treatment is not necessarily valued for its therapeutic efficacy. In a context where the traditional practitioner is considered as the intermediary between the ancestors and the living [44], it is forbidden to devalue their treatment. To do so would amount to devaluing the ancestors and running the risk of punishment, which could lead to death. The ancestor is incomparable [45] and therefore not criticizable. It can be dangerous to criticize the traditional treatment, as Jules emphasizes that it "alleviates" the fear and concerns the whole family.

Jules did not mention any consultation with a pastor, a priest or an imam. This is a problem in a context where families normally invest religious institutions (churches and mosques) to express their suffering and overwhelming misfortune [46]. It is possible that Jules, whose family is Christian, avoided talking about the care of his sister by the priest or by the pastor to a researcher whose family is of Muslim descent. He would have considered it disrespectful to talk about his religion to a researcher belonging to another religious denomination. It is also possible that, in not telling the researcher about his sister's consultation with priests or pastors, this young boy avoided hitting the researcher's religious sensitivity. He may not have talked to the researcher about this so as not to make him feel uncomfortable during the meeting.

In addition, this study showed that the traditional healer assigns, the uncle rather than the mother in the administration and follow-up of the care of the children and the family. This can be understood by the fact that the woman is often considered by traditional healers, as a being who can reduce the effectiveness of the treatment if she were to touch the patient [47]. Consequently, men are more often empowered to monitor and to enforce the prescriptions of traditional healers. It is also possible that the exclusion of women in this follow-up is motivated by the fact that they are considered to be responsible for the transmission of the disease to the child [14] and hence as a "stain" in family [4] and a hindrance to traditional treatment. In this case, it would be interesting to understand how mothers and fathers experience the care of their children with sickle cell anemia by hospital and traditional healers.

Jules's family agreed to participate in the research despite the fact that sickle cell anemia remains a taboo subject in African families [2]. It is possible that this family invested the research as a means of understanding the experience of the brothers and sisters of the sick child. The researcher can be considered a mediator who allows the family to talk indirectly about sickle cell anemia with the sick child and his siblings. The parents do not themselves talk with the children about this disease, but they prefer that someone else did it. Although this can be a coping mechanism due to the guilt they experience regarding the situation, they consider themselves as parents who have transgressed a cultural norm whose consequence is the child's illness. This behavior of the parents remains complex. Anyway, the participation of the family in this research shows the interest they had in understanding the experience of all the children in relation to the disease.

This research also allowed Jules to tell the researcher, his family and care professionals his experience with his sister's illness despite it being a taboo subject. It has therefore d upset the norm or violated the family taboo on sickle cell anemia. It would be interesting to understand the impact of Jules and his family's participation in this research on the mother, the sick child and Jules himself.

6. Conclusion

This article presents results similar to those of other works concerning the co-existence of traditional and modern representations of sickle cell anemia among sub-Saharan African families [9, 36] and their involvement in traditional and modern care systems [46]. Finally, Jules knows that in the event of seizures, only the hospital (where she is taken only for emergencies) can mitigate them and that there is a possibility that the treatment can fail and lead to her death, the brothers and sisters are then absent from this care. The traditional healers, meanwhile, intervene before crises in order to prevent them before they occur. This intervention protects the sick child and their family against the wizards, who are designated as responsible for the attacks and thereby the danger of a possible transmission of the disease to the patient's brothers and sisters.

This research indicates the need for spaces of speech within healthcare institutions that can enable families, parents and children to express their experiences with illness and care. It also indicates the need for professionals to take these experiences into account. It would therefore be interesting to question the experience of the sick child with the side by side existence of two care systems within the family.

Acknowledgements

Our heartfelt gratitude and thanks to Joy Gursky and Josephine Atieno for proofreading this work.

Conflict of interest

None.

Author details

Hassan Njifon Nsangou[1,2]* and Régine Scelles[2]

1 Département de Philosophie-Psychologie-Sociologie, Université de Dschang, Cameroon

2 Laboratoire Clipsyd, Université Paris Nanterre, France

*Address all correspondence to: hassannji75@yahoo.fr

References

[1] Josset-Raffet E, Yi MK, Benkerrou M. La trajectoire corporelle et psychique de la douleur chez l'enfant atteint de drépanocytose. Neuropsychiatrie de l'Enfance et de l'Adolescence. 2016;**64**(2):131-138. Disponible sur: http://www.sciencedirect.com/science/article/pii/S0222961716000040 [cité 8 sept 2017]

[2] Bonnet D. Rupture d'alliance contre rupture de filiation: Le cas de la drépanocytose. In: Dozon J-P, Fassin D, éditeurs. Critique de la santé publique: Une approche anthropologique. Paris: Balland; 2001. pp. 257-280. (Voix et Regards)

[3] World Health Organization. Sickle cell anaemia. Agenda item 11.4. 59th World Health Assembly [Internet]. 2006. Disponible sur: http://www.who.int/gb/ebwha/pdf_files/WHA59-REC1/e/WHA59_2006_REC1 [cité 12 juin 2012]

[4] Gernet S, Mestre C, Runel-Belliard C. Du pays d'origine au pays «d'accueil»: Perception de la maladie chez 26 familles drépanocytaires suivies au CHU de Bordeaux. Journal de pédiatrie et de puériculture. 2012;**25**(6):309-315. Disponible sur: http://www.em-consulte.com/en/article/771297 [cité 14 juill 2017]

[5] Njifon Nsangou H, Falck J, Scelles R. Culture familiale de la drépanocytose et image du corps chez les enfants atteints. Annales Médico-psychologiques, revue psychiatrique. 2019. Disponible sur: http://www.sciencedirect.com/science/article/pii/S0003448719302999 [cité 3 déc 2019]

[6] Organisation Mondiale de la Santé. Drépanocytose: Une stratégie pour la Région africaine de l'OMS: Rapport du Directeur régional. OMS. Bureau régional de l'Afrique 2011. Disponible sur: http://www.who.int/iris/handle/10665/1727 [cité 7 juill 2017]

[7] Weatherall DJ, Clegg JB. Inherited haemoglobin disorders: An increasing global health problem. Bulletin of the World Health Organization. 2001;**79**(8):704-712. Disponible sur: http://www.scielosp.org/scielo.php?script=sci_abstract&pid=S0042-96862001000800005&lng=en&nrm=iso&tlng=en [cité 9 juill 2017]

[8] Pradère J, Drain É, Taïeb O, Dutray B, Abbal T, Champion M, et al. Le travail de guérison d'une maladie chronique de l'enfant: Enjeux, processus et vulnérabilités. La Psychiatrie de l'Enfant. 2008;**51**(1):73-124. Disponible sur: http://www.cairn.info/revue-la-psychiatrie-de-l-enfant-2008-1-p-73.htm [cité 7 juill 2017]

[9] d'Autume C, Cavadini R, Giannica D, Drain É, Giraud F, Moro MR, et al. «Le sang de mon frère». Expérience de la greffe intrafamiliale à travers dessins et discours d'enfants drépanocytaires, « My brother's blood ». The experience of an intrafamilial transplant through drawings and the words of drepanocytic children. La Psychiatrie de l'Enfant. 2015;**57**(2):355-408. Disponible sur: http://www.cairn.info/revue-la-psychiatrie-de-l-enfant-2014-2-p-355.htm [cité 12 juill 2017]

[10] Mbassa Menick D, Ngoh F. Maltraitance psychologique d'enfants drépanocytaires au Cameroun: Description et analyse de cas. Médecine Tropicale. 2001;**61**:163-168

[11] Fotso-Djemo J-B. Le regard de l'autre: Médecine traditionnelle africaine. Paris: Agence de Coopération Culturelle et Technique EdSilex; 1982. 447 p

[12] Keita T. Phénoménologie traditionnelle de l'enfance en Afrique. In: Itoua F, Tettekpoe DA, Traoré A, Keita T,

M'Baye M, Kotto E, et al., éditeurs. Famille, enfant et développement en Afrique. Paris: Uneso; 1988. pp. 99-139

[13] Bonnet D. Au-delà du gène et de la culture. Hommes et Migrations. 2000;**1225**(1):23-38. Disponible sur: http://www.persee.fr/doc/homig_1142-852x_2000_num_1225_1_3508 [cité 3 juill 2017]

[14] Tsala Tsala J-P. Familles africaines en thérapie : Clinique de la famille camerounaise. Paris: Editions L'Harmattan; 2009. 268 p

[15] Bouchaud O. Intégrer les représentations culturelles dans la prise en charge des migrants. La Santé de l'Homme. 2007;**392**:25-27. Disponible sur: http://inpes.santepubliquefrance.fr/SLH/articles/392/03.htm [cité 7 mars 2017]

[16] Ndjiengwe F. Du stigmate physique au marquage symbolique: Évolution de la construction identitaire dans la drépanocytose. In: Lainé A, Bonnet D, Keclard L, Romana M, éditeurs. La drépanocytose Regards croisés sur une maladie orpheline. Paris: KARTHALA Editions; 2004. pp. 221-228

[17] Ohene-Frempong K, Weiner SJ, Sleeper LA, Miller ST, Embury S, MoohrJW,etal.Cerebrovascularaccidents in sickle cell disease: Rates and risk factors. Blood. 1998;**91**(1):288-294. Disponible sur: http://www.bloodjournal.org/content/91/1/288 [cité 7 juill 2017]

[18] Njamnshi AK, Mbong EN, Wonkam A, Ongolo-Zogo P, Djientcheu VD, Sunjoh FL, et al. The epidemiology of stroke in sickle cell patients in Yaounde, Cameroon. Journal of the Neurological Sciences. 2006;**250**(1):79-84. Disponible sur: http://www.sciencedirect.com/science/article/pii/S0022510X06003327 [cité 7 juill 2017]

[19] Kamdem A. L'évolution des pratiques dans la prise en charge de la drépanocytose chez l'enfant. In: 4ème symposium international du Réseau d'Etude de la Drépanocytose en Afrique Centrale (REDAC). Yaoundé; 2013. pp. 12-14

[20] Benkerrou M. Place de la greffe de cellules souches hématopoïétiques dans la drépanocytose. In: 4ème symposium international du Réseau d'Etude de la Drépanocytose en Afrique Centrale (REDAC). Yaoundé; 2013. pp. 30-33

[21] Lainé A. Parents d'enfants drépanocytaires face à la maladie et au système de soin. [Internet]. Paris; 2007. Disponible sur: https://hal.archives-ouvertes.fr/hal-00326056 [cité 13 juill 2017]

[22] Drain E, Pradère J, Taieb O, Dutray B, Champion M, Bonnet D, et al. Processus de guérison d'une maladie chronique: La drépanocytose traitée par allogreffe de cellules souches hématopoïétiques: Principaux résultats chez les adolescents. Neuropsychiatrie de l'Enfance et de l'Adolescence. 2008;**56**(4-5):305-310. Disponible sur: http://www.documentation.ird.fr/hor/fdi:010047377 [cité 4 juill 2017]

[23] Mboussou M. Soigner en rond : Sur le front du Partage de l'espace thérapeutique en Afrique noire. Nervure. 2002;**1**(15):22-25

[24] Mbassa Menick D. Les représentations sociales et culturelles du handicap de l'enfant en Afrique noire, Social and cultural perceptions of child disability in Subsaharian Africa. Perspectives Psy. 2015;**54**(1):30-43. Disponible sur: http://www.cairn.info/revue-perspectives-psy-2015-1-p-30.htm [cité 7 juill 2017]

[25] Menick DM, Simliwa DK. Nouvelles religiosités en Afrique: Des croyants à l'épreuve de la folie. Perspectives Psy. 2007;**46**(4):387-404. Disponible sur: http://www.cairn.info/revue-perspectives-psy-2007-4-p-387.htm [cité 7 juill 2017]

[26] Tsala Tsala J-P. Secret de famille et clinique de la famille africaine. Le Divan familial. 2010;**19**:31-46. Disponible sur: http://www.cairn.info/revue-le-divan-familial-2007-2-p-31.htm [cité 9 juill 2017]

[27] Ekomo Engolo C. Mutations socio-économiques et conditions de vie des ménages ruraux au Cameroun. Revue Française de Sociologie. 2001;**42**(2):281-294. Disponible sur: https://www.persee.fr/doc/rfsoc_0035-2969_2001_num_42_2_5355 [cité 21 mai 2018]

[28] Scelles R. Liens fraternels et handicap: De l'enfance à l'âge adulte, souffrances et ressources. Toulouse: Érès; 2010

[29] Scelles R. Frères et soeurs, complices et rivaux. Paris: Fleurus; 2003. 150 p (Le métier de parents)

[30] Evans RC, Burlew AK, Oler CH. Children with sickle-cell anemia: Parental relations, parent-child relations, and child behavior. Social Work. 1988;**33**(2):127-130. Disponible sur: https://academic.oup.com/sw/article/33/2/127/1897973/Children-with-Sickle-Cell-Anemia-Parental [cité 14 juill 2017]

[31] Adegoke SA, Kuteyi EA. Psychosocial burden of sickle cell disease on the family, Nigeria: Original research. African Journal of Primary Health Care and Family Medicine. 2012;**4**(1):1-6. Disponible sur: https://journals.co.za/content/phcfm/4/1/EJC133881 [cité 14 juill 2017]

[32] Assimadi JK, Gbadoé AD, Nyadanu M. L'impact familial de la drépanocytose au Togo. Archives de Pédiatrie. 2000;**7**(6):615-620. Disponible sur: http://www.sciencedirect.com/science/article/pii/S0929693X00801281 [cité 14 juill 2017]

[33] Burlew AK, Evans R, Oler C. The impact of a child with sickle cell disease on family dynamics. Annals of the New York Academy of Sciences. 1989;**565**:161-171

[34] Luboya E, Tshilonda J-CB, Ekila MB, Aloni MN. Répercussions psychosociales de la drépanocytose sur les parents d'enfants vivant à Kinshasa, République Démocratique du Congo: Une étude qualitative. The Pan African Medical Journal. 2014;**19**. Disponible sur: http://www.ncbi.nlm.nih.gov/pmc/articles/PMC4282867/ [cité 14 juill 2017]

[35] Gesteira ECR, Bousso RS, Misko MD, Ichikawa CRF, Oliveira PP. Families of children with sickle cell disease: An integrative review. Online Brazilian Journal of Nursing. 2016;**15**(2):276-290. Disponible sur: http://www.objnursing.uff.br/index.php/nursing/article/view/5289 [cité 14 juill 2017]

[36] Njifon Nsangou H, Scelles R. Drépanocytose et fratrie: Regard croisé du vécu d'une sœur et d'un frère d'un enfant malade. Journal de Pédiatrie et de Puériculture. 2019;**32**(2):75-84. Disponible sur: http://www.sciencedirect.com/science/article/pii/S0987798319300295 [cité 29 mars 2019]

[37] Souley A. «Emassi»: Discours autour de la drépanocytose en milieu Haoussa au Niger. In: Lainé A, Bonnet D, Keclard L, Romana M, éditeurs. La Drépanocytose: Regards croisés sur une maladie orpheline. Paris: Karthala; 2004. pp. 141-169

[38] Anate K. L'imaginaire de la communication à travers le concept de parole en Afrique et en Occident. Communication et organisation. 2002;**22**:12-21. Disponible sur: http://journals.openedition.org/communicationorganisation/2773 [cité 23 août 2018]

[39] Mappa S. Pouvoirs traditionnels et pouvoir d'Etat en Afrique: L'illusion universaliste. Paris: Karthala Editions; 1998. 210 p

[40] Ortigue MC, Ortigue E. Oedipe africain. Plon; 1973

[41] Jourdan C, Lachance J. Le dessin de famille: Présentation, grille de cotation, éléments d'interprétation. Paris: EAP Editions et Applications Psychologiques; 2000

[42] Tsala Tsala J-P. Test du dessin de famille et familles africaines. Le cas du Cameroun. Problèmes et méthodologie de la recherche. Annales de la Faculté des Arts. Lettres et Sciences Humaines. 1990;**VI**(1 et 2):201-216

[43] Bello MM, Giannotti A. Renaître en pays dendi. Couvade et possession au nord Benin. Paris: Le Grand Jardin; 2017. 164 p

[44] Burguet D. Au fil du récit d'un devin-guérisseur. Alliances avec les esprits ancestraux et de la nature (Vonizongo, Imerina). Études océan Indien. 2014;**51-52**. Disponible sur: http://journals.openedition.org/oceanindien/1560 [cité 13 oct 2018]

[45] Sow I. Les structures anthropologiques de la folie en Afrique Noire. Paris: Payot; 1978

[46] Mbassa Menick D. Famille, Foi, Folie et Soins en Afrique. Une pluralité des recours thérapeutiques complémentaires. Paris: Paari; 2018

[47] Faye SL. Quand les tradithérapeutes ouest-africains soignent l'infertilité conjugale à Dakar (Sénégal): Recompositions et dynamiques entrepreneuriales. Anthropologie & Santé Revue internationale francophone d'anthropologie de la santé. 2011;**3**. Disponible sur: http://journals.openedition.org/anthropologiesante/755 [cité 27 août 2018]

Chapter 3

Investigation and Management of Endocrinopathies in Thalassaemia Major

Kinda Al-Hourani, Jessica Lee Siew Hua and Parijat De

Abstract

A combination of sub-therapeutic chelation and subsequent iron overload are regarded as the principal drivers of endocrine dysfunction in thalassaemia. The clinical presentation of endocrine complications and their timing of onset can be highly variable, in part due to population heterogeneity but also variation in chelation strategies. Endocrinopathies commonly associated with thalassaemia include: growth delay; pubertal delay; gonadal dysfunction; thyroid disorders; parathyroid and adrenal gland impairment; impaired bone metabolism; and type 2 diabetes mellitus. In this chapter we summarise the main presentations of endocrine disorder in thalassaemia, summarising their epidemiology, clinical presentation and pathophysiologic basis. Furthermore, we review screening, monitoring and treatment strategies, with particular regard to the UK Thalassaemia Society's 2016 National Standards.

Keywords: thalassaemia major, beta thalassaemia, endocrinopathy, endocrine dysfunction, iron overload, puberty, thyroid, adrenal, diabetes mellitus, bone density

1. Introduction

The inherited haemoglobinopathy thalassaemia major (also known as beta thalassaemia major) results from homozygous carriage of mutations at the beta-globin locus, resulting in defective haemoglobin synthesis and a severe hypochromic, microcytic anaemia. Epidemiologically, the largest incidence of thalassaemia major is in the Mediterranean countries and the Middle East, but demographic change and international migration have resulted in it posing a global health issue. Life expectancy has been radically increased by the advent of combined transfusion and chelation therapy, but this regimen is complicated by both citrate toxicity and the development of endocrine complications secondary to destructive haemosiderin deposition in glandular tissues, particularly during adolescence and young adulthood [1]. Pathologic iron deposition is concentrated in cardiac tissue, the liver parenchyma and endocrine glands [2], with the development of multiple endocrinopathies first being reported by Bannerman and colleagues in 1967 [3]. Determining the prevalence and onset patterns of endocrine disease in thalassaemia major remains a challenge, despite their high frequency; primarily, this related to variation in exposure to chelation therapy, compliance with chelation, and improved survival shedding light on new disease phenomena [4–8].

Chronic anaemia—and subsequent tissue hypoxia—results in compensatory increases in erythropoiesis and gastrointestinal iron absorption. In conjunction with regular blood transfusion, these processes conspire to produce massive iron deposition in thalassaemia. Iron is regulated exclusively at the level of absorption, with no excretory mechanism. Chelation therapies are available, but challenges in their administration, including via the parenteral route, and need for regular

	Routine: annual	**Routine: other interval**	**Specific circumstances**
Glycaemic Control	Non-DM patients[*]: OGTT and fructosamine DM: fructosamine and review as per NICE 9 Key Care Processes[**]	DM: home capillary blood glucose as per individual management plan	• IFG or IGT: fructosamine at 6-monthly intervals • Symptomatic hyperglycaemia: random plasma glucose ± ketones to exclude DKA
Thyroid Function	Thyroid Function Tests (TFTs)[†]: free TSH, free T3, free T4		• Clinical evidence of thyroid dysfunction: random TFTs
Puberty	Systematic clinical assessment from age 10: Tanner staging		
Gonadal Function	Annual clinical assessment[‡] Men: annual morning testosterone Women: if normal menstrual history, no further investigations indicated	Male: if low testosterone ➔ measure LH/FSH/SHBG	Female: if oligomenorrhoea/amenorrhoea develop ➔ measure LH/FSH/oestradiol. Specialist endocrine review advised before initiation of hormone replacement.
Growth		6-monthly: height/weight/height velocity from diagnosis to attainment of final adult height	If concerns regarding growth delay: bone age estimation (wrist plain radiographs) at 1–2 year intervals Faltering height velocity: growth hormone stimulation test
Bone Metabolism	Vitamin D level[•]	6-monthly[••]: calcium/phosphate/ALP ➔ PTH if calcium level low	
Adrenal Function	Annual morning cortisol level		

Key: OGTT: oral glucose tolerance test DM: diabetes mellitus IFG: impaired fasting glycaemia IGT: impaired glucose tolerance DKA: diabetic ketoacidosis PTH: parathyroid hormone.
ALP: alkaline phosphatase LH: luteinizing hormone FSH: follicle-stimulating hormone SHBG: sex-hormone binding globulin.
[*] *From puberty, or age 10 years if family history of DM.*
[†] *From age 12 years.*
[••] *From age 12 years.*
[**] *NICE 9 Key Care Processes: glycaemic control (via Fructosamine); blood pressure; cholesterol level; retinal screening; foot checks; urinary albumin testing; serum creatinine testing; weight monitoring; smoking status check.*
[‡] *Including, for female patients, menstrual history; for male patients: history of impotence.*
[•] *From age 2 years. UKTS (2016) guidelines recommend ~80 nmol/L optimal target following supplementation.*

Table 1.
Summary of endocrine investigations in thalassaemia major [after UK Thalassaemia Standards, 2016].

blood monitoring, hamper their acceptability. The primary endocrine complications found in thalassaemia, in the order reviewed in this chapter, are: disorders of growth; sexual development and fertility; abnormal bone mineralisation; diabetes mellitus; hypothyroidism; and hypoadrenalism [9].

We have previously published an online Review of Endocrine Disorders in Thalassaemia in 2014 (Open Journal of Endocrine and Metabolic Diseases, 2014, 4, 25–34). In this book chapter, we have updated all the latest evidence and discuss current thoughts & details of the multi-system endocrine involvement in Thalassaemia. Finally, **Tables 1** and **2** summarise the investigations and treatment of such patients.

Glycaemic Control	• Impaired glucose regulation (IFG/IGT) or Non-insulin treated Diabetes: Intensify chelation therapy, consider using combination chelation regimens • Diabetes: Referral to diabetes specialist. Managed according to NICE treatment targets and recommendations for type 1 and type 2 diabetes	In patients with symptoms/signs of Diabetic Ketoacidosis (DKA) who are acutely unwell and plasma glucose>12 mmol; measure blood or urinary ketones
Thyroid Function	• Hypothyroidism: thyroxine replacement	✦Hypothyroidism may impair cardiac function/rhythm
Puberty	• Suspicion of pubertal delay: Referral to paediatric endocrinologist	
Gonadal Function	• Hypogonadism: hormone (oestrogen/testosterone) replacement • Females: combined oral contraceptive pill (when contraception is also required, or "post-menopausal" replacement regime)	✦Specialist endocrine review advised before initiation of hormone replacement.
Growth	• Positive growth hormone stimulation test: may consider GH therapy in childhood✣	
Bone Metabolism	• Vitamin D replacement if required • Bisphosphonates: considered for patients with low BMD for age‣, fragility fractures and/or falling BMD despite adequate vitamin D levels • Denosumab▹: advisable that treatment is supervised by a clinical with experience and interest in osteoporosis	• Bisphosphonate: should be reviewed after a maximum of 5 years for oral agents and 3 years for IV agents. Bisphosphonate 'holiday': is recommended after the above intervals for a period of 2–3 years
Adrenal Function	• Adrenal insufficiency: Hydrocortisone supplementation	✦Adrenal dysfunction may be subacute (during acute illness), consider adrenal support, even before formal proof of insufficiency is available

Key: DM: diabetes mellitus IFG: impaired fasting glycaemia IGT: impaired glucose tolerance DKA: diabetic ketoacidosis BMD: Bone Mineral Density GH: growth hormone.
✦*Note.*
‣*Z-score < −2.0 if premenopausal or under 50, t-score < −2.5 if post-menopausal or over 50.*
▹*Anti-RANKL monoclonal antibody.*
✣*some evidence for GH therapy in childhood only.*

Table 2.
Summary of endocrine treatments in thalassaemia major [after UK Thalassaemia Standards, 2016].

2. Growth and development in thalassaemia

From the foetal, through to infantile, pre-pubertal period and puberty, children with thalassaemia exhibit delayed growth [9]. It is estimated that 20–30% of these children and adolescents are affected by growth hormone (GH) deficiency [10]. In the remainder of thalassaemic patients without overt growth hormone deficiency, provocative testing—for example clonidine or glucagon stimulation tests—suggests that peak GH levels are lower than seen in constitutive short stature. Dhouib et al. recently showed a 35% incidence of GH deficiency in a Tunisian paediatric cohort [11]. Multiple causes for growth failure have been posited. These include features directly related to iron overload, including free radical toxicity [12]; damage to other endocrine axes, including the GH/Insulin-like growth factor (IGF-1) axis [13], pubertal delay and hypothyroidism; and complications of therapy, including chelation agent, particularly desferrioxamine, toxicity [14]. Hepatic cirrhosis, anaemia and zinc deficiency have also been implicated [15].

The anterior pituitary gland is particularly vulnerable to oxidative stress caused by free radicals, with even modest levels of iron deposition, detected by magnetic resonance imaging (MRI), disrupting its function [12]. Comparative studies of diurnal hormone secretion suggest that the 24-hour profile of GH secretion, and the response growth hormone releasing hormone (GHRH, secreted by the arcuate nucleus of the hypothalamus), in thalassaemic patients is similar that of children with idiopathic short stature [16]. It is posited that thalassaemia major may be associated with increased somatostatin tone, with subsequent disruption of GH secretion [17].

Thalassaemia major may be characterised by relative growth hormone deficiency, implied by the low levels of serum IGF-1 but normal GH reserve seen in patients. The positive therapeutic response seen with exogenous GH supplementation implies that, at the post-receptor level, this resistance may only be partial [18]. Anaemia, ineffecient erythropoiesis and chelation therapy also inhibits linear growth in children with thalassaemia major. Desferrioxamine and pathologic iron deposition are proposed to disrupt local IGF-1 production and paracrine signalling at the growth plate [14], resulting in inhibition of cellular proliferation and mineral deposition. Truncal shortening and abnormal body proportions are frequently observed, and have been attributed to the disease process itself, compounded by iron and desferrioxamine toxicity [18]. Limited evidence is emerging that these phenomena may be at least partly contingent on the timing of initiation of chelation and its route of administration. Soliman and colleagues reported a cross-sectional cohort analysis of beta thalassaemia patients commenced on oral iron chelation (OIC) with desferoxamine either before ($n = 15$) or after ($n = 40$) attaining final adult height. In this small study, pre-pubertal initiation of OIC was correlated with increased final adult height, in parallel with a lower overall incidence of endocrinopathies and reduced hepatic iron deposition [19].

Karamifar et al. have demonstrated that 62.9% of girls and 69% of boys affected with thalassaemia were less than 2SD below the mean for normal height [20]. Sharma et al. studied an Indian cohort of beta-thalassaemic children on oral desferiprone, of whom 55% were of short stature and 27% had a height z-score less than −3 SD. In the subset with height z-score < −3 SD, 17 of 19 patients also had severely impaired GH induction in response to dynamic testing with clonidine [21]. In one cohort from Germany, 40.6% of patients were defined as being short in stature (final adult height < 3rd percentile/below 2 standard deviations [SD] from the mean) [22]. Soliman and colleagues replicated this observation, reporting short stature (<2SD) in 49% of their thalassaemic patients [23], whereas Borgna-Pignatti et al. reported short stature in 37% of their patients [24]. Moayeri et al. showed that

62% were less than 2SD and 49% were 3SD below the mean and also confirmed decreased growth hormone response to two provocative tests and low levels of IGF-1 in a majority of their thalassaemic patients[24]. Similar reduced responses to provocative tests have been reported in studies led by Gulati et al. (51%) and Theodiris et al. (20%) [10, 25]. Interestingly, Soliman et al. report that in a small sample of adult patients on oral chelation therapy, IGF-1 expression levels did not differ significantly between those with normal GH levels and those with GH deficiency, despite significantly lower final adult height in the GH deficient group [19].

Although the results of short term GH therapy are encouraging, the impact of treatment on final height of non-GH deficient thalassaemic children remains uncertain [18] and often GH produces uncertain clinical response [26, 27]. Ngim et al. have undertaken a Cochrane Systematic Review of GH replacement in thalassaemia. A single non-randomised trial was eligible, which enrolled 20 Turkish children with beta-thalassaemia major, receiving either daily subcutaneous GH or standard care. It presented tentative evidence that height velocity may be increased with GH, but reported no significant differences in the height standard deviations between groups at the study end-point [28]. Most patients lack the pubertal spurt and have reduced GH peak amplitude [29], hence responses to recombinant human GH therapy is poor when compared with that of children with GH deficiency, idiopathic short stature or Turner Syndrome.

The 2016 United Kingdom Thalassemia Society (UKTS) guidelines recommend stringent assessment of growth during childhood. This includes recording of height (both sitting and standing), weight and height velocity at six-monthly intervals until final adult height is attained [30]. Height deficits should prompt referral to a paediatric endocrinologist. Plain hand/wrist radiographs at 1–2 year intervals until fusion of the epiphyses may aid investigation of faltering height velocity [30]. Reduced height velocity, particularly around age 8–12 years, should prompt consideration of both desferrioxamine toxicity and GH deficiency, requiring GH stimulation testing and supplementation if deficient [30].

In contrast to GH deficiency in childhood, GH abnormalities in adults with thalassaemia are less well characterised. Recent data from an I-CETA survey (International Network of Clinicians for Endocrinopathies in Thalassemia and Adolescent Medicine) covering 3314 adult thalassaemia major patients across 15 international centres, reported a GH deficiency incidence of 3% [31]. The discrepancy between this figure and earlier estimates from paediatric cohorts is multifactorial. Unlike childhood growth failure, there is no obvious pathological correlate of adult growth hormone deficiency to prompt investigation. Adult GH deficiency can manifest with neuropsychiatric symptoms; abnormal body composition; and cardiac features, including both reduced exercise performance [32] and altered myocardial structure [33]. Soliman and colleagues have proposed criteria for GH deficiency screening in adults with thalassaemia major. These include individuals with high iron loads, short stature (height < −2.5 SDS), low serum IGF-1 (< −2 SDS) or existing cardiomyopathy [34]. Given increasing survival of patients with thalassaemia major into adulthood, this topic remains in need of further investigation.

3. Hypogonadism and puberty in thalassaemia

Sexual immaturity is a profound complication of severe thalassaemia [35]. Disruption of the hypothalamic–pituitary-gonadal axis (HPG) may result in infertility [36]. While hypogonadism can occur as a result of primary or secondary hypogonadism or as a combination of both, multiple studies have shown gonadotropin failure (hypogonadotropic hypogonadism) is the commonest complication [36, 37]. Primary gonadal failure is caused by iron deposition on gonadal tissue [37]. Secondary hypogonadism occurs as a result of pituitary gland gonadotrophic cell iron deposition, as evidenced by GnRH stimulation which demonstrates inadequate FSH and LH response [38–40]. Failure of pubertal onset has a very high incidence rate, with studies varying between 50–100% [9]. In female patients, delayed puberty is defined as a lack of breast development in girls by age 13 and in male patients, by a lack of testicular development by age 14 [30].

Delayed puberty in patients with beta thalassaemia major occurs as a result of multiple factors. Evidence suggests that the accumulation of excess iron from multiple transfusions leads to tissue damage in multiple organs (e.g. the liver, heart, endocrine organs), and the presence of free radicals leads to oxidative stress [41]. Delays in sexual maturation has been shown to be a result of impaired synthesis of leptin caused by the deposition of iron on adipose tissue [42]. Adipose cells response to the expression of the *ob* gene to produce leptin which functions as an indicator to instigate puberty. Despite chelation therapy, iron accumulation continues to occur in the pituitary, hypothalamus and gonads [43]. The lack of response to gonadotropin releasing hormone in patients with low gonadotropin levels is synonymous with hypothalamic and pituitary damage [44].

While MRI assessment of the pituitary gland for iron accumulation has been studied with promising results, it is currently not part of routine assessment [45]. In terms of growth velocity, patients with thalassaemia were found to have distinctly lower or completely absent annual growth rates [46]. Short stature was found in up to 20% of such patients [14] and the lack of pubertal growth spurt in puberty, whether spontaneous or induced, ultimately adversely affected the attainment of a normal final height [18]. Impairment of truncal growth [47] is also compounded by disproportionate body ratios and variation in spinal growth. As a result, failure of pubertal growth spurt, delayed or absence of sexual development and infertility are common sequelae among patients with beta thalassaemia major [36].

Hypogonadism as an endocrine complication in patients with thalassaemia major has been reported in multiple studies [36]. A high incidence of hypogonadotropic hypogonadism has been found by Chern et al. in their study population [48]. A 45% prevalence was found in male patients and 39% in female patients, with an overall prevalence of 72%. Of note were significant delays or cessation in development of secondary sexual characteristics and the menstrual cycle. These findings were reiterated in a cross-sectional study set up in Hong Kong, in which 75% of female patients and 62% of male patients were found to have diminished gonadal function [13]. In a study conducted of by Saffari et al., hypogonadism was found to be the most common endocrine complication. From a study population of 77 patients, 36 (46.8%) patients were found to have hypogonadism, 28 (36.4%) had delayed puberty and in 8 (10.4%) patients there was absence of pubertal progression [49]. In this study, it was also noted that there was 'significant correlation between bone mineral density and pubertal status ($p = 0.001$). This study demonstrates the effects of hypogonadism not only on the reproductive system, but also on bone mineral density as well [49].

Failure of puberty was reported by Moayeri et al. in 69% of patients with thalassaemia with suppressed FSH and LH levels (73.2% in male patients and 64.8% in female patients) [50]. Similar findings were reported in a separate Italian multicentre study, which described hypogonadism 47% of female patients and 51% of male patients. Hagag et al. demonstrated that in males testosterone levels and testicular volume were significantly lower in thalassaemic patients with iron overload [51]. A similar study conducted by Hagag et al. in female patients, they showed that FSH, LH and oestrogen levels were significantly lower in thalassaemic patients with iron overload [52].

Pubertal failure has also been described in 73% of male and 42% of female patients under the age of 21 years old by Soliman et al. [23]. Similar findings were noted by Borgna-Pignatti and colleagues with 67% of males and 38% of females experiencing puberty failure [24]. Remarkably, successful conception may still be achieved by women who receive adequate chelation therapy.

Bone growth, growth velocity and puberty may be assisted by administration of chelation therapy before the commencement of sexual maturation and the use of low dose sex steroids in adolescence [9].

Current Standards for the Clinical Care of Children and Adults with Thalassaemia UK Guidelines recommend that assessment of gonadal function should be done annually throughout adulthood [30]. In men, this would include an annual morning testosterone level alongside LH/FSH and SHBG if testosterone levels are low. In women, no testing is required in the presence of a normal menstrual history. However, in the presence of menstrual disturbances, further testing (LH/FSH and oestradiol) is recommended [30]. Deficiency should be replaced with oestrogen/testosterone while bearing in mind that under-replacement contributes to a low bone mineral density. Management is best achieved through a joint multidisciplinary consultation between the endocrinologist and thalassaemia team [30].

4. Glucose intolerance and diabetes mellitus

Effective management of patients suffering from homozygous beta thalassaemia has led to improved life expectancy and hence manifestations of haemosiderosis related complications, notably, disturbances of the exocrine and endocrine function of the pancreas [53]. The prevalence of glucose intolerance and diabetes mellitus (DM) in patients with homozygous beta thalassaemia has been found to be variable. A retrospective analysis of 92 patients performed by Ang et al. showed that diabetes mellitus was one of the most common endocrinopathies with 41% of the study population affected [54] while a study conducted by Kanbour et al. reported a prevalence of 16.7% for impaired fasting glucose and 12.5% for diabetes mellitus [55]. Recently, a meta-analysis conducted by He et al. which included 44 studies with 16,605 cases showed that diabetes mellitus was present in 6.54%, impaired fasting glucose (IGF) in 17.21% and impaired glucose tolerance (IGT) in 12.46% [56]. While the prevalence of glucose intolerance and diabetes mellitus is undoubtedly high, many risk factors have also been identified. There was evidence of increased risk of diabetes mellitus with co-infection with hepatitis C [55–57], longer duration of disease [57–59] and with increased pancreatic iron deposition [58, 60].

Li et al. have found that in addition, patients with diabetes mellitus were characterised by higher ferritin levels, smaller pancreas volume, lower cardiac T2 magnetic resonance signal (MRI) than patients without diabetes, and higher prevalence of hypogonadism. Interestingly, patients with diabetes were found to be young (median age was 22 years [range of 10 to 34 years]) and non-obese (BMI of 20.1 ± 2.8 kg/m^2) [58]. This may explain why the classical association between diabetes and increased prevalence of arteriosclerotic cardiovascular disease is not a feature in this population [30].

Poor compliance with desferrioxamine therapy ($p < 0.05$), older age commencing intensive chelation therapy, liver cirrhosis and severe fibrosis were found to be risk factors for glucose intolerance and diabetes mellitus. Risk factors for impaired glucose tolerance (IGT) also included male sex [61], poor compliance with desferrioxamine therapy and high hepatic iron concentration.

Current UK guidelines recommend annual monitoring for impaired glucose tolerance and diabetes from the onset of puberty, or from the age of 10 years if there is a family history of diabetes [30]. Screening is carried out with the oral glucose tolerance test (OGTT) [30]. However, OGTT compliance is often poor. This makes the development of adjunct or alternative screening tests of particular interest, as detecting pre-clinical diabetes is crucial because the development of clinical diabetes can possibly be slowed down or halted. Pancreatic iron overload can be assessed by MRI [62] but does not seem to correlate with siderosis in other organs. Currently, the relationship between MRI detectable iron and pancreatic beta cell dysfunction is not well characterised and MRI of the pancreas for iron deposition monitoring is not used clinically [30, 63]. However, there may be scope to use cardiac and liver MRI which already have established protocols, for the purpose of screening for impaired glucose tolerance or diabetes. Ang et al. found that abnormal myocardial T2 signal may indicate the development of diabetes mellitus and other prediabetic states [54]. Li et al. showed similar findings whereby Cardiac T2 MRI values were higher in patients with normal fasting glucose levels ($P = 0.03$) [58]. Kanbour et al. found that patients with very high liver iron concentration (LIC) (>30 mg Fe/gm dry liver) were more likely to have a higher prevalence of impaired fasting glucose when compared to those with lower LIC ($p = 0.044$) [55]. The use of continuous glucose monitoring (CGMS) in detecting glucose intolerance and diabetes mellitus has also been studied, with CGMS found to be superior when compared to OGTT ($p = 0.012$) [64]. El-Samahy et al. studied 20 beta thalassaemia patients with random blood glucose >7.8 mmol, who then had OGTT and CGMS. OGTT detected 6/20 patients (30%) who had impaired glucose tolerance and 7/20 (35%) patients who were in the diabetic range, while CGMS found that 7/20 (35%) patients had IGT and 13/20 (65%) had frank diabetes mellitus [64].

In terms of determining overall glycaemic control, UK guidelines recommend that serum fructosamine should be used. Fructosamine is a circulating glycated protein which measures overall glucose control in the previous 2–3 weeks. HbA1c or glycated haemoglobin should be avoided in thalassaemia as it is unreliable in any haemoglobinopathy and also after transfusion [30].

Although inadequate insulin release has been reported by several groups [60, 65, 66]. Other aetiologies identified include hyperinsulinemia, reduced insulin sensitivity [67] and reduction of hepatic insulin release. A study by Siklar et al. suggested that development of insulin impairment occurs prior to insulin resistance [68]. Furthermore, autoimmunity results in selective oxidative damage to beta cells of the pancreas [68]. Beta cells retain their function up to the later stages of the disease [9], however insulin sensitivity was found to be inversely related to iron overload and age [69]. Fasting pro-insulin and pro-insulin to insulin ratios was found to be considerably elevated and have a positive correlation with hepatic iron [70], however C-peptide levels were found to be inconsistent, thus reflecting fluctuating beta cell function [71, 72]. A reduction in serum trypsin and lipase levels were found, alongside regular alpha amylase activity. It was also found that the development of other endocrine and cardiac complications were followed by the onset of diabetes mellitus [73]. A 50% decline beta cell function was found to be correlated with glucose intolerance, and beta cell function was not entirely recovered even after intensive iron chelation. Moreover, high transfusion regimes that were not paired with appropriate iron chelation could advance the prevalence of diabetes mellitus further.

The prevalence of abnormal glucose metabolism has gradually increased over the last 20 years [55]. Therefore, the topic of glucose intolerance and diabetes mellitus in patients with thalassaemia major continues to be of significant clinical importance.

5. Thyroid dysfunction

Thyroid dysfunction is a frequently occurring endocrine complication in thalassaemia major [39]. Hypothyroidism occurs either as a results of primary gland failure, or insufficient thyroid gland stimulation [74]. Hypothyroidism is thought to be a graded phenomenon and many types of hypothyroidism have been described: (1) sub-biochemical hypothyroidism: which consists of an exaggerated TSH response to TRH test in the presence of normal TSH and FT4; (2) sub-clinical hypothyroidism: elevated serum TSH with normal serum FT4 levels; (3) overt (clinical) hypothyroidism: High TSH with low FT4 level and (4) central Hypothyrodism: an inappropriately low or normal TSH with a low free T4 level [74]. The lack of autoimmune thyroiditis in thalassaemia patients continues to be supported by multiple studies [75, 76].

Subclinical hypothyroidisim was found to be the most prevalent thyroid dysfunction in many studies [77, 78]. In a study of 144 thalassaemia patients by by Saleem et al., hypothyroidism was found in 31.2% of patients. Subclinical hypothyroidism was found to be the most prevalent thyroid dysfunction (31.2%; 45 patients), whilst only 6.7% [3] patients were found to have overt hypothyroidism. Interestingly, 76% of the patients with subclinical hypothyroidism were in the first decade of life [77].

The study conducted by Yassouf et al. demonstrated that out of the 82 cases of thalassaemia studied, subclinical hypothyroidism was once again found to be the most prevalent thyroid disorder - 29.27% of patients [24] had subclinical hypothyroidism while only one patient (1.22%) had overt hypothyroidism. In contrast to other studies, no case of central hypothyroidism was found [78].

There is a general consensus that central hypothyroidism is underestimated as there are only a handful of studies on the topic currently. The diagnosis of central hypothyroidism remains difficult from a clinical perspective, as its non-specific symptoms means that symptoms are usually attributed to another cause. From a biochemical perspective, central hypothyroidism is diagnosed based on a low to normal TSH level, in the presence of low levels of free T4 [74].

De Sanctis et al. explored the prevalence of central hypothyroidism in their thalassaemia population (339 patients). They found that central hypothyroidism was present in 6% of patients aged less than 21 years old, and 7.9% in patients above 21 years of age. Delaporta et al. showed that 16% of 114 studied patients (mean age 20.9 ± 7.8 years) had central hypothyroidism [79].

A prospective study carried out by Soliman et al. followed a total of 48 patients over a period of 12 years. In this duration, hypothyroidism was diagnosed in 35% [17] of patients - central hypothyrodisim was found in 13/17 (76%) patients [75]. Unexpectedly, this paper also found that the mean serum ferritin level did not differ significantly between patients with or without central hypothyroidism. This in turn did not support the hypothesis that iron overload of the HPA axis had resulted in central hypothyroidism thus concluding that the precise underlying aetiology of central hypothyroidism was unclear. However, due to the susceptibility of the pituitary gland to excess iron, central hypothyroidism due to iron overload of the HPA axis still remains a possibility [74].

Belhoul et al. found an increase in prevalence of hypothyroidism in splenectomised patients [80]. In non-splenectomised thalassemic patients, the spleen was thought to have a scavenging effect on free iron fractions. However, further studies are needed to evaluate this hypothesis [74].

Thyroid failure was found to correlate with age at which iron chelation therapy started. When iron chelation therapy was started late, thyroid dysfunction was found to occur earlier [74]. A study published in 2018 by Upadya et al. showed that of a population of 83 children with thalassaemia, 4.8% had evidence of subclinical hypothyroidism. In this study, the mean ferritin level was 3983.0 ± 169,830 ng/ml. However, while the severity of thyroid dysfunction was statistically significantly associated with higher serum TSH value in children in the second decade of life ($p = 0.001$), it is important to note that no significant correlation was found between the severity of thyroid dysfunction and serum ferritin levels [76].

These findings were also echoed in the study conducted by Yassouf et al. They found that serum ferritin was directly correlated with TSH levels ($r = 0.414$; $p < 0.001$). However, there was no correlation between serum ferritin and FT4 levels ($r = 0.027$; $p > 0.05$) [78]. This study also demonstrated that the risk of thyroid dysfunction was increased by non-compliance of chelation therapy by 6.38 fold as compared with compliant patients (RR = 6.385 l 95% CI, 2.40–16.95) [78].

In another study a total of 72 thalassaemia patients were followed for 8 years. The study endpoint was defined as the incidence of thyroid dysfunction, and aim of the study was to analyse ferritin as a prognostic maker. It found that that patients with thyroid dysfunction had higher ferritin levels in contrast to those with normal thyroid function (1500 (872–2336)) vs. (513 (370–698) ug/l; $P < 0.0001$). The study also found patients with ferritin values above 1800ug/L had a more rapid progression towards the endpoint of thyroid dysfunction [81].

However, as a single value, ferritin may not always be reliable. Ferritin, as an acute phase protein, is subject to fluctuations caused by other variables such as inflammation and malignancy. However, ferritin may still be the most convenient way to assess iron overload, especially when used as part of a serial measurement [81]. Ferritin may be of value as a prognostic maker and may be used to identify patients at risk of developing thyroid dysfunction [81]. This begs the question as to whether the value of ferritin in determining the severity of thyroid dysfunction is over-appreciated [76].

Currently, the UK Thalassaemia Society Standards for the clinical care of children and adults with thalassaemia in the UK (2016) recommend thyroid functions tests annually in patients with thalassaemia from age of 12 years, or if there are any suggestive symptoms of thyroid deficiency between times [30].

6. Hypoparathyroidism

Hypoparathyroidism, resulting in hypocalcaemia, is a late complication of iron overload, typically manifesting after the age of 10 years and with a higher incidence in men [46]. The first sign of incipient hypoparathyroidism is loss of the diurnal pattern of parathyroid hormone (PTH) secretion [9]. The typical biochemical profile is low serum calcium, low serum PTH, low serum vitamin D and elevated serum phosphate levels [82]. Clinical signs of the disorder are most frequently noted from the second decade of life onwards [15].

A recent survey of clinicians by the International Network of Clinicians for Endocrinopathies in Thalassemia and Adolescence Medicine (ICET-A) published in 2018 reported a prevalence of 6.8% among 3023 thalassaemia major patients from 17 centres [83]. 42.2% of hypoparathyroid patients in this study were described as asymptomatic at diagnosis. The most common presenting symptom was paraesthesia and/or cramping seen in 37.6% patients [83]. In the ICET-A study, 49.8% of [83] hypoparathryoid individuals were also noted to have serum ferritin level > 2.500 ng/ml[8]. Chirico and colleagues also noted a significant association between elevated ferritin and incidence of hypoparathyroidism in thalassaemia major, proposing its use a prognostic marker for development of endocrinopathy [84].

Inconsistencies in case definition of hypoparathyroidism have complicated estimates of prevalence. In a cohort of transfusion-dependent thalassaemia major patients, 13.5% were shown to have hypoparathyroidism, characterised by low serum PTH, total and ionised calcium levels [85]. In contrast, a multicentre study in Italy, encompassing 25 units, showed the prevalence to be 3.6% [46]. A French study from 1993 showed the prevalence of hyperparathyroidism to be as high as 22.5% [86]; similarly Aleem and colleagues reported a prevalence of 20% [87]. Shamshirsaz and colleagues showed a prevalence of 7.6% [1] with male:female ratio of 4:1, a higher ratio than has been described elsewhere [46, 83]. Further studies in Iran by Bordbar et al. and Bazi et al. reported prevalences of 13.2% [88] and 18% [89] respectively among their thalassaemia patient cohorts. Interestingly, Tangngam and colleagues reported a prevalence of asymptomatic hypoparathyroidism of 38% in their cohort of 66 transfusion-dependent thalassaemia patients, with significantly lower serum FGF-23, a major regulator of phosphate, detected in hypoparathyroid patients [90].

A small study by Even and colleagues suggests loss of normal diurnal variation in PTH secretion in thalassaemia patients, even in individuals with normal daytime calcium levels [91].

In the UK, annual screening of parathyroid function and bone profile is recommended in thalassaemia patients [30]. Limited data [92, 93] shows that early supplementation with Vitamin D or calcitriol treatment for three months is sufficient to normalise plasma calcium and phosphate levels. 2016 UKTS guidelines recommend treatment with activated vitamin D preparations in the case of primary hypoparathyroidism secondary to iron overload. In order to avoid nephrocalcinosis, adjusted calcium levels should be targeted towards the lower reference range [30].

With regard to other complications, tetany, seizures or cardiac failure due to severe hypocalcaemia is rare and requires immediate correction with intravenous administration of calcium. Koutsis and colleagues report a rare case of Fahr's syndrome—striatopallidodentate calcinosis—in a 42 year-old woman with thalassaemia major with erratic compliance with oral vitamin D/calcium supplementation. Her hyperkinetic symptoms resolved with resumption of adequate oral supplementation [94].

7. Adrenal dysfunction

Histological and imaging studies have shown that iron deposits in the adrenal cortex of thalassaemic patients are mainly confined to the zona glomerulosa with rare involvement of the zona fascicularis [95]. Most studies have revealed intact pituitary adrenal axis in thalassaemia patients [35, 60, 65, 66, 96]. Prevalence of adrenal insufficiency is variable and depends both on the degree of iron overload, cut off values for cortisol measurement and diagnostic test used [97, 98].

Poggi et al. used a low dose synacthen test with adrenal insufficiency determined by cortisol <500 nmol/L and found a prevalence of 13.7% in the study population [97]. Huang et al. used a glucagon stimulation test, followed by corticotrophin-releasing hormone and found a prevalence of 61% [98].

Raised ACTH levels were found by McIntosh which suggests primary adrenal failure [66], however Costin et al. found suppressed ACTH levels and reduced adrenal reserve despite the lack of clinical signs [5]. The diminished ability of the adrenal cortex to react to further pulses of ACTH may be reflected in the fact that baseline serum and urinary cortisol levels are usually normal [99].

Low serum Dihydroepiandrostenedione (DHEA), Dihydroepiandrostenedione Sulphate (DHEAS), androstenedione and testosterone levels were found to be caused by the dissociation between androgen, cortisol and aldosterone synthesis. This may be the reason adrenarche is usually absent in these patients [100]. Dysfunctions in ACTH secretion circadian patterns but unaffected cortisol and aldosterone secretory were seen in these patients [101]. In addition to that, falsely low serum cortisol levels may be found in thalassaemic patients with chronic liver disease because cortisol is usually bound to cortisol binding globulin (CBG) which is produced by hepatocytes [102]. Currently, there are no reports on CBG levels in thalassaemic patients. Nonetheless, the role of CBG in adrenal insufficiency is excluded by a normal CBG level in the presence of low cortisol. In female patients, oestrogen may cause a rise in CBG levels resulting in inaccurate cortisol levels.

Current research shows female gender to be a protective factor [97]. Huang et al. have found that there was a significant prevalence of adrenal insufficiency in males when compared to females (92% vs. 29%, p = 0.049) in their study cohort [98]. Imaging studies by Drakonaki et al. using MRI scan have frequently identified adrenal hypointensity without alteration of morphology in thalassaemia patients and verified autopsy findings of correlation between adrenal iron and liver iron [103]. However a study by Guzelbey et al., found that, on the contrary, there was no statistically significant correlation between iron deposition in the adrenal glands and liver [104]. Another study suggests that imaging from Cardiac MRI T2 could be used as a surrogate of adrenal hypofunction, with a sensitivity of 81% and specificity of 78% [105]. However, despite high sensitivity, histology still remains the gold standard for diagnosis of iron deposition.

Currently, routine cortisol monitoring does not form part of the recommended routine investigations to screen for adrenal dysfunction in patients with thalassaemia [30]. However, the UK standards for thalassaemia guidelines acknowledges that annual monitoring of cortisol may allow for trends in decline to be noted, but also stress that normal cortisol levels does not exclude partial adrenal insufficiency when the patient is unwell. While current literature is very contradictory, adrenal dysfunction can be life-threatening in an acutely unwell patient. Therefore, hydrocortisone supplementation should be considered even before formal proof of insufficiency is available, if clinically relevant [30].

8. Osteoporosis

Beta thalassaemia is associated with marrow expansion, osteopaenia with cortical thickening, trabecular coarsening and bone deformity [106]. Osteoporosis—defined as a microarchietctual deterioration in bone tissue leading to an increased fracture risk [107]—is the predominant bone disease in beta thalassaemia. The prevalence of osteoporosis in thalassaemia is variably estimated from 13.6–50% [108]. In a cohort of well-treated thalassaemia patients, Baldini and colleagues reported demineralization—.osteoporotic or osteopaenic bone—in 92.7% [109].

Factors implicated in its cause include hypogonadism, diabetes mellitus, hypothyroidism, hypoparathyroidism, iron overload and its treatment [108, 110]. Malnutrition, inadequate exercise and absence of adrenal sex hormones during adrenarche and gonadal hormones during puberty are other contributory factors [111]. Excessive erythropoesis may also impair bone formation [112]. Iron chelation therapy is further linked to hypercalciuria, with consequential nephrolithiasis and reduced bone mineral density (BMD) [113]. Desferrioxamine is also linked to bone dysplasia, independently of osteoporosis [114].

Spine and hip osteoporosis is common in both sexes, with spinal osteoporosis more common in women and the lumbar vertebrae and femoral neck affected more frequently in men [110]. Osteoporosis is characterised by significant decreases in bone mineral density, both cortical and trabecular. In an Italian case series, pathological fractures were reported in 19.7% of transfusion-dependent patients with thalassaemia major [115]. With regard to putative mechanisms, significantly lower osteoprotegerin/RANKL ratios have been observed in thalassaemia patients. Excessive RANKL activity favours osteoclastic bone resorption, leading to reduced BMD [116]. Sapunarova and colleagues report 10-fold higher serum levels of sclerostin, a secreted glycoprotein with anti-osteoblastic properties, in adults with transfusion-dependent beta thalassaemia compared to controls [117]. Given its correlation with both lumbar spine/femoral neck Z-scores and incidence of fragility fractures, it has been proposed to act as a biomarker of severe osteoporosis in advanced beta thalassaemia. In Tehran, Shamishiraz et al. [1] demonstrated similar prevalence of that osteoporosis and osteopaenia in the lumbar spine (50.7% and 39.4% respectively) of patients with thalassaemia. In the same cohort, osteoporosis and osteopaenia prevalences were 10.8% and 36.9% at the femoral neck. These prevalences have been replicated in other cohorts [118, 119]. Jensen amd colleagued reported "severely low" bone mass in 51% of thalassaemia patients, with "low bone mass" in 45% [110]. Among 31 thalassaemic patients studied by Vogiatzi and colleagues (5 of whom with the milder thalassaemia intermedia phenotype), 22.6% had reduced bone mass (defined as Z score = −1 to −2 on DXA analysis) and 61.3% had a low bone mass (Z score ≤ −2) [93].

Early diagnosis requires accurate estimation of BMD via densitometry. Interpretation of dual-energy X-ray absorptiometry (DXA) may be confounded in thalassaemia due to short stature and spinal deformities caused by medullary expansion, bone dysplasia and the increased rate of degenerative vertebral disc disease in TM patients [120, 121]. Artefact from hepatic iron loading might also derange DXA analysis [122]. Alternative modalities for assessing bone microarchitecture in thalassaemia include trabecular bone structure (TBS) analysis—a textural assessment derived from DXA images—and quantitative computed tomography (QCT). These alternative methods remain limited by the distinctive profile of thalassaemia osteopathy and, in the case of QCT, by the amount of vertebral iron deposition [121, 123].

Prevention, early diagnosis and effective chelation therapy are most effective in arresting the progression of bone disease in thalassaemia. Tight adherence to recommended chelation treatment is required during childhood to prevent desferroximine-asssociated bone pathologies, including "pseudo-rickets" and cartilaginous dysplasia [30]. Diets rich in calcium and Vitamin D and exercise can improve the outcome [69]. The role of lifestyle interventions is particularly prominent during childhood. If deficient, calcium, vitamin D and zinc supplementation are advised, preferably via the oral route [119]. 2016 UKTS guidelines advise that many patients will require maintenance vitamin D3 supplementation [30]. Annual monitoring of vitamin D levels are recommended from age 2 years, aiming for a level of approximately 80 nmol/L. Intramuscular depot injection of vitamin D are not recommended by UKTS, nor are activated vitamin D preparations (for example alfacalcidol) in the absence of proven hypoparathyroidism secondary to iron deposition [30].

In terms of anti-osteoclastic treatments, the human anti-RANKL monoclonal antibody denosumab has shown promise in a Phase 2b RCT, increasing both lumbar spine and wrist BMD in transfusion-dependent TM patients [119]. Data from both Indian and Iranian cohorts suggest a role for zolendronic acid in increasing lumbar spine BMD [124, 125]. Alendronate and vitamin D regimen showed promise in an Italian Phase 2b RCT [126]. Prior to this, Morabito and colleagues showed that daily oral alendronate increased BMD in a two-year study of young adults with thalassaemia [127]. A 2016 Cochrane review of both bisphosphonates and zinc supplementation for thalassaemia-associated osteoporosis acknowledges an accretion of evidence in favour of their use, but suggests that further RCT evidence is required [128].

Current UKTS guidelines advocate consideration of anti-osteoclastic agents for individuals with low age-adjusted BMD or in whom fragility fractures have occurred despite appropriate vitamin D/calcium or hormone supplementation. Bisphosphonate initiation should occur following consultation with a specialist in osteoporosis, given that no definite evidence exists for fracture reductions with bisphosphonates in thalassaemia patients, despite the evidence for improved BMD. Burden of adverse effects, including atypical femoral fractures and osteonecrosis of the jaw, are significant [30].

Hormone replacement therapy is beneficial in patients with concomitant osteoporosis and hypogonadism but may not offer complete resolution, due to the multifactorial nature of bone pathology in thalassaemia [129, 130]. Patients with concomitant hypogonadism require hormone replacement therapy [108].

9. Conclusions

There is a high incidence of endocrinological abnormalities in patients with thalassaemia. Thalassaemic patients have been shown to have an elevated frequency of endocrinopathies in several research centres. The role of regular follow-up to allow early detection and proper management of complications is vital. The care and quality of life of thalassaemic patients can be positively impacted by advancements in transfusion protocols and chelating therapy. Early recognition of endocrinopathies in patients with thalassaemia is crucial apart from the fact that life expectancy is increased, at the same time morbidity and mortality as a result of complications can be decreased with routine monitoring, appropriate interventions and follow-up in thalassaemia-endocrine join care clinics.

Author details

Kinda Al-Hourani[1], Jessica Lee Siew Hua[2] and Parijat De[3]*

1 Haematology, NHS Greater Glasgow and Clyde, UK

2 Sandwell and West Birmingham NHS Trust, UK

3 Diabetes and Endocrinology, Sandwell and West Birmingham NHS Trust, UK

*Address all correspondence to: p.de@nhs.net

References

[1] Shamshirsaz AA, Bekheirnia MR, Kamgar M, Pourzahedgilani N, Bouzari N, Habibzadeh M, et al. Metabolic and endocrinologic complications in beta-thalassaemia major: A multicenter study in Tehran. BMC Endocrine Disorders. 2003 Aug 12;**3**(1):4

[2] Al-Elq AH, Al-Saeed HH. Endocrinopathies in patients with thalassaemias. Saudi Medical Journal. 2004 Oct;**25**(10):1347-1351

[3] Bannerman RM, Keusch G, Kreimer-Birnbaum M, Vance VK, Vaughan S. Thalassemia intermedia, with iron overload, cardiac failure, diabetes mellitus, hypopituitarism and porphyrinuria. The American Journal of Medicine. 1967 Mar;**42**(3):476-486

[4] Cappellini M-D, Cohen A, Eleftheriou A, Piga A, Porter J, Taher A. Guidelines for the Clinical Management of Thalassaemia: Thalassaemia International Federation. In: Guidelines for the Clinical Management of Thalassaemia [Internet]. 2nd Revised. Nicosia (CY): Thalassaemia International Federation; 2008 [cited 2020 May 9]. p. 41-9. Available from: http://www.ncbi.nlm.nih.gov/books/NBK173968/

[5] Costin G, Kogut MD, Hyman CB, Ortega JA. Endocrine abnormalities in thalassaemia major. American Journal of Diseases of Children. 1979 May;**133**(5):497-502

[6] Brezis M, Shalev O, Leibel B, Bernheim J, Ben-Ishay D. Phosphorus retention and hypoparathyroidism associated with transfusional iron overload in thalassaemia. Mineral and Electrolyte Metabolism. 1980;**4**:57-61

[7] Sabato AR, de Sanctis V, Atti G, Capra L, Bagni B, Vullo C. Primary hypothyroidism and the low T3 syndrome in thalassaemia major. Archives of Disease in Childhood. 1983 Feb;**58**(2):120-127

[8] De Sanctis V, Vullo C, Katz M, Atti G, Capra L, Di Palma A, et al. Endocrine complications in thalassaemia major. In: In advances and controversies in thalassaemia therapy. New York, NY, US: Alan R. Liss, Inc. (Publishers); 1989. p. 77-83.

[9] Tiosano D, Hochberg Z. Endocrine complications of thalassaemia. Journal of Endocrinological Investigation. 2001 Oct 1;**24**(9):716-723

[10] Theodoridis C, Ladis V, Papatheodorou A, Berdousi H, Palamidou F, Evagelopoulou C, et al. Growth and management of short stature in thalassaemia major. Journal of Pediatric Endocrinology & Metabolism. 1998;**11**(Suppl 3):835-844

[11] Dhouib NG, Ben Khaled M, Ouederni M, Besbes H, Kouki R, Mellouli F, Bejaoui M. Growth and Endocrine Function in Tunisian Thalassemia Major Patients. Mediterr J Hematol Infect Dis. 2018 May 1;10(1):e2018031. doi: 10.4084/MJHID.2018.031. PMID: 29755708; PMCID: PMC5937976.

[12] De Sanctis V. Growth and puberty and its management in thalassaemia. Hormone Research. 2002;**58**(Suppl 1):72-79

[13] Kwan E, Lee A, Li A, Tam S, Chan C, Lau Y, et al. A cross-sectional study of growth, puberty and endocrine function in patients with thalassaemia major in Hong Kong. Journal of paediatrics and child health. 1995 Apr;**31**(2):83-87

[14] Raiola G, Galati MC, De Sanctis V, Caruso Nicoletti M, Pintor C, De Simone M, et al. Growth and puberty

in thalassaemia major. Journal of Pediatric Endocrinology & Metabolism. 2003 Mar;**16**(Suppl 2):259-266

[15] De P, Mistry R, Wright C, Pancham S, Burbridge W, Gangopadhayay K, et al. A Review of Endocrine Disorders in Thalassaemia. Open Journal of Endocrine and Metabolic Diseases [Internet]. 2014 Feb 18 [cited 2020 Jun 27];2014. Available from: http://www.scirp.org/journal/PaperInformation.aspx?PaperID=42952

[16] Leger J, Girot R, Crosnier H, Postel-Vinay MC, Rappaport R. Normal growth hormone (GH) response to GH-releasing hormone in children with thalassaemia major before puberty: A possible age-related effect. The Journal of Clinical Endocrinology and Metabolism. 1989 Aug;**69**(2):453-456

[17] DeLuca G, Maggiolini M, Bria M, Caracciolo M, Giorno A, Salerno M, et al. GH secretion in thalassaemia patients with short stature. Hormone Research. 1995;**44**(4):158-163

[18] Low LC. Growth, puberty and endocrine function in beta-thalassaemia major. Journal of Pediatric Endocrinology & Metabolism. 1997 Apr;**10**(2):175-184

[19] Soliman AT, Yassin MA, De Sanctis V. Final adult height and endocrine complications in young adults with β-thalassaemia major (TM) who received oral iron chelation (OIC) in comparison with those who did not use OIC. Acta Bio-Medica. 2018;**89**(Suppl 2):27-32

[20] Karamifar H, Shahriari M, Amirhakimi GH. Failure of puberty and linear growth in beta-thalassaemia major. Turkish Journal of Haematology. 2005 Jun 5;**22**(2):65-69

[21] Sharma R, Seth A, Chandra J, Gohain S, Kapoor S, Singh P, et al. Endocrinopathies in adolescents with thalassaemia major receiving oral iron chelation therapy. Paediatr Int Child Health. 2016 Feb;**36**(1):22-27

[22] Roth C, Pekrun A, Bartz M, Jarry H, Eber S, Lakomek M, et al. Short stature and failure of pubertal development in thalassaemia major: Evidence for hypothalamic neurosecretory dysfunction of growth hormone secretion and defective pituitary gonadotropin secretion. European Journal of Pediatrics. 1997 Oct;**156**(10):777-783

[23] Soliman AT, elZalabany M, Amer M, Ansari BM. Growth and pubertal development in transfusion-dependent children and adolescents with thalassaemia major and sickle cell disease: A comparative study. Journal of Tropical Pediatrics 1999;45(1):23-30.

[24] Borgna-Pignatti C, De Stefano P, Zonta L, Vullo C, De Sanctis V, Melevendi C, et al. Growth and sexual maturation in thalassaemia major. The Journal of Pediatrics. 1985 Jan;**106**(1):150-155

[25] Gulati R, Bhatia V, Agarwal SS. Early onset of endocrine abnormalities in beta-thalassaemia major in a developing country. Journal of Pediatric Endocrinology & Metabolism. 2000 Jun;**13**(6):651-656

[26] Bridge N. Disorders of puberty: Pubertal delay and pubertal failure. In: Clinical Pediatric Endocrinology. 4th ed. London: Blackwell Science; 2001. p. 173-5.

[27] Britton RS, Ramm GA, Olynyk J, Singh R, O'Neill R, Bacon BR. Pathophysiology of iron toxicity. Advances in Experimental Medicine and Biology. 1994;**356**:239-253

[28] Ngim CF, Lai NM, Hong JY, Tan SL, Ramadas A, Muthukumarasamy P, et al.

Growth hormone therapy for people with thalassaemia. Cochrane Database Syst Rev. 2017 18;9:CD012284.

[29] Shehadeh N, Hazani A, Rudolf MCJ, Peleg I, Benderly A, Hochberg Z. Neurosecretory dysfunction of growth hormone secretion in thalassemia major. Acta Paediatrica. 1990 Aug 1;**79**(8-9):790-795

[30] United Kingdom Thalassaemia Society 2016, Yardumian A, Telfer P, Shah F, Ryan K, Darlison M, et al. Standards for the Clinical Care of Children and Adults with Thalassaemia in the UK, 3rd Edition. Third Edition.

[31] De Sanctis V, Soliman AT, Canatan D, Tzoulis P, Daar S, Di Maio S, et al. An ICET-A survey on occult and emerging endocrine complications in patients with β-thalassaemia major: Conclusions and recommendations. Acta Biomed. 2019 15;89(4):481-9.

[32] Colao A, Cuocolo A, Di Somma C, Cerbone G, Della Morte AM, Nicolai E, et al. Impaired cardiac performance in elderly patients with growth hormone deficiency. The Journal of Clinical Endocrinology and Metabolism. 1999 Nov;**84**(11):3950-3955

[33] Thomas JDJ, Dattani A, Zemrak F, Burchell T, Akker SA, Gurnell M, et al. Characterisation of myocardial structure and function in adult-onset growth hormone deficiency using cardiac magnetic resonance. Endocrine. 2016;**54**(3):778-787

[34] De Sanctis V, Soliman A, Candini G, Campisi S, Anastasi S, Iassin M. High prevalence of central hypothyroidism in adult patients with β-thalassaemia major. Georgian Medical News. 2013 Sep;**222**:88-94

[35] Kuo B, Zaino E, Roginsky MS. Endocrine function in thalassemia major. The Journal of Clinical Endocrinology and Metabolism. 1968 Jun 1;**28**(6):805-808

[36] De Sanctis V, Soliman AT, Yassin MA, Di Maio S, Daar S, Elsedfy H, et al. Hypogonadism in male thalassaemia major patients: pathophysiology, diagnosis and treatment. Acta Biomed. 2018 16;89(2-S):6-15.

[37] Srisukh S, Ongphiphadhanakul B, Bunnag P. Hypogonadism in thalassaemia major patients. Journal of Clinical & Translational Endocrinology. 2016 Sep;**5**:42-45

[38] Anoussakis C, Alexiou D, Abatzis D, Bechrakis G. Endocrinological investigation of pituitary Conadal Axis in thalassemia major. Acta Paediatrica. 1977;**66**(1):49-51

[39] Landau H, Matoth I, Landau-Cordova Z, Goldfarb A, Rachmilewitz EA, Glaser B. Cross-sectional and longitudinal study of the pituitary-thyroid axis in patients with thalassaemia major. Clinical Endocrinology. 1993 Jan;**38**(1):55-61

[40] Kletzky OA, Costin G, Marrs RP, Bernstein G, March CM, Mishell DR. Gonadotropin insufficiency in patients with thalassemia major. The Journal of Clinical Endocrinology and Metabolism. 1979 Jun 1;**48**(6):901-905

[41] Castaldi MA, Cobellis L. Thalassemia and infertility. Human Fertility (Cambridge, England). 2016 Jun;**19**(2):90-96

[42] Moshtaghi-Kashanian G-R, Razavi F. Ghrelin and leptin levels in relation to puberty and reproductive function in patients with beta-thalassaemia. Hormones (Athens, Greece). 2009 Sep;**8**(3):207-213

[43] Chatterjee R, Katz M, Cox TF, Porter JB. Prospective study

of the hypothalamic-pituitary axis in thalassaemic patients who developed secondary amenorrhoea. Clinical Endocrinology. 1993 Sep;**39**(3):287-296

[44] Danesi L, Scacchi M, De Martin M, Dubini A, Massaro P, Majolo AT, et al. Evaluation of hypothalamic-pituitary function in patients with thalassaemia major. Journal of Endocrinological Investigation. 1992 Mar;**15**(3):177-184

[45] Bozdağ M, Bayraktaroğlu S, Aydınok Y, Çallı MC. MRI assessment of pituitary iron accumulation by using pituitary-R2 in β-thalassaemia patients. Acta Radiologica. 2018 Jun;**59**(6):732-739

[46] Multicentre study on prevalence of endocrine complications in thalassaemia major. Italian working group on endocrine complications in non-endocrine diseases. Clinical Endocrinology. 1995 Jun;**42**(6):581-586

[47] Caruso-Nicoletti M, De Sanctis V, Capra M, Cardinale G, Cuccia L, Di Gregorio F, et al. Short stature and body proportion in thalassaemia. Journal of Pediatric Endocrinology & Metabolism. 1998;**11**(Suppl 3):811-816

[48] Chern JPS, Lin K-H, Tsai W-Y, Wang S-C, Lu M-Y, Lin D-T, et al. Hypogonadotropic hypogonadism and hematologic phenotype in patients with transfusion-dependent beta-thalassaemia. Journal of Pediatric Hematology/Oncology. 2003 Nov;**25**(11):880-884

[49] Saffari F, Mahyar A, Jalilolgadr S. Endocrine and metabolic disorders in β-thalassaemiamajor patients. Caspian Journal of Internal Medicine. 2012;**3**(3):466-472

[50] Moayeri H, Oloomi Z. Prevalence of growth and puberty failure with respect to growth hormone and gonadotropins secretion in beta-thalassaemia major. Archives of Iranian Medicine. 2006 Oct;**9**(4):329-334

[51] Hagag AA, Badraia IM, Elfarargy MS, El-Enein AMA. Study of male sex hormone levels in male Egyptian children with Beta-thalassemia: Correlation with iron load. Endocrine, Metabolic & Immune Disorders Drug Targets. 2016;**16**(2):124-130

[52] Hagag AA, Badraia IM, Elfarargy MS, Abo El-Enein AM. Gonadal hormones in adolescent females with β-thalassemia in relation to iron load. Endocrine, Metabolic & Immune Disorders Drug Targets. 2016;**16**(2):148-153

[53] Karahanyan E, Stoyanova A, Moumdzhiev I, Ivanov I. Secondary diabetes in children with thalassaemia major (homozygous thalassaemia). Folia Med (Plovdiv). 1994;**36**(1):29-34

[54] Ang AL, Tzoulis P, Prescott E, Davis BA, Barnard M, Shah FT. History of myocardial iron loading is a strong risk factor for diabetes mellitus and hypogonadism in adults with β thalassaemia major. European Journal of Haematology. 2014 Mar;**92**(3):229-236

[55] Kanbour I, Chandra P, Soliman A, De Sanctis V, Nashwan A, Abusamaan S, et al. Severe liver iron concentrations (LIC) in 24 patients with β-thalassemia major: Correlations with serum ferritin, liver enzymes and endocrine complications. Mediterr J Hematol Infect Dis. 2018;**10**(1):e2018062

[56] He L-N, Chen W, Yang Y, Xie Y-J, Xiong Z-Y, Chen D-Y, et al. Elevated prevalence of abnormal glucose metabolism and other endocrine disorders in patients with β-thalassemia major: A meta-analysis. BioMed Research International. 2019;**2019**:6573497

[57] Chern JP, Lin KH, Lu MY, Lin DT, Lin KS, Chen JD, et al. Abnormal glucose tolerance in transfusion-dependent beta-thalassemic patients. Diabetes Care. 2001 May;**24**(5):850-854

[58] Li M-J, Peng SS-F, Lu M-Y, Chang H-H, Yang Y-L, Jou S-T, et al. Diabetes mellitus in patients with thalassaemia major. Pediatric Blood & Cancer. 2014 Jan;**61**(1):20-24

[59] Gomber S, Dabas A, Bagmar S, Madhu SV. Glucose homeostasis and effect of chelation on β cell function in children with β-thalassemia major. Journal of Pediatric Hematology/Oncology. 2018;**40**(1):56-59

[60] Lassman MN, O'Brien RT, Pearson HA, Wise JK, Donabedian RK, Felig P, et al. Endocrine evaluation in thalassemia major*. Annals of the New York Academy of Sciences. 1974;**232**(1):226-237

[61] Pes GM, Tolu F, Dore MP. Anti-thyroid peroxidase antibodies and male gender are associated with diabetes occurrence in patients with Beta-thalassemia major. Journal Diabetes Research. 2016;**2016**:1401829

[62] de Assis RA, Ribeiro AAF, Kay FU, Rosemberg LA, Nomura CH, Loggetto SR, et al. Pancreatic iron stores assessed by magnetic resonance imaging (MRI) in beta thalassemic patients. European Journal of Radiology. 2012 Jul;**81**(7):1465-1470

[63] Noetzli LJ, Mittelman SD, Watanabe RM, Coates TD, Wood JC. Pancreatic iron and glucose dysregulation in thalassaemia major. American Journal of Hematology. 2012 Feb;**87**(2):155-160

[64] El-Samahy MH, Tantawy AA, Adly AA, Abdelmaksoud AA, Ismail EA, Salah NY. Evaluation of continuous glucose monitoring system for detection of alterations in glucose homeostasis in pediatric patients with β-thalassaemia major. Pediatric Diabetes. 2019;**20**(1):65-72

[65] Toccafondi R, Maioli M, Meloni T. Plasma insulin response to oral carbohydrate in Cooley's anemia. Rivista di Clinica Medica. (70):96-101.

[66] McIntosh N. Endocrinopathy in thalassaemia major. Archives of Disease in Childhood. 1976 Mar 1;**51**(3):195-201

[67] Cavallo-Perin P, Pacini G, Cerutti F, Bessone A, Condo C, Sacchetti L, et al. Insulin resistance and hyperinsulinemia in homozygous beta-thalassaemia. Metabolism, Clinical and Experimental. 1995 Mar;**44**(3):281-286

[68] Siklar Z, Citak FE, Uysal Z, Oçal G, Ertem M, Engiz O, et al. Evaluation of glucose homeostasis in transfusion-dependent thalassemic patients. Pediatric Hematology and Oncology. 2008 Sep;**25**(7):630-637

[69] Vichinsky EP. The morbidity of bone disease in thalassaemia. Annals of the New York Academy of Sciences. 1998 Jun 30;**850**:344-348

[70] Cario H, Holl RW, Debatin K-M, Kohne E. Disproportionately elevated fasting proinsulin levels in normoglycemic patients with thalassaemia major are correlated to the degree of iron overload. Hormone Research. 2003;**59**(2):73-78

[71] Dmochowski K, Finegood DT, Francombe W, Tyler B, Zinman B. Factors determining glucose tolerance in patients with thalassaemia major. The Journal of Clinical Endocrinology and Metabolism. 1993 Aug;**77**(2):478-483

[72] Arrigo T, Crisafulli G, Meo A, Sturiale M, Lombardo F, Miceli M, et al. Glucose tolerance, insulin secretion and peripheral sensitivity in thalassaemia major. Journal of pediatric

endocrinology & metabolism : JPEM. 1998;**11**(Suppl 3):863-866

[73] De Sanctis V, Zurlo MG, Senesi E, Boffa C, Cavallo L, Di Gregorio F. Insulin dependent diabetes in thalassaemia. Archives of Disease in Childhood. 1988 Jan;**63**(1):58-62

[74] De Sanctis V, Soliman AT, Canatan D, Yassin MA, Daar S, Elsedfy H, et al. Thyroid disorders in homozygous β-thalassemia: Current knowledge, emerging issues and open problems. Mediterr J Hematol Infect Dis. 2019;**11**(1):e2019029

[75] Soliman AT, Al Yafei F, Al-Naimi L, Almarri N, Sabt A, Yassin M, et al. Longitudinal study on thyroid function in patients with thalassaemia major: High incidence of central hypothyroidism by 18 years. Indian J Endocrinol Metab. 2013 Nov;**17**(6):1090-1095

[76] Upadya SH, Rukmini MS, Sundararajan S, Baliga BS, Kamath N. Thyroid function in chronically transfused children with Beta thalassemia major: A cross-sectional hospital based study. International Journal Of Pediatrics. 2018;**2018**:9071213

[77] Saleem M, Ghafoor MB, Anwar J, Saleem MM. Hypothyroidism in beta thalassaemia major patients at Rahim Yar Khan. JSZMC. 2016;**7**:1016-1019

[78] Yassouf MY, Alquobaili F, Kabalan Y, Mukhalalaty Y. Compliance with Deferoxamine therapy and thyroid dysfunction of patients with β-thalassemia major in Syria. Hemoglobin. 2019 May;**43**(3):218-221

[79] Delaporta P, Karantza M, Boiu S, Stokidis K, Petropoulou T, Papasotiriou I, et al. Thyroid function in Greek patients with thalassemia major. Blood. 2012 Nov 16;**120**(21):5176-5176

[80] Belhoul KM, Bakir ML, Saned M-S, Kadhim AMA, Musallam KM, Taher AT. Serum ferritin levels and endocrinopathy in medically treated patients with β thalassaemia major. Annals of Hematology. 2012 Jul;**91**(7):1107-1114

[81] Chirico V, Valeria C, Lacquaniti A, Antonio L, Salpietro V, Vincenzo S, et al. Thyroid dysfunction in thalassaemic patients: Ferritin as a prognostic marker and combined iron chelators as an ideal therapy. European Journal of Endocrinology. 2013 Dec;**169**(6):785-793

[82] Zamboni G, Marradi P, Tagliaro F, Dorizzi R, Tatò L. Parathyroid hormone, calcitonin and vitamin D metabolites in beta-thalassaemia major. European Journal of Pediatrics. 1986 Apr;**145**(1-2):133-136

[83] De Sanctis V, Soliman AT, Canatan D, Elsedfy H, Karimi M, Daar S, et al. An ICET- A survey on Hypoparathyroidism in Patients with Thalassaemia Major and Intermedia: A preliminary report. Acta Biomed. 2018 16;88(4):435-44.

[84] Chirico V, Rigoli L, Lacquaniti A, Salpietro V, Piraino B, Amorini M, et al. Endocrinopathies, metabolic disorders, and iron overload in major and intermedia thalassaemia: Serum ferritin as diagnostic and predictive marker associated with liver and cardiac T2* MRI assessment. European Journal of Haematology. 2015 May;**94**(5):404-412

[85] Angelopoulos NG, Goula A, Rombopoulos G, Kaltzidou V, Katounda E, Kaltsas D, et al. Hypoparathyroidism in transfusion-dependent patients with beta-thalassaemia. Journal of Bone and Mineral Metabolism. 2006;**24**(2):138-145

[86] Pérignon F, Brauner R, Souberbielle JC, de Montalembert M, Girot R. Growth and endocrine function in major thalassaemia.

Archives Françaises de Pédiatrie. 1993 Oct;**50**(8):657-663

[87] Aleem A, Al-Momen AK, Al-Harakati MS, Hassan A, Al-Fawaz I. Hypocalcemiaduetohypoparathyroidism in beta-thalassaemia major patients. Annals of Saudi Medicine. 2000 Nov;**20**(5-6):364-366

[88] Bordbar M, Bozorgi H, Saki F, Haghpanah S, Karimi M, Bazrafshan A, et al. Prevalence of endocrine disorders and their associated factors in transfusion-dependent thalassaemia patients: A historical cohort study in southern Iran. Journal of Endocrinological Investigation. 2019 Dec;**42**(12):1467-1476

[89] Bazi A, Harati H, Khosravi-Bonjar A, Rakhshani E, Delaramnasab M. HypothyroidismandHypoparathyroidism in thalassemia major patients: A study in Sistan and Baluchestan Province. Iran. Int J Endocrinol Metab. 2018 Apr;**16**(2):e13228

[90] Tangngam H, Mahachoklertwattana P, Poomthavorn P, Chuansumrit A, Sirachainan N, Chailurkit L, et al. Under-recognized Hypoparathyroidism in thalassemia. Journal of Clinical Research in Pediatric Endocrinology. 2018 Dec;**10**(4):324-330

[91] Even L, Bader T, Hochberg Z. Nocturnal calcium, phosphorus and parathyroid hormone in the diagnosis of concealed and subclinical hypoparathyroidism. European Journal of Endocrinology. 2007 Jan 1;**156**(1):113-116

[92] Goyal M, Abrol P, Lal H. Parathyroid and calcium status in patients with thalassemia. Indian Journal of Clinical Biochemistry. 2010 Oct;**25**(4):385-387

[93] Vogiatzi MG, Autio KA, Mait JE, Schneider R, Lesser M, Giardina PJ. Low bone mineral density in adolescents with beta-thalassaemia. Annals of the New York Academy of Sciences. 2005;**1054**:462-466

[94] Koutsis G, Karadima G, Panas M. Symptomatic striopallidodentate calcinosis (Fahr's syndrome) in a thalassemic patient with hypoparathyroidism. Annals of Hematology. 2015 May 1;**94**(5): 897-899

[95] Bhamarapravati N, Na-Nakorn S, Wasi P, Tuchinda S. Pathology of abnormal hemoglobin diseases seen in Thailand. American Journal of Clinical Pathology. 1967 Jun 1;**47**(6):745-758

[96] Canale VC, Steinherz P, New M, Erlandson M. Endocrine function in thalassemia major. Annals of the New York Academy of Sciences. 1974;**232**(1):333-345

[97] Poggi M, Samperi I, Mattia L, Di Rocco A, Iorio C, Monti S, et al. New insights and methods in the approach to thalassemia major: The lesson from the case of adrenal insufficiency. Frontiers in Molecular Biosciences. 2019;**6**:162

[98] Huang KE, Mittelman SD, Coates TD, Geffner ME, Wood JC. A significant proportion of thalassaemia major patients have adrenal insufficiency detectable on provocative testing. Journal of Pediatric Hematology/Oncology. 2015 Jan;**37**(1):54-59

[99] Scacchi M, Danesi L, Cattaneo A, Valassi E, Pecori Giraldi F, Radaelli P, et al. The pituitary-adrenal axis in adult thalassaemic patients. European Journal of Endocrinology. 2010 Jan;**162**(1):43-48

[100] Sklar CA, Lew LQ, Yoon DJ, David R. Adrenal function in thalassaemia major following long-term treatment with multiple transfusions and chelation therapy. Evidence for dissociation of cortisol and

adrenal androgen secretion. American Journal of Diseases of Children. 1987 Mar;**141**(3):327-330

[101] Pasqualetti P, Colantonio D, Collacciani A, Casale R, Natali G. Circadian pattern of circulating plasma ACTH, cortisol, and aldosterone in patients with beta-thalassaemia. Acta Endocrinologica. 1990 Aug;**123**(2):174-178

[102] Poomthavorn P, Isaradisaikul B, Chuansumrit A, Khlairit P, Sriphrapradang A, Mahachoklertwattana P. High prevalence of "biochemical" adrenal insufficiency in Thalassemics: Is it a matter of different Testings or decreased cortisol binding globulin? The Journal of Clinical Endocrinology and Metabolism. 2010 Oct 1;**95**(10): 4609-4615

[103] Drakonaki E, Papakonstantinou O, Maris T, Vasiliadou A, Papadakis A, Gourtsoyiannis N. Adrenal glands in beta-thalassaemia major: Magnetic resonance (MR) imaging features and correlation with iron stores. European Radiology. 2005 Dec;**15**(12):2462-2468

[104] Guzelbey T, Gurses B, Ozturk E, Ozveren O, Sarsilmaz A, Karasu E. Evaluation of iron deposition in the adrenal glands of β thalassemia major patients using 3-tesla MRI. Iranian Journal of Radiology. 2016 Jul;**13**(3):e36375

[105] Uçar A, Öner N, Özek G, Çetinçakmak MG, Abuhandan M, Yıldırım A, et al. Evaluation of the glucocorticoid, mineralocorticoid, and adrenal androgen secretion dynamics in a large cohort of patients aged 6-18 years with transfusion-dependent β-thalassaemia major, with an emphasis on the impact of cardiac iron load. Endocrine. 2016 Jul;**53**(1):240-248

[106] De Sanctis V, Stea S, Savarino L, Granchi D, Visentin M, Sprocati M, et al. Osteochondrodystrophic lesions in chelated Thalassemic patients: An histological analysis. Calcified Tissue International. 2000 Aug 1;**67**(2):134-140

[107] WHO Scientific Group on the Prevention and Management of Osteoporosis (2000): Geneva S. Prevention and management of osteoporosis : report of a WHO scientific group [Internet]. World Health Organization; 2003 [cited 2020 Apr 27]. Available from: https://apps.who.int/iris/handle/10665/42841

[108] De Sanctis V, Soliman AT, Elsedfy H, Yassin M, Canatan D, Kilinc Y, et al. Osteoporosis in thalassaemia major: An update and the I-CET 2013 recommendations for surveillance and treatment. Pediatric Endocrinology Reviews. 2013 Dec;**11**(2):167-180

[109] Baldini M, Forti S, Marcon A, Ulivieri FM, Orsatti A, Tampieri B, et al. Endocrine and bone disease in appropriately treated adult patients with beta-thalassaemia major. Annals of Hematology. 2010 Dec;**89**(12):1207-1213

[110] Jensen CE, Tuck SM, Agnew JE, Koneru S, Morris RW, Yardumian A, et al. High prevalence of low bone mass in thalassaemia major. British Journal of Haematology. 1998 Dec;**103**(4):911-915

[111] Filosa A, Di Maio S, Saviano A, Vocca S, Esposito G. Can Adrenarche influence the degree of osteopenia in Thalassemic children? Journal of Pediatric Endocrinology and Metabolism. 1996 May 1;**9**(3):401-406

[112] Valderrábano RJ, Wu JY. Bone and blood interactions in human health and disease. Bone. 2019 Feb 1;**119**:65-70

[113] Wong P, Fuller PJ, Gillespie MT, Kartsogiannis V, Strauss BJ, Bowden D, et al. Thalassemia bone disease: The association between nephrolithiasis, bone mineral density and fractures.

Osteoporosis International. 2013 Jul;**24**(7):1965-1971

[114] Chan Y-L, Pang L-M, Chik K-W, Cheng JCY, Li C-K. Patterns of bone diseases in transfusion-dependent homozygous thalassaemia major: Predominance of osteoporosis and desferrioxamine-induced bone dysplasia. Pediatric Radiology. 2002 Jul;**32**(7):492-497

[115] Ruggiero L, De Sanctis V. Multicentre study on prevalence of fractures in transfusion-dependent thalassaemic patients. Journal of Pediatric Endocrinology & Metabolism. 1998;**11**(Suppl 3):773-778

[116] Morabito N, Gaudio A, Lasco A, Atteritano M, Pizzoleo MA, Cincotta M, et al. Osteoprotegerin and RANKL in the pathogenesis of thalassemia-induced osteoporosis: New pieces of the puzzle. Journal of Bone and Mineral Research. 2004;**19**(5):722-727

[117] SapunarovaK,Goranova-MarinovaV, Georgiev P, Deneva T, Tsvetkova S, Grudeva-Popova Z. Associations of serum sclerostin with bone mineral density, markers of bone metabolism and thalassaemia characteristics in adult patients with transfusion-dependent beta-thalassaemia. Annals of Medicine. 2020 Mar;**26**:1-15

[118] Molyvda-Athanasopoulou E, Sioundas A, Karatzas N, Aggellaki M, Pazaitou K, Vainas I. Bone mineral density of patients with thalassaemia major: Four-year follow-up. Calcified Tissue International. 1999 Jun;**64**(6):481-484

[119] Voskaridou E, Kyrtsonis MC, Terpos E, Skordili M, Theodoropoulos I, Bergele A, et al. Bone resorption is increased in young adults with thalassaemia major. British Journal of Haematology. 2001 Jan;**112**(1):36-41

[120] Desigan S, Hall-Craggs MA, Ho C-P, Eliahoo J, Porter JB. Degenerative disc disease as a cause of back pain in the thalassaemic population: A case-control study using MRI and plain radiographs. Skeletal Radiology. 2006 Feb 1;**35**(2):95-102

[121] Pellegrino F, Zatelli MC, Bondanelli M, Carnevale A, Cittanti C, Fortini M, et al. Dual-energy X-ray absorptiometry pitfalls in thalassemia major. Endocrine. 2019;**65**(3):469-482

[122] Allard HM, Calvelli L, Weyhmiller MG, Gildengorin G, Fung EB. Vertebral bone density measurements by DXA are influenced by hepatic iron overload in patients with Hemoglobinopathies. Journal of Clinical Densitometry. 2019 Sep;**22**(3):329-337

[123] Mylona M, Leotsinides M, Alexandrides T, Zoumbos N, Dimopoulos PA. Comparison of DXA, QCT and trabecular structure in β-thalassaemia. European Journal of Haematology. 2005;**74**(5):430-437

[124] Naithani R, Seth T, Tandon N, Chandra J, Choudhry VP, Pati H, et al. Zoledronic acid for treatment of Low bone mineral density in patients with Beta thalassemia major. Indian J Hematol Blood Transfus. 2018 Oct;**34**(4):648-652

[125] Darvishi-Khezri H, Kosaryan M, Akbarzadeh R, Aliasgharian A, Fazli M. Administration of Intravenous Zoledronic Acid every 3 months vs. annually in β-thalassaemia patients with Low bone mineral density: A retrospective comparison of efficacy. Med Arch. 2018 Jun;**72**(3):170-173

[126] Forni GL, Perrotta S, Giusti A, Quarta G, Pitrolo L, Cappellini MD, et al. Neridronate improves bone mineral density and reduces back pain in β-thalassaemia patients with osteoporosis: Results from a phase 2, randomized, parallel-arm, open-label study. British Journal of Haematology. 2012 Jul;**158**(2):274-282

[127] Morabito N, Lasco A, Gaudio A, Crisafulli A, Di Pietro C, Meo A, et al. Bisphosphonates in the treatment of thalassaemia-induced osteoporosis. Osteoporosis International. 2002 Aug;**13**(8):644-649

[128] Bhardwaj A, Swe KMM, Sinha NK, Osunkwo I. Treatment for osteoporosis in people with ß-thalassaemia. Cochrane Database of Systematic Reviews. 2016 Mar 10;**3**:CD010429

[129] Anapliotou ML, Kastanias IT, Psara P, Evangelou EA, Liparaki M, Dimitriou P. The contribution of hypogonadism to the development of osteoporosis in thalassaemia major: New therapeutic approaches. Clinical Endocrinology. 1995 Mar;**42**(3):279-287

[130] Chatterjee R, Katz M, Bajoria R. Use of hormone replacement therapy for correction of high turnover bone disease in hypogonadal β-thalassemia major patients presenting with osteoporosis: Comparison with idiopathic premature ovarian failure. Hemoglobin. 2011;**35**(5-6):653-658

Section 2

Blood Groups

Chapter 4

The Duffy Blood Group System

Fatima A. Aldarweesh

Abstract

The Duffy group system includes six known antigens that reside on a glycoprotein which acts as a receptor for chemokines. It is also a receptor for some malaria species. There are significant racial variations in expression of Duffy antigens. Approximately 68% of Blacks lack both Fy^a and Fy^b antigens. Individuals with this unique phenotype are resistant to two malaria species. Antibodies formed against the Duffy antigens are of IgG subclass and are clinically significant as they can be implicated in acute and delayed hemolytic transfusion reactions as well as hemolytic disease of fetus and newborn. Patients who form anti-Fya or anti-Fy^b must receive antigen negative blood units in the future.

Keywords: Duffy, RBC antigens, FYA, FYB, DARC, hemolysis, fetus, HDFN

1. Introduction

The Duffy blood group system, ISBT number 008/symbol (FY), was published for the first time in 1950 when anti-Fya was identified in a suspected hemolytic transfusion reaction in a 43-year-old patient with hemophilia who received 3 packed red blood cell (PRBC) units for treatment of spontaneous bleeding and who developed jaundice 1 day after transfusion [1, 2]. Approximately, 1 year later, anti-Fyb was discovered in a postpartum blood sample from a patient who gave birth to her third child [3].

Chromosome 1 has both FY and RH gene loci. The FY locus is located on the long arm at position 1q22-q23 where it consists of two exons distributed over 1.5 kbp of gDNA, whereas RH resides on the short arm. The Duffy system is N-glycosylated multi-pass transmembrane glycoprotein (**Figure 1**) [4] also known as the atypical chemokine receptor 1 (ACKR1, CD234). The protein is composed of 336 amino acids. There are two possible Duffy mRNAs which are translated from the Duffy antigen gene, a less abundant α form (338 amino acids) and a major β form (336 amino acids) which differ by 2 amino acids in the N-terminus. Approximately 6000–13,000 copies of the Duffy protein are found on the surface of RBCs [5].

The Duffy blood group includes six known antigens that differ by amino acid sequence. The Duffy antigen prevalence varies between racial groups.

ACKR1 (previously known as DARC) is a receptor for a variety of chemokines, including interleukin-8, monocyte chemotactic protein-1, and melanoma growth stimulatory activity. Also, this glycoprotein is a receptor for *Plasmodium vivax* and *Plasmodium knowlesi*; thus red cells with Fy(a-b-) phenotype are resistant to invasion by these malarial species. Antibodies formed against the Duffy antigens show a dosage effect and are a cause of both hemolytic transfusion reactions and hemolytic disease of fetus and newborn. The Duffy protein is also found on the endothelial cells of capillary and postcapillary venules, the epithelial cells of kidney collecting ducts, lung alveoli, and Purkinje cells of cerebellum [6].

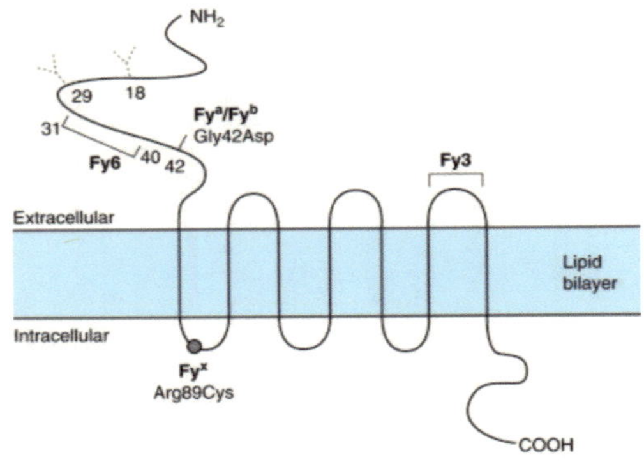

Figure 1.
The predicted seven-transmembrane domain structure of the Duffy protein. The amino acid change responsible for Fya/Fyb polymorphism, the mutation responsible for Fyx, and the glycosylation sites and the regions where Fy3 (and Fy6) map are indicated (reproduced with permission).

2. Duffy antigens

There are six known antigens with four main phenotypes; Fy(a+b+), Fy(a−b+), Fy(a+b−), and Fy(a−b−) (**Table 1**) [5]. The most common antigens are, two polymorphic and antithetical, Fya (FY1) and Fyb (FY2) which differ by one amino acid at position 42 on the extracellular domain, with glycine resulting in Fya expression and aspartic acid resulting in Fyb expression [5, 7]. They are sensitive to destruction when RBCs are treated with proteolytic enzymes such as papain or ficin, whereas, there is no RBCs destruction with trypsin treatment [8].

Fya antigen has a prevalence of 66% in Caucasians, 10% in Blacks, and 99% in Asians. It has been identified on fetal RBCs as early as 6 weeks gestation and reaches adult levels in approximately 12 weeks after birth. Fyb has a prevalence of 83% in Caucasians, 23% in Blacks, and 18.5% in Asians. It is expressed on cord blood cells. Fy3 antigen is expressed in 100% of Caucasians, 32% of Blacks, and 99.9% of Asians. It is also expressed on cord cells and demonstrates increased expression after birth. Fy5 antigen is expressed on 32% of Blacks and 99.9% of Caucasians and Asians. It is not expressed on Rh null RBCs. Fy6 is expressed in 100% of most populations and 32% of Blacks. The Fy(a–b–) phenotype is the major phenotype in approximately 70% Blacks, but is very rarely found in other populations. This phenotype is characterized by the

Red cell phenotype	Prevalence (%)		Allele
	Caucasians	Blacks	
Fy (a+b−)	17	9	FY*01/FY*01 or FY*A/FY*A
Fy (a−b+)	34	22	FY*02/FY*02 or FY*B/FY*B
Fy (a+b+)	49	1	FY*A/FY*B
Fy (a−b−)	Rare	68	FY*/N.01–05, FY*/N.01–02‡
Fy^3	100	32	
Fy^5	99.9	32	
Fy^6	100	32	

‡Nomenclature pending approval by the ISBT working party on terminology for red cell surface antigens.

Table 1.
Duffy blood group system phenotypes and prevalence. Reproduced with permission and modification.

absence of the Fyb antigen on RBCs and its presence on non-erythroid cells. Duffy mRNA is not detected in the bone marrow of Fy(a–b–) individuals; however, it is detected in other tissues including the colon, lung, and spleen. This unique phenotype is caused by a single amino acid substitution at position 46 in the Duffy (Fyb) gene. This mutation impairs the promotor activity in erythroid cells by disrupting the binding site for GATA1 erythroid transcription factor. Furthermore, some individuals with this phenotype do not make anti-Fyb. This is believed to be due to a mutation in the, erythroid promoter, GATA-1 binding motif. Interestingly, the same Fy(a–b–) phenotype rarely found in Caucasians is characterized by absence of Duffy antigens expression in both erythroid and non-erythroid tissues due to possibly presence of mutations which prevent formation of Duffy protein. These individuals can form anti-Fy3. The have high prevalence antigens; Fy3, Fy5, and Fy6 are conformational epitopes as opposed to specific sequence epitopes with Fy5 hypothesized to be a combined conformational epitope of Duffy and Rh protein [9–12].

3. Duffy antibodies

Anti-Fya and -Fyb are clinically significant RBC alloantibodies which can cause immediate and delayed hemolytic transfusion reactions (HTRs) as well as hemolytic disease of the fetus and newborn (HDFN). They often result from previous exposure such as after transfusion or pregnancy. They are not usually naturally occurring. The Duffy antibodies are predominantly of the IgG subclass whereas the IgM form is rare.

The mechanism of extravascular hemolysis (EH) in both HDFN and HTR is similar. In HDFN, the mother lacks a certain red cell antigen which the fetus is positive for, thus the mother is allo-immunized (i.e., made a new antibody) during the first pregnancy. If she gets exposed to the same antigen in subsequent pregnancy (ies), the fetus (es) is/are at risk of HDFN. Similarly, if a patient lacks a certain red cell antigen but receives red cell transfusion with a unit that has such antigen, the patient is at risk for allo-immunziation after the transfusion and HTR in subsequent transfusion (s). EH is typically induced by IgG red cell antibodies. EH consists of consumption of antibody and/or C3b-bound red cells by phagocytes in the reticulo-endothelial system (RES) causing a delayed hemolytic transfusion reaction (DHTR). DHTRs can be clinically significant leading to morbidity and possibly mortality. To avoid DHTR, patients with known clinically significant antibodies, receive red cell units that lack antigen (s) to their the cognate antibody (ies). The Duffy antibodies are usually associated with a moderate DHTR and mild HDFN [13].

Anti-Fya is identified more than anti-Fy3, anti-Fy5, or anti-Fyb. Fya is 20 times more immunogenic than Fyb. Some of anti-Fya can bind and activate complements [14]. Anti-Fy3 is also clinically significant antibody which can cause mild HDFN and HTRs. Serologically, it can react with enzyme treated Fy(a+) or Fy(b+) RBCs, but fails to react with Fy(a−b−) RBCs [15]. Anti-Fy4 shows lack of consistent test results. It was found to be reactive with Fy(a−b−), some Fy(a+b−), some Fy(a−b+) RBCs but shows no reaction with Fy(a+b+) RBCs [16]. Anti-Fy5 reacts with enzyme treated Fy(a+) or Fy(b+) RBCs with no reaction with Fy(a−b−) RBCs or Rh null RBCS. It has been reported in sickle cell patients with delayed HTRs in the presence of other clinically significant alloantibodies [17]. A human anti-Fy6 has not been identified [18].

4. The Duffy glycoprotein as a receptor for chemokines

The Duffy glycoprotein can bind to a variety of chemokines and is known commonly as the Duffy antigen receptor for chemokines (DARC) or more recently atypical chemokine receptor 1 (ACKR1). Chemokines are proteins secreted by immune cells as a mean to communicate signals to guide their interactions. The exact function of DARC is not fully clear. One postulated function is that DARC permits erythrocyte to act a chemokine scavenger to limit leukocyte activation. The importance of this function in inflammatory diseases is not well established [6, 19].

5. Duffy and malaria

The Duffy glycoprotein plays an important role in malaria transmission by acting as the erythroid receptor for *Plasmodium vivax* through binding to the Fy6 epitope (previously known as *P. vivax* Duffy-binding protein (PvDbp)) and for Plasmodium knowlesi. Individuals with Fy(a−b−) phenotype were resistant to parasitic invasion in a study performed on 11 volunteers, whereas those who contracted malaria were Fy(a+) or Fy(b+). Fy6 is present on all erythroid cells with an Fy(a+) or Fy(b+) phenotype. Thus it is absent on red cells with Fy(a−b−) phenotype. In west Africa, individuals with Fy(a−b−) phenotype are found in greater frequency than in areas where *P. vivax* is absent. The protective effect of Fy(a−b−) phenotype does not extend to *P. falciparum* which can infect red cells of all Duffy phenotype [20].

Acknowledgements

I want to thank the department of Pathology at the University of Chicago, Chicago, IL, United States.

Conflict of interest

The author declares no conflict of interest.

Author details

Fatima A. Aldarweesh
Department of Pathology, Biological Sciences Division, Blood Bank and Transfusion Service, The University of Chicago, Chicago, IL, USA

*Address all correspondence to: faldarweesh@uchicago.edu

References

[1] Cutbush M, Mollison PL. The Duffy blood group system. Heredity. 1950;**4**:383-389

[2] Cutbush M, Mollison PL, Parkin DM. A new human blood group. Nature. 1950;**165**:188-189

[3] Ikin EW, Mourant AE, Pettenkofer JH, Blumenthal G. Discovery of the expected haemagglutinin, anti-Fyb. Nature. 1951;**168**:1077-1078

[4] Shaz BH, Hillyer CD, Gil MR. Transfusion Medicine and Hemostasis. 3rd ed. Amsterdam, Netherlands: Elsevier; 2019

[5] Pogo AO, Chaudhuri A. The Duffy protein: A malarial and chemokine receptor. Seminars in Hematology. 2000;**37**:122-129

[6] Rot A, von Andrian UH. Chemokines in innate and adaptive host defense: Basic chemokinese grammar for immune cells. Annual Review of Immunology. 2004;**22**:891-928

[7] Chaudhuri A, Zbrzezna V, Johnson C, et al. Purification and characterization of an erythrocyte protein complex carrying Duffy blood group antigenicity. Possible receptor for *Plasmodium vivax* and *Plasmodium knowlesi* malaria parasite. The Journal of Biological Chemistry. 1989;**264**:13770-13774

[8] Daniels G. Duffy blood group system. In: Human Blood Groups. 2nd ed. Malden, MA: Blackwell Science; 2002. pp. 324-341

[9] Tournamille C, Colin Y, Cartron JP, Le Van Kim C. Disruption of a GATA motif in the Duffy gene promoter abolishes erythroid gene expression in Duffy-negative individuals. Nature Genetics. 1995;**10**:224-228

[10] Albrey JA, Vincent EE, Hutchinson J, et al. A new antibody, anti-Fy3, in the Duffy blood group system. Vox Sanguinis. 1971;**20**:29-35

[11] Mallinson G, Soo KS, Schall TJ, Pisacka M, Anstee DJ. Mutations in the erythrocyte chemokine receptor (Duffy) gene: The molecular basis of the Fya/Fyb antigens and identification of a deletion in the Duffy gene of an apparently healthy individual with the Fy(a−b−) phenotype. British Journal of Haematology. 1995;**90**:823-829

[12] Rios M, Chaudhuri A, Mallinson G, et al. New genotypes in Fy(a−b−) individuals: Nonsense mutations (Trp to stop) in the coding sequence of either FY a or FY B. British Journal of Haematology. 2000;**108**:448-454

[13] Issitt PD, Anstee DJ. Applied Blood Group Serology. 4th ed. Durham, NC: Montgomery Scientific Publications; 1998

[14] Klein HG, Anstee DJ. Mollison's Blood Transfusion in Clinical Medicine. 11th ed. Malden, MA: Blackwell Publishing; 2005

[15] Olteanu H, Gerber D, Partridge K, Sarode R. Acute hemolytic transfusion reaction secondary to anti-Fy3. Immunohematology. 2005;**21**:48-52

[16] Behzad O, Lee CL, Gavin J, Marsh WL. A new antierythrocyte antibody in the Duffy system: Anti-Fy4. Vox Sanguinis. 1973;**24**:337-342

[17] Colledge KI, Pezzulich M, Marsh WL. Anti-Fy5, an antibody disclosing a probable association between the rhesus and Duffy blood group genes. Vox Sanguinis. 1973;**24**:193-199

[18] Waśniowska K, Blanchard D, Janvier D, et al. Identification of the Fy6

epitope recognized by two monoclonal antibodies in the N-terminal extracellular portion of the Duffy antigen receptor for chemokines. Molecular Immunology. 1996;**33**:917-923

[19] Pruenster M, Rot A. Throwing light on DARC. Biochemical Society Transactions. 2006;**34**:1005-1008

[20] Miller LH, Mason SJ, Clyde DF, McGinniss MH. The resistance factor to Plasmodium vivax in blacks. The Duffy-blood-group genotype, FyFy. The New England Journal of Medicine. 1976;**295**:302-304

Chapter 5

Post-Transfusion Haemolytic Reactions

Jolanta Korsak and Anna Piotrowska

Abstract

Haemolytic post-transfusion reaction is caused by accelerated destruction of erythrocytes by immunological incompatibility between the donor and the recipient. It also occurs for non-immunological reasons: thermal, osmotic or mechanical damage and bacterial infection. Haemolysis can be endogenous (usually acute) and exogenous with macrophages in the reticuloendothelial system of spleen or liver (delayed). The pathophysiology: antibody binding erythrocyte antigens, antibody-coated erythrocytes interaction with monocytes/macrophages activating phagocytosis or antibody-dependent cytotoxicity and the production of inflammatory mediators. Antibodies destroying transfused blood cells are called clinically relevant antibodies that are active in vitro at 37°C. An interesting mechanism is the "bystander immune cytolysis".

Keywords: haemolytic reaction, haemolysis, transfusion reaction, HTR

1. Introduction

Haemolytic transfusion reaction (HTR) is the result of accelerated destruction of red blood cells. The most common cause is immunological incompatibility between a donor and a blood recipient. It is mainly haemolysis that is responsible for the destruction of transfused donor blood cells by antibodies present in the recipient, but in rare cases, destruction may be caused in recipient blood cells by donor antibodies present in transfused plasma or platelet concentrate [1]. Haemolysis may also occur due to non-immunological reasons, such as thermal, osmotic or mechanical damage to the transfused blood; bacterial infection or extremely rare and blood transfusion from a donor with congenital haemolytic anaemia due to deficiency of glucose-6-phosphate dehydrogenase [2].

2. The incidence of haemolytic transfusion reactions

Currently, the incidence of haemolytic transfusion reactions is difficult to estimate. Most data come from retrospective studies that do not include reactions not reported by clinicians. In contrast, prospective studies also contain errors due to reaction symptoms often remaining unrecognised or masked by associated diseases, for example, bleeding or liver disease [1]. The frequency of reporting haemolytic transfusion reactions may also depend on other factors, such as patient population, transfusion response reporting system and medical staff education. Historical research results indicate that the frequency of haemolytic transfusion reactions falls

IntechOpen

between 1:10,000 and 1:50,000 transfused blood components [3, 4]. In contrast, the incidence for patients receiving a transfusion is estimated to be higher (about 1:500–1:800 patients) because most recipients receive more than one blood unit. It is worth noting that the estimation of the frequency of haemolytic reactions depends on the number of transfusions in a given centre. Thus, in large clinical centres, where severely ill patients are treated, more of these events are recorded [4]. A report issued by the Quebec Haemovigilance System covering 5 years of observation described 47 ABO incompatibility reactions, 55 cases of acute haemolytic transfusion reaction and 91 cases of delayed transfusion reaction in reference to 7059 all reported transfusion reactions. It was estimated that the frequency of reactions resulting from the ABO incompatibility was 1:27,318, acute haemolytic transfusion reactions 1:14,901 and delayed haemolytic transfusion reactions 1:9313 per unit of transfused red blood cell concentrate [5].

The most common reaction among the acute (approximately 30%) was haemolysis resulting from ABO incompatibility [5]. In the annual report Serious Hazards of Transfusion (SHOT), published in England, in 2017, 42 haemolytic transfusion reactions were reported in reference to 3230 of all reactions observed following transfusion of blood components, of which 13 cases of acute haemolytic transfusion reaction and 29 cases of delayed haemolytic reaction (including 6 cases of hyperhemolysis) were reported. The number of reported cases of delayed haemolytic transfusion reaction was higher than in 2016, but comparable with previous years [6]. Factors that can affect the increase in the number of delayed haemolytic reactions include correctness in carrying out serological tests, longer survival of patients after transfusions and an increase in the number of transfused blood components. Since most patients receive more than one unit of red blood cell concentrate, the estimated incidence of delayed haemolytic transfusion reactions is from 1:854 to 1:524 per patient who has been transfused and is higher than per transfused unit [7]. In the population, delayed haemolytic transfusion reactions occur with a frequency of 1.69/100,000 per year [7].

3. Mechanisms of haemolytic transfusion reactions

Red blood cells undergo haemolysis in the intravascular mechanism, in blood or extravascular vessels, that is, organs involving cells of the reticuloendothelial system, primarily spleen and/or liver. Clinically significant differences between the above mechanisms of red blood cells destruction are based on the time of onset of haemolysis and the destruction rate of red blood cells. Intravascular haemolysis is characterised by the destruction of red blood cells at a rate of about 200 ml of transfused cells within 1 h of transfusion. It is manifested by a rapid decrease in haemoglobin, haemoglobinemia and haemoglobinuria and can potentially be life threatening [2]. In contrast, extravascular haemolysis is less dramatic, with a rate of destruction of red blood cells of approximately 0.25 ml/h/1 kg of recipient's body weight. For example, for 70 kg recipient, about 18 ml of transfused red blood cells are destroyed per hour. However, it is worth noting that despite the low intensity of haemolysis, the survival time of red blood cells after transfusion is significantly reduced [2]. In general, intravascular haemolysis is called as an early acute haemolytic transfusion reaction. It can occur during transfusion or up to 24 h after transfusion of red blood cells. In comparison extravascular haemolysis is called delayed haemolytic transfusion reaction and usually occurs 24 h or days after the end of the transfusion. The quoted breakdown of reactions is somewhat artificial, because the symptoms associated with haemolytic reactions sometimes overlap [1].

The occurrence and severity of individual clinical symptoms can vary widely and are often non-specific [1, 8].

Red blood cell transfusion can also stimulate the production of alloantibodies without the occurrence of haemolysis. This phenomenon is called delayed serologic transfusion reaction (DSTR) and should be differentiated from delayed haemolytic transfusion reaction [9].

3.1 Intravascular haemolysis

Most often intravascular haemolysis is the result of the destruction of red blood cells by the complement system, stimulated by the presence of alloantibodies or autoantibodies. Among alloantibodies, such haemolysis is induced by anti-A and anti-B, rarely anti-Jka, anti-Jkb, anti-Vel, anti-P, anti-Lea and very unique antibodies with other specificities [10, 11]. In all these cases, haemolysis takes place via the classical pathway of complement activation. Its occurrence and severity, in addition to the class of antibodies, is also affected by the number of antigenic determinants with which the antibodies react. The reaction is most severe in the case of antigens A and B, because their number is estimated at about 5×10^5 per cell [12, 13]. In contrast, the presence of antigens from the Rh, Kell, Kidd and Duffy systems on the surface of red blood cells is determined in the range of 10^3–10^4 per cell [12]. **Table 1** shows the number of antigenic determinants on the cell surface for selected red blood cell antigens.

Antibodies combined with antigens by triggering the complement cascade lead to cell lysis. This mechanism is called the classic pathway for complement activation and is shown in **Figure 1**.

The starting point is the antigen-antibody complex present on the surface of the cell membrane [14, 15]. Antibodies of the IgM and IgG class (outside the IgG4 subclass) bind the C1q protein in the initial stage of activation. The condition for complement activation is the binding of the C1q molecule by two Fc fragments of adjacent IgG antibodies or by one IgM molecule. It should be noted here that the IgM class is more efficient in starting the process of complement activation than the IgG class [2, 15]. The C1qrs complex is created and activates the C_2 and C_4 components and their distribution into C2a and C2b as well as C4a and C4b. The C4b2a

Blood group system	Antigens	The number of antigenic determinants on the surface of the cell membrane
ABO	A_1	8.5×10^5
	A_2	2.5×10^5
	B	7.5×10^5
Rh	D	$1–2 \times 10^5$
	C	$7–8 \times 10^4$
	e	$1.8–2.4 \times 10^4$
Kell	K	6.1×10^3
Duffy	Fy^a	1.7×10^4
Kidd	Jk^a	1.4×10^5
MNSs	S	1.2×10^4

Table 1.
Number of antigenic determinants on the cell surface of the red blood cell (according to [12, 13]).

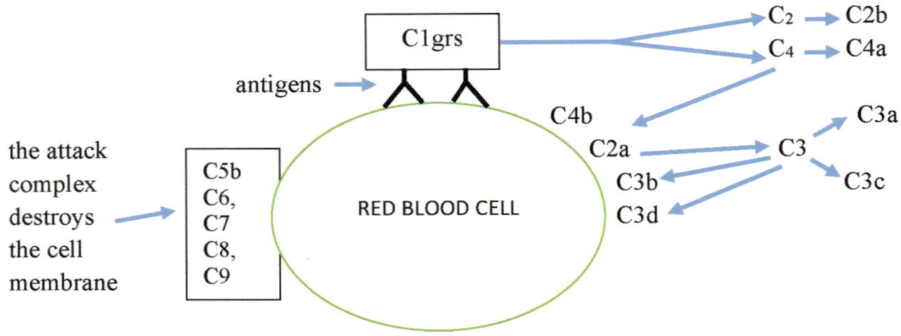

Figure 1.
The classic pathway for complement.

complex has proteolytic properties and is called C3 convertase. Convertase breaks down molecules of C3 into C3a, C3b, C3c and C3d. The C3b and C3d components bind with the red blood cell membrane and in many cases the complement cascade process ends. In other cases, the C3b component activates C5 and C5a and C5b are formed. C5b binds to C6, then to C7. This creates a complex of three C5b-6-7 particles, which is partially incorporated into the cell membrane and further binds C8. The C5b-8 complexes create holes in the cell membrane that increase when exposed to the C9 component. The C5B-C9 complex called membrane attack complex (MAC) creates pores in the cell membrane of a red blood cell that are 1/700 of its size. Haemoglobin escapes from the cells into the plasma, and the effects of haemolysis are visible macroscopically in the plasma of the blood sample [15].

The alternative path of complement activation and the lectin path of complement activation do not play a role in the destruction of red blood cells. Although the mechanism of the lectin route may be the reason for the in vivo ineffectiveness of the use of monoclonal and recombinant antibodies, which are thus eliminated from the body before they fulfil their function, for example, anti-D Ig for prevention purposes in RhD maternal-foetal conflict [16].

However, the complement system does not work specifically. The safety of body cells is enabled by factors that regulate complement activity present in plasma and on cells of various tissues, including red blood cells. Membrane inhibitor of reactive lysis (MIRL) (CD59) and decay accelerating factor (DAF) (CD55) are essential to protect red blood cells from haemolysis. The expression of these membrane inhibitors is associated with Cromer group system and CD59. On blood cells with the Cromer mull phenotype, known as Inab, DAF inhibitor expression is absent [17, 18]. DAF regulates C3a-converting activity. MIRL inhibits membrane attack complex [15, 17]. Lack of these particles may increase the susceptibility of red blood cells to intravascular haemolysis due to complement activation [19].

3.2 Extravascular haemolysis

In a situation in which, despite activation of the complement system, through antigen-antibody reaction, there is no intravascular haemolysis, red blood cells with detectable C3b component remain in the circulation. This kind of mechanism of red blood cell destruction occurs for IgG antibodies with complement system [13]. They may interact with CR1 and CR3 receptors on macrophages and consequently undergo phagocytosis. Most of the cells coated by the complement C3b component are destroyed by liver macrophages, that is, by Kupffer cells, while the cells coated with antibody molecules are mainly destroyed by spleen macrophages. They have surface receptors that recognise antibody classes and subclasses, and complement components, of which the Fc R1 receptor is specific for red cells coated with antibodies [1]. Blood cells connected to this receptor are destroyed in the process of antibody-dependent cytotoxicity. Red blood cells can be absorbed and completely "digested" inside the macrophage. They can also be partially absorbed and then the integrity of the cell membrane is disturbed by the loss of proteins and lipids, which changes its osmotic properties. Such a blood cell, after being released from the macrophage, circulates in the blood as a spherocyte, whose survival is short. The macrophage cytotoxins are another mechanism that plays a role in the destruction of red blood cells. As a consequence of antibody-dependent cell-mediated cytotoxicity (ADCC) haemoglobinemia and haemoglobinuria may occur similarly to intravascular haemolysis, although the antibodies that caused it do not bind complement components.

4. Mediators of inflammatory reactions in haemolytic transfusion reactions

Receptors for complement activation products C3a and C5a are found on many cells: monocytes, macrophages, neutrophils, platelets, endothelium and smooth muscle. Their release causes an increase in the concentration of oxygen radicals, leukotrienes, nitric oxide and cytokines. The increase in cytokine release may also be due to the interaction of Fcγ R1 receptors with IgG molecules associated with red blood cells. Udani et al. [20] showed in vitro that in the case of ABO incompatibility, monocytes are directly involved in the formation of acute haemolytic transfusion reaction [15]. Incompatible red blood cells reduce CD14 expression and increase CD44 expression on monocytes in whole blood. After 24 incubations with incompatible red blood cells, monocytes show a significant increase in CD44 levels. The results of these studies indicate a critical role of monocyte activation in the development of intravascular haemolytic transfusion reaction [15].

In ABO incompatibility, in which anti-A, anti-B and anti-AB antibodies activate complement leading to intravascular haemolysis, a large amount of tumour necrosis factor-α (TNF) and interleukins CXCL8 (IL-8) and CCL2 are released into the plasma (MCP-1) [19–21]. TNF-α is released first, its elevated concentration is already detected within first 2 h. It carries a pro-inflammatory potential that is responsible for fever, leukocyte activation, stimulation of procoagulant activity, increased antibody production and vascular wall permeability [22]. TNF-α also stimulates endothelial cells to synthesise adhesion molecules and chemotactic cytokines [22]. CXCL8 and CCL2 produced in the blood during ABO incompatibility will appear later than TNF-α in very high concentrations. CXCL8 primarily activates neutrophils, which leads to the accumulation of leukocytes in the lung vessels of small diameter and damage to the endothelium of blood vessels and their higher permeability [1, 12]. CCL2 is mainly a chemotactic and activating factor for monocytes [1, 12].

In incompatibility, in which non-complement IgG antibodies cause extravascular haemolysis, cytokines belonging to two categories differing in response rates are produced: (1) synthesised at a concentration higher than 1 μg/ml within 24 h and (2) synthesised at a concentration of about 100 pg/ml. Low concentration cytokines include IL-1β, IL-6 and TNF-α. CXCL8 concentration is similar to that in intravascular haemolysis, whereas TNF-α is synthesised at low concentration, estimated at <100 pg/ml [1, 2]. IL-1ra (receptor antagonist) is produced in extravascular haemolysis, which is an IL-1 receptor antagonist. Its presence to some extent affects some clinical differences between extravascular and intravascular haemolysis [23]. IL-1β concentration and IL-6 produced by monocytes in response to red blood cells coated with IgG antibodies increase progressively within 24 h to a concentration of 100 pg/ml. Since IL-1β and IL-6 affect proliferation and differentiation of β-lymphocytes, the synthesis of these two cytokines enhances the synthesis of allo- and autoantibodies, which are often involved in the formation of delayed haemolytic transfusion reaction [1, 24, 25].

5. Complications of haemolytic transfusion reactions

5.1 Disseminated intravascular coagulation associated with haemolytic transfusion reaction

The key pathogenetic phenomenon in DIC is excessive thrombin generation in the tissue factor (TF)-dependent pathway and activated factor VII (FVIIa-activated factor VII) [26]. In the pathogenesis of DIC, interactions between the blood coagulation system and mediators of the inflammatory response are also of great importance [27]. Proinflammatory cytokines affect blood coagulation and fibrinolysis, for example, TNF-α and IL-1 increase TF expression and inhibit thrombomodulin (TM) expression on vascular endothelial cells [28]. On the one hand, these processes lead to the production of a large amount of thrombin that converts fibrinogen to fibrin. Fibrin creates blood clots in the light of small vessels trapping the platelets. If the activation of coagulation is not timely inhibited, the resulting clots will block the blood supply to vital organs, which will be manifested in their failure. On the other hand, the formation of a large amount of blood clots will "consume" blood coagulation factors and platelets, which will manifest as a haemorrhagic diathesis. In addition, their degradation products (fibrinogen/fibrin degradation products (FDP)) resulting from the breakdown of fibrinogen and fibrin exhibit anticoagulant properties, inhibit platelet function, act as cytotoxic vascular endothelium and increase capillary permeability, further disrupting haemostasis mechanisms [26].

Clinically, this is manifested by unexpected bleeding and/or a decrease in blood pressure. The course is acute, dynamic, with thrombocytopenia, increased concentration of fibrin degradation products, prolonged prothrombin time (PT), extended partial thromboplastin time after activation (activated partial thromboplastin time (APTT)) and hypofibrinogenaemia. **Table 2** presents the point algorithm for the diagnosis of acute disseminated intravascular coagulation.

However, this complication is rare and predominantly accompanies intravascular haemolysis, but in recipients who have received non-compliant blood in the ABO system, it occurs even in 25% of cases [1].

5.2 Hypotension and shock

Hypotension occurs in about 1 in 10 cases of intravascular haemolytic transfusion reaction, but is also sometimes observed in extravascular haemolysis. Complement activation appears to be the most important determining factor in these cases. During the haemolytic reaction, C3a, C4a, C5a and C5a-des-arg anaphylatoxins are released. Furthermore, consumption of a C1-esterase inhibitor contributes to the activation of the kinin pathway associated with the release of bradykinin [32]. In addition, tumour necrosis factor (TNF) and interleukin-1 (IL-1), released by phagocytes during haemolytic transfusion reaction may also contribute to hypotension and shock [32].

5.3 Impaired renal function

Impaired renal function is observed in both intravascular and extravascular haemolytic transfusion reactions, although definitely more frequently in the case of

Test	Result	Score
Platelet count ($\times 10^9$/l)	>100	0
	>50, ale ≤ 100	1
	≤50	2
Concentration of fibrinogen/fibrin degradation markers (FDP; D-dimery)	Normal	1
	Moderate	2
	Growth significant increase	3
Prothrombin time extended	o < 3 s	0
	o ≥ 3 s, ale < 6 s	1
	o ≥ 6 s	2
Fibrinogen concentration (g/l)	>1.0	0
	≤1.0	1
DIC acute diagnosis	≥5	

Table 2.
Point algorithm for the diagnosis of acute disseminated coagulation Intravascular [29–31].

intravascular. The severity of this abnormality varies greatly—from asymptomatic increase in urea (BUN) and serum creatinine up to complete anuria. Concomitant hypotension and intravascular coagulation syndrome may increase renal impairment. Blood clots that form in the renal arterioles cause cortical kidney attacks. Haemoglobin released from red blood cells also reacts nephrotoxically with nitric oxide (NO), damaging the epithelial cells of the renal tubules and the stroma that remains after their breakdown [33, 34].

Intravascular haemolysis modulates blood pressure and local blood flow through changes in the metabolism of the physiological vasodilator—nitric oxide (NO). NO can bind to thiol groups and haemoglobin haeme [35]. The connection of NO with haeme Fe^{2+} impairs oxygen transport through Hb. The presence of O_2 leads to oxidation of NO to NO_3 and oxidation of Fe^{2+} to Fe^{3+} and the formation of methaemoglobin. The interaction between Hb and NO is regulated by the allosteric transition of haemoglobin R (oxyHb) to the T form (deoxyHb). In oxyHb, cysteine is exposed at position 93 of the haemoglobin amino acid chain (Cys 93β). It is known that a significant proportion of NO does not immediately bind to $HbFe^{2+}$ heme, instead it binds to cysteine, resulting in the formation of the S-nitrosothiol derivative Hb (SNO-Hb). This process is reversible, so SNO-Hb releases NO, which is transported to endothelial receptors, where it participates in the regulation of vascular wall tone and blood flow. In the case of haemolysis of red blood cells, the free haemoglobin released from them reacts with NO much faster and more strongly than Hb inside cells [35]. The effect of intravascular haemolysis described above may be very similar to the side effect caused by transfusion of first-generation stromal haemoglobin solutions. This has been tested for its use as a substitute for red blood cells. It had vasoconstrictive and, as a result, hypertensive effect. This effect is largely attributed to the binding nitric oxide by free haemoglobin (NO) [36].

6. Clinical symptoms of transfusion haemolytic reactions

Intravascular haemolysis is accompanied by haemoglobinaemia and usually also haemoglobinuria, whereas extravascular haemolysis can only be

Initial symptoms of haemolytic transfusion reactions	Complications
Intravascular haemolysis Nausea or vomiting Ache Dyspnoea Decrease in RR and/or tachycardia Dark urine	Kidney failure Disseminated intravascular coagulation (DIC)
Extravascular haemolysis Fever and/or chills Nausea or vomiting Ache Dyspnoea	Kidney failure disseminated intravascular coagulation (DIC)

Table 3.
Initial symptoms of haemolytic transfusion reactions.

accompanied by anaemia. In both cases, the patient's serum bilirubin increases, but it depends on the degree of haemolysis as well as liver function [1]. Elevated LDH is always observed with intravascular haemolysis, not always with extravascular haemolysis. Reduced haptoglobin levels usually occur in both types of haemolysis. Drop in blood pressure is much more common in patients with intravascular than extravascular haemolysis. Renal failure and DIC are also more commonly associated with intravascular haemolysis. Some patients may experience organ failure such as the pancreas, heart and even multiple organ failure that threatens the patient's life.

In unconscious patients and patients under general anaesthesia, it may be difficult to recognise a haemolytic transfusion reaction, as some symptoms may go unnoticed (e.g. pain and nausea). Pain, which is described as a symptom of haemolytic reactions, is located at the puncture site, back, chest, groin and head. The occurrence of pain in the haemolytic transfusion reaction is not clear. It is probably the result of direct stimulation of nociceptive nerves in perivascular tissue by bradykinin, which, in turn, is released during sudden activation of complement [37]. Clinical manifestations are shown in **Table 3**.

7. Causes of haemolytic transfusion reactions

7.1 Haemolytic transfusion reactions caused by alloantibodies

The most common cause of haemolytic transfusion reactions is the immunological destruction of red blood cells resulting from the reaction of antibodies in the recipient's blood and the antigens present on the transfused donor's blood cells to which these antibodies are made.

Antibodies capable of destroying transfused blood cells are called clinically relevant antibodies, and the transfusion reaction in the event of immunological incompatibility depends on: (1) specificity of antibodies; (2) thermal amplitude of the antibodies; (3) IgG classes and IgG subclasses; (4) number, density and spatial configuration of antigenic sites on red blood cells; (5) the ability of antibodies to activate the complement system; (6) plasma concentrations of antibodies and (7) volumes of transfused red blood cells. A very important feature of all antibodies responsible for causing a haemolytic transfusion reaction is its in vitro activity at 37°C.

Antibodies detected at a lower temperature are not considered clinically relevant, for example, anti-A1, anti-M and anti-P1, whose optimal reaction is usually at low temperature, but if detected at 37°C, they can cause destruction of red blood cells with the appropriate antigen. They then become clinically significant.

Features of antibodies (specificity, class and heat amplitude) and antigens (density of antigenic sites and their distribution) against which the antibodies directed are interconnected. In different people, antibodies with a particular specificity most often occur in the same class of immunoglobulins and have a similar heat amplitude, for example, anti-A, anti-B and anti-AB from the ABO system often belong to both IgM and IgG classes, they bind complement and have an extended thermal amplitude of up to 37°C.

A and B antigens are highly immunogenic. Anti-A, anti-B and anti-AB antibodies are involved in causing an early intravascular transfusion reaction, and transfusion of incompatible blood in the ABO system poses a threat to the recipient's life, especially when group A red blood cells are transfused to a patient with group O. Sixty-one (61%) of all haemolytic transfusion-related fatal reactions are associated with the ABO incompatibility [38, 39]. A contrasting example is the Lua antigen and anti-Lua antibodies. They are usually IgM molecules, are rarely active at 37°C and usually do not bind complement. Lua antigens have uneven distribution on red blood cells and are weakly immunogenic. No cases of acute haemolytic reaction caused by anti-Lua antibodies have been reported, delayed transfusion haemolytic reaction is rare and occurs only in mild form.

Not all detectable alloantibodies that react with red blood cells can cause a haemolytic reaction. The specificity of the antibodies potentially responsible for intravascular and extravascular haemolysis is shown in **Table 4**.

Similar reactions to anti-A and anti-B come from anti-PP_1P^k, anti-P1 and anti-Vel. Other antibodies cause intravascular haemolysis, but sometimes they may be accompanied by intravascular haemolysis. Such reactions were observed in the following blood group systems: Rh, MNSs, Lutheran, Kell, Duffy, Diego and Lewis. The mechanism of appearance of intravascular symptoms has not been fully explained, because although some of the antibodies bind complement components,

Blood group system	Intravascular haemolysis	Extravascular haemolysis
ABO, H	Anti-A, -B, -AB, -H in the Bombay phenotype	
Rh		All
Kell	Anti-K	All
Kidd	Anti-Jk^a	Anti-Jk^a, -Jk^b, -Jk^3
Duffy		Anti-Fy^a, -Fy^b
MNS		Anti-M, -S, -s, -U
Lutheran		Anti-Lu^b
Lewis	Anti-Le^a	
Cartwright		Anti-Yt^a
Vel	Anti-Vel	
Colton		Anti-Co^a
Dombrock		Anti-Do^a, -Do^b

Table 4.
Specificity of selected antibodies associated with haemolytic transfusion reactions.

their reactions end with C3 components. Only in the case of rare haemolytic reactions due to anti-Lea it was shown that the coated cells are destroyed by the spleen macrophages very slowly and in the event of transfusion of large volumes of red blood cells, they become inefficient. Then intravascular haemolysis coincides with visible haemoglobinuria [40, 41]. Interesting clinical point of view are antibodies from the Kidd system. They activate the complement system to the stage of binding of the C3b component, causing extravascular haemolysis. However, the symptoms in some recipients, or the occurrence of a reaction already during a blood transfusion and haemoglobinuria, indicate that the destruction of blood cells also takes place inside the vessel. In the laboratory setting, anti-Jka antibodies are called "insidious" antibodies because they are often difficult to detect due to their low concentration, and yet they can cause a severe haemolytic complication [41].

Patients with antibodies found to be clinically insignificant may theoretically be given a blood transfusion from a donor with the antigen to which they are directed. In clinical practice, however, such antibodies can sometimes destroy donor blood cells. Therefore, if possible, blood without this antigen should be selected [41].

Another cause for haemolytic transfusion reaction may be a secondary immune response in patients who have developed alloantibodies during previous transfusions of blood components or pregnancy. This is called delayed haemolytic transfusion reaction (DHTR) in which current blood transfusion stimulates memory lymphocytes and stimulates the production of alloantibodies directed at incompatible antigen found on transfused blood cells [21, 42]. In approximately 50% of cases, alloantibodies produced after transfusion or pregnancy cease to be detected after a few months, and this period of time depends on the specificity of the antibodies and the individual characteristics of the immune system. Schonewille et al. found that, using current laboratory methods, 25% of red blood cell antibodies become indeterminate on average after about 10 months from production [43]. Therefore, pre-transfusion tests may not always detect the presence of antibodies. Antibodies stimulated for synthesis may cause symptoms of haemolysis after 3–10 days, usually very mild and their presence can be detected after 10–21 days. **Table 5** presents features of delayed haemolytic transfusion reaction and the time of their occurrence.

Antibodies that cause a delayed haemolytic transfusion reaction are IgG molecules that are binding or non-binding for complementary components. Their specificity is most often directed to the antigens of the Rh, Kidd, Duffy, MNS and Kell systems [14]. In approximately 11% of cases, more than one antibody specificity is

Time (days)	Occurrence	Explanation
0	Negative pre-transfusion test	Antibody titres below detection threshold
1	Red blood cell transfusion	
3–10	Clinical symptoms of haemolysis	Acceleration of transfused blood cells destruction
10–21	Post-transfusion testing of blood samples: DAT and screen of antibodies positive	Increase in antibody titre; donated blood cells coated with antibodies
>21	DAT can be negative	Destruction of donor blood cells in reticuloendothelial system and/or liver
>21–300	DAT may be positive, eluate testing may show presence of alloantibodies or panagglutination	Alloantibodies not specifically associated with autologous red blood cells or produced warm antibodies

DAT—direct antiglobulin test.

Table 5.
Features of late hemolytic transfusion reaction and time of their occurrence [21].

detected. In rare cases, the result of transfusion alloimmunity in DHTR may be the production of autoantibodies (warm IgG autoantibodies or cold autoagglutinins). This phenomenon occurs in patients with sickle cell disease [44–46].

7.2 Haemolytic transfusion reactions due to passive transmission of alloantibodies in blood components or in blood products

Transfusion of plasma, platelet or granulocyte concentrate from donors incompatible in the ABO system with the recipient may lead to acute haemolytic transfusion reaction and even death. The severity of the reaction depends on the titre of anti-A and/or anti-B antibodies in the transfused plasma or in the blood component containing the plasma, and on its volume [47–49]. Tests on the ABO system titre in group O apheresis concentrates of platelets show that 26% of samples have an anti-A or anti-A, B antibody titre of 64 or higher. This concentration may be responsible for causing a haemolytic reaction [50]. In turn, the results of studies by Coolig et al. [51] carried out in pooled platelet concentrates of whole blood groups showed that 60% of them had anti-A titres of at least 64 [51]. Repeated transfusions of ABO incompatible platelet concentrate may lead to accumulation of anti-A antibodies in the recipient's plasma, which may result in severe haemolytic reactions [52]. Unfortunately, despite many studies, it has not been possible to determine the critical titre of anti-A and/or anti-B antibodies that would be safe in the event of transfusion of ABO incompatible platelet concentrates, and in many countries, proprietary haemolysis prevention programs have been developed for recipients of incompatible platelets [48–50, 53].

Haemolytic transfusion reactions due to passively transferred anti-A and/or anti-B antibodies have also been observed in patients after intravenous immunoglobulin administration [54]. Spath et al. [55] analysed reports available in the literature describing cases of haemolysis in patients treated with intravenous immunoglobulins [55]. They showed that the haemolytic reaction is induced by IgG anti-A/B antibodies present in immunoglobulin products. The reaction generally occurs in high-dose IVIG recipients [55].

7.3 Haemolytic reaction associated with the "bystander immune cytolysis"

The haemolytic transfusion reactions may have a different immunological origin than the reactions of antibodies in the recipient's blood and the antigen present on the donor's blood cells. This additional mechanism occurs when recipient's red blood cells are destroyed by a reaction called "bystander immune cytolysis". It is defined as the immunological destruction of red blood cells by antibodies whose specificity corresponds to antigens found on other cells/blood cells (e.g. HLA antigens found on leukocytes and plasma proteins), while red blood cells are only close to this immunological "confusion" [56]. They are destroyed by the complement system, although they did not participate directly in the antigen-antibody reaction. One of the reasons for this haemolytic reaction is the binding of the C567 complement complex, activated in an immune reaction, to the membrane of red blood cells not participating in the reaction but located in the vicinity [56]. Blood cells are destroyed as a result of the activation of the binding of the remaining components of C8 and C9 complement and the formation of the MAC complex on the blood cells [56]. The mechanism of "bystander" haemolysis is similar to the destruction of blood cells in patients with paroxysmal nocturnal haemoglobinuria [57, 58]. A characteristic feature of the cell membrane of these blood cells is the lack or weak expression of the CD55 (DAF) and CD 59 (MIRL) proteins, which are complement inhibitors. This makes the subject more susceptible to haemolysis. It was found that when red blood cells became the "bystander" of leukocyte reactions and antibodies directed to them, they underwent haemolysis. The reaction of anti-HLA antibodies with leucocytes caused complement activation, which resulted in haemolysis of the patient's red blood cells sensitive to the complement [59]. It is noteworthy that in patients with a haemolytic reaction associated with the immune cytolysis of the "bystander" not only transfused red blood cells but also autologous blood cells of the patient were destroyed.

8. Differentiation

Early haemolytic transfusion reactions should be differentiated with septic shock due to bacterial contamination of the blood component, as well as anaphylaxis and bleeding. In addition, immune haemolysis of nocturnal paroxysmal haemoglobinuria or autoimmune anaemia should also be considered. The cause of an early haemolytic reaction may also be congenital haemolytic anaemia, for example, glucose-6-phosphate dehydrogenase deficiency or microangiopathic haemolytic

- Alloantibodies responsible for haemolysis
- Delayed serological transfusion reaction
- Autoimmune haemolytic anaemia
- Cold agglutinins disease
- Non-immune haemolysis
    - use of inappropriate fluids
    - improper storage of blood components
    - defects in the blood-heating devices
    - needle diameter too small, haematocrit of transfused red blood cells too high
    - an inappropriate method of freezing/thawing red blood cells
    - using the wrong infusion pumps
    - bacterial infection of blood components
    - mechanical damage to blood cells, artificial valves
- Congenital haemolytic anaemia
- Haemoglobinopathies
- Drug-induced haemolysis of red blood cells
- Microangiopathic haemolytic anaemia
    - thrombocytopenic thrombosis (TTP)
    - haemolytic uremic syndrome
    - HELLP syndrome
- Bleeding
- Nocturnal paroxysmal haemoglobinuria
- Polyagglutination
- Infections
    - *Clostridium perfringens*
    - Malaria
    - Babesiosis

Table 6.
Differential diagnosis of haemolytic transfusion reactions [1].

anaemia (TTP, HUS and HELLP). In differential diagnosis, attention should also be paid to non-immune reasons related to improper blood storage, transfusion of red blood cells through a small needle diameter, etc.

Differential diagnosis of delayed haemolytic transfusion reactions includes latent sources of infection, autoimmune haemolytic anaemia, cold agglutinin disease, nocturnal paroxysmal haemoglobinuria, bleeding, mechanical destruction of red blood cells, for example, artificial heart valves and TTP.

It should be noted that an increase in body temperature and white blood cell count, typical for DHTR, can be interpreted as a sign of infection. In some patient groups, it may be difficult to recognise a delayed haemolytic transfusion reaction. Patients with liver failure are a special problem. Haemoglobinemia is not diagnosed in the serum of these patients due to jaundice, often direct antiglobulin reaction (DTA) is positive and elevated bilirubin and LDH are found.

Another group are patients with absorbing haematomas. They may be similar to delayed haemolytic reactions. Elevated unbound bilirubin, LDH and decreased haptoglobin are observed. The presence of fibrinogen degradation products from an absorbing haematoma can be interpreted as a DIC symptom. DHTR can be identified in these patients by the presence of antigen on the transfused red blood cells to which the antibodies may be directed. **Table 6** presents the differential diagnosis of haemolytic transfusion reactions.

9. Diagnosis of transfusion haemolytic reactions

If a haemolytic transfusion reaction is suspected, medical personnel should immediately stop transfusing a blood component. The blood unit should be checked at the patient's bedside, whether it was properly administered. Often, the clinical manifestations of haemolytic reactions are not clear, and the cause of the complication should be differentiated with bacterial infection. Therefore, prior to conducting laboratory tests of donor blood, bacteriological examination of the component remaining after the transfusion cessation should be conducted.

9.1 Tests carried out in case of suspected early hemolytic transfusion reaction

Laboratory tests—mainly serological—are crucial for the diagnosis of an early haemolytic reaction. The type of laboratory tests performed for early transfusion haemolytic reactions is shown in **Table 7**.

The basic serological examination consists of direct antiglobulin testing (DAT); determination of blood group and RhD in donor and recipient; repetition of the serological compliance test. A test should be performed for the presence of antibodies in the recipient before and after the transfusion. Positive DAT indicates haemolysis of red blood cells of immunisation origin. A negative DAT result does not exclude haemolysis, it may mean that the transfused blood cells have been destroyed by alloantibodies or the method used is not very sensitive. Alvarez et al. [60] compared the sensitivity of DAT performed by technique using monospecific IgG antiglobulin, flow cytometry and antibody elution. The study showed that DAT could only indicate 10% of antibody coated cells [61]. Performing DAT in the red blood cell eluate, its sensitivity was 1%. Flow cytometry proved to be a similarly sensitive method.

The re-determination of the ABO and RhD blood group of the recipient before and after the transfusion and in the donors' blood will exclude errors in the identification of the recipient or blood sample (wrong blood in tube (WBIT)). Test results carried out by Biomedical Excellence for Safer Transfusion Working Party of The International Society for Blood Transfusion in 10 countries with 62 institutions,

Blood product	Confirm ABO, Rh Confirm other antigen types, if indicated
Blood bank laboratory	Direct antiglobulin test (DAT) Confirm ABO, RH, antibody screen and identification Post-transfusion haemolysis check
Clinical laboratory	Complete blood count, platelet count Urinalysis for haemoglobin Serum bilirubin, creatinine, urine quantitation, coagulation profile DIC evaluation

Table 7.
Type of laboratory tests and the location of their performance in the case of early transfusion reaction.

Laboratory indicators	Frequency (%)
Low haptoglobin 92	92
Positive DAT	89*
Increased bilirubin concentration medium/slow	80
The presence of haemoglobin in plasma and/or urine	88 vs. 52**

**Negative DAT mainly associated with HTR in ABO incompatibility.*
***IHTR vs. DHTR.*

Table 8.
Changes in laboratory indicators in haemolytic transfusion reactions [56].

which examined a total of 690,000 blood samples, showed that the frequency of WBIT is 1 in 165. In two countries, Sweden and Finland, which have implemented national identification systems, this frequency was 1 for 1986 samples [61].

All-antibody screening for recipients is generally performed using routine testing on standard blood cells. A panel of standard cells should contain clinically important antigens in a homozygous form to detect the presence of weak antibodies. The test should be performed on serum/plasma samples taken before and after transfusion. If positive results indicate alloantibodies are present, they should be identified. Detection of a specific antigen on the donor's blood cells is the confirmation that the detected alloantibodies were responsible for the haemolytic transfusion reaction. If negative results are obtained, additional tests should be performed, for example, PTA PEG, polybrene test and PTA NaCl test. If negative results persist, the test should be repeated after a week and after 2 weeks, as in some patients, the antibodies may have been consumed to destroy transfused incompatible red blood cells.

Laboratory tests that help to differentiate haemolysis include determination of free haemoglobin in the blood and urine, haptoglobin and lactate dehydrogenase (LDH) and bilirubin. While interpreting the obtained test results, it should be kept in mind that haemolysis or shortening the survival time of red blood cells can be caused by non-immunological factors, for example, adding hypotonic fluids to red blood cells, inefficient heating or freezing devices, etc. [62]. **Table 8** presents changes in laboratory indicators in transfusion haemolytic reactions [56].

9.2 Tests carried out in case of suspected delayed haemolytic transfusion reaction

Laboratory tests show anaemia, increased LDH and bilirubin, decreased haptoglobin and higher white blood cell counts in post-transfusion haemolytic reactions. Bilirubin concentration depends on the severity of haemolysis and liver function.

Serological tests show positive DAT and the presence of all red blood cell antibodies that were not detected prior to transfusion. This means that after transfusion of red blood cells, the production of alloantibodies directed to the antigen found on the transfused blood cells occurs.

Positive DAT with anti-IgG reagents or with anti-IgG and anti-C3 reagents is generally seen as two red blood cell populations. It has been observed that in some patients, the coating of blood cells includes not only transfused, but also autologous red blood cells. Positive DAT with anti-IgG and anti-C3d reagents may persist for several months [9].

Alloantibody testing should be performed in the intermediate antiglobulin test (IAT) and enzyme test. In both methods, in addition to the reference blood cells, the patient's autologous blood cells should be included. Depending on the specificity, alloantibodies responsible for the delayed transfusion reaction activate in characteristic tests, for example, antibodies from the Rh system react in an enzymatic test, often also in anti-globulin testing. In contrast, anti-K, anti-Fya antibodies react in an anti-globulin test. Positive reactions with allogeneic blood cells are accompanied by positive auto control of the patient's red blood cells. Ness et al. [9] showed that the formation of warm autoantibodies after the onset of DHTR is relatively common. Approximately one-third of patients who were examined 25 days after the onset of the reaction presented a positive DAT due to autoantibodies with broad specificity [9]. The incidence of autoantibodies after DHTR may be even higher because autoantibodies may mimic the specificity of alloantibodies.

Usually, plasma alloantibodies are detectable at 4–7 days after the transfusion and reach maximum activity between 10 and 15 days after the transfusion. When examining recipient red blood cells using a diagnostic reagent with a specificity corresponding to alloantibodies detected in the patient, mixed agglutination is observed, which indicates the presence of two blood cell populations in the patient's circulation. One of them, which does not react with diagnostic antibodies, is the recipient's autologous blood cells, the other population is antigenically incompatible transfused donor cells, not yet removed from the recipient's circulation.

10. Treatment of transfusion haemolytic reactions

Treatment of early haemolytic transfusion reactions depends mainly on the patient's condition, which must be closely monitored. It is most important to observe the clinical symptoms of the recipient and stop the blood transfusion at the right moment. Particular attention should be paid to the patient's circulation. In the event of a marked decrease in blood pressure, make-up fluids should be transfused and pressure amines should be administered. However, it is important to avoid overloading the circulation with fluids, especially in patients with heart or kidney failure. Catheterisation of the pulmonary artery helps to monitor the situation.

In some cases, an exchange transfusion should be considered, bearing in mind that the haemolysis intensity depends mainly on the volume of incompatible blood transfused. For exchange transfusion, red blood cells without an antigen should be used against which the patient has developed alloantibodies. The decision to carry it out must be balanced and the course carefully monitored. It should be emphasised that in patients with an early reaction due to ABO incompatibility, exchange transfusion may reduce the risk of serious complications or death. For patients with ongoing haemorrhage choosing a blood for transfusion may be difficult. However, it should be remembered that these difficulties must not cause risk of haemorrhage. Often the way out of this situation is transfusion of O RhD negative red blood cells.

Therapeutic intervention	Indication	Typical dose
Hydration	Prevent renal impairment Maintain urine output >100 ml/h	Normal saline and/or 5% dextrose 200 ml/m^2/h
Alkalinisation of urine	Prevent renal impairment Maintain urine pH > 7.5	NaH_2CO_3 40–70 mEq
Diuresis	Prevent renal impairment	Mannitol 20% 100 ml/m^2 Furosemide 40–80 mg
Vasodilation	Increase renal blood flow	Dopamine 1–5 μg/kg/min
Anticoagulant	Treat DIC	Heparin 5–10 u/kg/h
Red cells exchange transfusion	Decrease load of incompatible red cells	Exchange of one estimated red cells mass
Plasma or platelet transfusion	Treat haemorrhagic complications of DIC	Platelet—1 unit platelet/10 kg or 1 unit apheresis platelet FFP—10 ml/kg
Intravenous immunoglobulin (not standard therapy)	Prevent extravascular haemolysis	0.4 mg/kg

DIC—disseminated intravascular coagulation; FFP—fresh frozen plasma.

Table 9.
Therapeutic options in haemolytic transfusion reactions [1].

The prevention of renal failure is aided by an early prevention of hypotension. A fluid balance should be maintained, the use of dehydrating agents (mannitol and furosemide) is helpful, but their oliguria should be closely monitored. Low doses of dopamine (1–5 μg/kg/min) may be used to maintain renal circulation, but this may not be effective.

Treatment and prevention of DIC during haemolytic transfusion reaction is controversial. Heparin is recommended because it additionally acts as an inhibitor of the complement activity and limits haemolysis. However, there is a danger of bleeding. Another method of treating early haemolytic transfusion reaction is to use a high dose of 0.4/kg intravenous immunoglobulin per 24 h after blood transfusion.

Delayed haemolytic transfusion reactions are well tolerated by most patients. Additional fluid and diuretic therapy are usually not necessary. Depending on the severity of the anaemia, transfusion of blood components should be avoided until the antibodies responsible for the reaction have been identified and the appropriate selection of blood cells has been made. Attempts have been made to use high doses of intravenous immunoglobulins to prevent haemolytic reactions in patients who have been immunised for winter and for whom compatible red blood cells have not been selected [63]. The main procedure for subsequent transfusions is to select red cells that do not contain the antigen for which all antibodies have been detected. **Table 9** summarises the treatment options used in haemolytic transfusion reactions.

11. Prevention of haemolytic transfusion reactions

Data on the incidence of haemolytic transfusion reactions vary from country to country and change over time. There are several causes. One of them was the use of improved techniques for detecting clinically relevant alloantibodies, which reduce the number of haemolytic transfusion reactions observed in blood recipients.
In addition, the widespread introduction of automation and computerisation to

pre-transfusion studies, which significantly limits the possibility of errors in serology laboratories and blood banks.

The above improvements, however, did not significantly affect the elimination of mistakes made in hospitals leading to transfusion of inappropriate blood to the patient. These include, among others, errors in collecting blood samples from patients and blood transfusions to a wrong patient. These errors are the most common cause of ABO incompatible transfusions, threatening the patient's life.

The introduction of haemovigilance transfusiological surveillance systems has enabled the analysis of all fatal and severe transfusion reactions. It allows to identify malfunctioning procedures leading to transfusion reactions. It enforces the introduction of procedures eliminating further errors.

12. Summary

Preventing haemolytic transfusion reactions by focusing on advances in serology and transfusion medicine has significantly reduced their incidence. Progress in understanding reaction pathophysiology has helped clinically assess patients and treat them effectively. It is possible that technological progress enabling modification of red blood cells and the use of red blood cell substitutes will significantly change transfusion practice in the future and eliminate the occurrence of haemolytic transfusion reactions. But until then, HTRs will remain the most important adverse post-transfusion reaction.

Author details

Jolanta Korsak* and Anna Piotrowska
Military Institute of Medicine, Poland

*Address all correspondence to: jkorsak@wim.mil.pl

References

[1] Davenport RD. Hemolytic transfusion reactions. In: Simon L, Snyder EL, Solheim BG, Stowell RG, Strauss RG, Petrides M, editors. Rossi's Principles of Transfusion Medicine. 4th ed. Bethesda: AABB; 2009. pp. 811-825

[2] Flegel WA. Pathogenesis and mechanisms of antibody-mediated hemolysis. Transfusion. 2015;**55**:S47-S58. DOI: 10.1111/trf.13147

[3] Pineda AA, Brzica SM Jr, Taswell HF. Hemolytic transfusion reactions: Recent experience in a large blood bank. Mayo Clinic Proceedings. 1978;**53**:378

[4] Lichtiger B, Perry-Thorton E. Haemolytic transfusion reactions in oncology patients: Experience in a large cancer center. Journal of Clinical Oncology. 1984;**25**:438

[5] Robillard P, Itay KN, Chapdelaine A. Five-year trends in the incidence of serious adverse transfusion reactions in the Quebec Hemovigilance system (abstract). Transfusion. 2006;**46**(Suppl):86A

[6] Annual SHOT Report 2017. Manchester, UK; 2018

[7] Vamvalcas EC, Pineda AA, Reisner R, et al. The differentiation of delayed hemolytic and delayed hemolytic and delayed serologic transfusion reactions: Incidence and predictors of hemolysis. Transfusion. 1995;**35**:26-32

[8] Ambruso DR. Acute hemolytic transfusion reactions. In: Hillyer CD, Silberstein LE, Ness PM, Anderson KC, editors. Blood Banking and Transfusion Medicine—Basic Principles and Practice. Philadelphia: Churchill Livingstone; 2003. pp. 391-394

[9] Ness PM, Shirey RS, Thoman SK, Buck SA. The differentiation of delayed serologic and delayed hemolytic transfusion reactions: Incidence, long-term serologic findings and clinical significance. Transfusion. 1990;**30**:688-693

[10] Roback JD, Corubs MR, Grossman BJ, Hillyer CHD. Technical Manual. XVI ed. Bathesda: AABB; 2008. pp. 715-750

[11] Danfi L, Rondell P. Universality of anti-A and anti-B human isolysins. Vox Sanguinis. 1971;**21**:81-85

[12] Mollison PL, Engelfriet CP, Contreras PM. Blood Transfusion in Clinical Medicine. 9th ed. Oxford Blackwell Scientific Publication; 1993. p. 487

[13] Strobel E. Hemolytic transfusion reactions. Transfusion Medicine and Hemotherapy. 2008;**36**:346-353

[14] Davenport RD. Management of transfusion reactions. In: Mintz PD, editor. Transfusion Therapy Clinical Principles and Practice. III ed. Bethesda: AABB; 2011. pp. 757-784

[15] Brodsky RA. Complement in haemolytic anaemia. Blood. 2015;**126**:2459-2465

[16] Kumpel BM. Efficacy of RhD monoclonal antibodies in clinical trias as replacement therapy for prophylactic anti-D immunoglobulin: More questions than answers. Vox Sanguinis. 2007;**93**:99-111

[17] Telen MJ, Green AM. The Inab phenotype: Characterization of the membrane protein and complement regulatory defect. Blood. 1989;**74**:437-441

[18] Pandey P, Anani WQ, Grotschal JL, Donomme GA. Potential impact of complement regulator deficiencies

on haemolytic reactions due to minor ABO-mismatched transfusions. Blood Advances. 2017;**1**:1977-1982

[19] Frazer-Abel A, Sepiashvili L, Mbughuni MM, Willrich MA. Overview of laboratory testing and clinical presentations of complement deficiencies and dysregulation. Advances in Clinical Chemistry. 2016;**77**:1-75

[20] Udani M, Rao N, Telen MJ. Leukocyte phenotypic changes in an in vitro model of ABO hemolytic transfusion reaction. Transfusion. 1997;**37**:904-909

[21] Shirey RS, King KE, Ness PM. Hemolytic transfusion reactions: Acute and delayed. In: Hillyer CD, Silbestein LE, Ness PM, Anderson KC, Roback JD, editors. Blood Banking and Transfusion Medicine. Philadelphia: Elsevier; 2007. pp. 668-676

[22] Davenport RD, Strieter MM, Kunkel SL. Red cell ABO incompatibility and production of tumour necrosis factor-alpha. British Journal of Haematology. 1991;**78**:540-544

[23] Davenport RD, Strieter MM, Standiford TJ, Kunkel SL. Interleukin-8 production in red blood cell incompatibility. Blood. 1990;**76**:2439-2442

[24] Esmon CT. The impact of the inflammatory response on coagulation. Thrombosis Research. 2004;**114**:321-327

[25] Davenport RD, Burdick MD, Strieter RM, Kunkel SL. In vitro interleukin-1 receptor antagonist in IgG mediated red cell incompatibility. Transfusion. 1994;**34**:297-303

[26] Levi M, ten Cate H. Disseminated intravascular coagulation. The New England Journal of Medicine. 1999;**341**:586-592

[27] van der Poll T, de Jonge E, Levi M. Regulatory role of cytokines in disseminated intravascular coagulation. Seminars in Thrombosis and Hemostasis. 2001;**27**:639-651

[28] de Jonge E, Friederich PW, Levi M, van der Poll T. Activation of coagulation by administration of recombinant factor VIIa elicits interleukin-6 and interlukin-8 release in healthy human subjects. Clinical and Diagnostic Laboratory Immunology. 2003;**10**:495-497

[29] Taylor FB, Toh CH, Hoots WK, Wada H, Levi M. Towards definition, clinical and laboratory criteria and a scoring system for disseminated intravascular coagulation. Thrombosis and Haemostasis. 2001;**86**:1327-1330

[30] Toh CH, Hoots WK, On behalf of the SSC on Disseminated Intravascular Coagulation of the ISTH. The scoring system of scientific and standardization committee on disseminated intravascular coagulation of the international society on thrombosis and haemostasis: A 5-year overview. Journal of Thrombosis and Haemostasis. 2007;**5**:604-606

[31] Toh CH, Downey C. Performance and prognostic importance of a new clinical and laboratory scoring system for identifying non-overt disseminated intravascular coagulation. Blood Coagulation & Fibrinolysis. 2005;**16**:69-74

[32] Joseph K, Kaplan AP, Frederick WA. Formation of bradykinin: A major contributor to the innate inflammatory response. Advances in Immunology. 2005;**86**:159-208

[33] Chan WL, Tang NL, Yim CC, et al. New features of renal lesion induced by stroma free hemoglobin. Toxicologic Pathology. 2000;**28**:635-642

[34] Patel RP. Biochemical aspects of the reaction of haemoglobin and

NO: Implications for Hb-based blood substitutes. Free Radical Biology & Medicine. 2000;**28**:1518-1525

[35] Vaughn MW, Huang KT, Kuo L, Liao JC. Erythrocytes possess an intrinsic barrier to nitric oxide consumption. The Journal of Biological Chemistry. 2000;**275**:2342-2348

[36] Gould SA, Moss GS. Clinical development of human polymerized hemoglobin as a blood substitute. World Journal of Surgery. 1996;**20**:1200-1207

[37] Kindgen-Milles D, Klement W, Arndt JO. The nociceptive systems of skin, poravascular tissue and hand veins of humans and their sensitivity to bradykinin. Neuroscience Letters. 1994;**181**:39-42

[38] Linden JV. Errors in transfusion medicine. Scope of the problem. Archives of Pathology & Laboratory Medicine. 1999;**123**:563-565

[39] Janatpour KA, Kalmin ND, Jensen HM, Holland PV. Clinical outcomes of ABO-incopatible RBC transfusion. American Journal of Clinical Pathology. 2008;**129**:276-281

[40] Arnold PA, Garraty G. A retrospective analysis of the allue of monocyte monolayer assay result for predicting the clinical significance of blood group alloantibodies. Transfusion. 2004;**44**:1273-1281

[41] Zimring JC, Spitalnik SL. Alloimmunization to red cell antigens and management of alloimmunized patients. In: Mintz P, editor. Transfusion Therapy Clinical Principles and Practice. 3rd ed. Bethesda, MD: AABB Press; 2011. pp. 631-642

[42] Unni N, Peddingghous M, Tormey CA, Stack G. Record fragmentation due to transfusion at multiple health care facilities: A risk factor for delayed hemolytic transfusion reactions. Transfusion. 2014;**54**:98-103

[43] Schonewille H, Haak HL, van Zijl AM. RBC antibody persistence. Transfusion. 2000;**40**:1127-1131

[44] King KE, Shirey RS, Lankiewicz MW, et al. Delayed hemolytic transfusion reactions in sickle cell disease: Simultaneous destruction of recipients' cells. Transfusion. 1997;**37**:376-381

[45] Ahrens N, Pruss A, Kahne A, et al. Coexistence of autoantibodies and alloantibodies to red blood cells due to blood transfusion. Transfusion. 2007;**47**:813-816

[46] Talano JA, Hilley CA, Gottschall JL, Baylerian DM, Scott JP. Delayed hemolytic transfusion reaction/hyperhemolysis syndrome in children with sickle cell disease. Pediatrics. 2003;**40**:e661-e665

[47] Larson LG, Welsh VJ, Ladd DJ. Acute intravascular hemolysis secondary to out-of-group platelet transfusion. Transfusion. 2000;**40**:902-906

[48] Josephson CD, Castillejo MI, Grima K, et al. ABO-mismatched platelet transfusions: Strategies to mitigate patient exposure to naturally occurring hemolytic antibodies. Transfusion and Apheresis Science. 2010;**42**:83-88

[49] Ikebe E, Matsuoka S, Tanaka A, et al. Reduction in adverse transfusion reactions with increased use of washed platelet concentrates in Japan—A retrospective multicenter study. Transfusion and Apheresis Science. 2019;**58**:162-168

[50] Josephson CD, Mullis NC, Van Demark C, Hillyer CD. Significant numbers of apheresis-derived group O

platelet units have "high-titer" anti A/AB: Implications for transfusion policy. Transfusion. 2004;**44**:805-808

[51] Cooloing LW, Butch S, Downs T, Davenport R. Isoagglutinin titers in pooled group O platelets are comparable to apheresis platelets (abstract). Transfusion. 2007;**47**(Suppl):78A

[52] Sadani DT, Urbanaiak SJ, Bruce M, Tighe JE. Repeat ABO-incompatible platelet transfusions leading to hamolytic transfusion reaction. Transfusion Medicine. 2006;**16**:375-379

[53] Cooling L. ABO and platelet transfusion therapy. Immunohematology. 2007;**23**:2033

[54] Cherin P, Marrie J, Michallet M, Pelus E, et al. Management of adverse events in the treatment of patients with immunoglobulin therapy: A review of evidence. Autoimmunity. 2016;**15**:71-81

[55] Spath PJ, Granata G, La Marra F, Knijpers TW, Quinti I. On the dark side of therapies with immunoglobulin concentrates: The adverse events. Frontiers in Immunology. 2015;**6**:11

[56] Petz LD, Garatty G. Immune Hemolytic Anemia. 2nd ed. Philadelphia: Churchill Livingstone; 2004

[57] Mota M, Bley C, Aravectia MG, et al. Autoantibody formation after alloimmunization inducing bystander immune hemolysis. Immunohematology. 2009;**25**:9-12

[58] Petz LD. The axpanding boundaries of transfusion medicine. In: Nance LTS, editor. Clinical Basic Science Aspects of Immunohematology. AABB: Arlington; 1991. pp. 73-113

[59] Garraty G. Severe reactions associated with transfusion of patients with sickle disease (editorial). Transfusion. 1997;**37**:357-361

[60] Alvarez A, Rivers S, Montoto S, et al. Relative sensitivity of direct antiglobulin test, antibody elution and flow cytometry in the serologic diagnosis of immune hemolytic transfusion reactions. Haematologica. 2000;**85**:181-188

[61] Dzik W, Murphy A, Andreu G, et al. An international study of performance of sample collection from patients. Vox Sanguinis. 2003;**85**:40-47

[62] Davenport RD. Haemolytic transfusion reactions. In: Popovsky MA, editor. Transfusion Reactions. 3rd ed. Bethesda, MD: AABB Press; 2007. pp. 1-55

[63] Win N, Yeghen T, Needs M, et al. Use of intravenous immunoglobulin and intravenous methylprednisolone in hyperhaemolysis syndrome in sickle cell disease. Haematology. 2004;**9**:433-441

Chapter 6

Distribution of Clinically Relevant Blood Group Antigens among Nigerians and the Management of Rhesus D Negative Pregnancies: Implications for Haemolytic Disease of the Foetus and Newborn and Haemolytic Transfusion Reactions

Osaro Erhabor, Tosan Erhabor, Teddy Charles Adias and Iwueke Ikechukwu Polycarp

Abstract

The ABO and Rhesus blood group systems are the most clinically relevant blood group systems from haemolytic disease of the foetus and newborn (HDFN) and haemolytic transfusion reaction (HTR) perspectives. Other clinically relevant blood group systems include the Kell, Duffy, Kidd and MNSs blood group systems. The clinical relevance of a blood group system depends on the ability of antibodies of the system to cause HDFN and HTR. This chapter discusses the distribution of ABO, Rhesus and other clinically relevant red cell antigens among Nigerians and implications for HDFN and HTR. There are several challenges associated with the management of Rhesus negative pregnancies, pregnancies associated with clinically significant alloantibodies, implementation of policy on routine antenatal anti-D prophylaxis (RAADP), management of Rhesus negative women that require termination of pregnancy (TOP), provision of antigen negative blood for certain patient groups and the management of pregnant and non-pregnant patients with clinically significant alloantibodies. This chapter highlights the need for Nigeria and other African countries to implement best practices to optimize the care offered to pregnant women as well as patients in whom red cell transfusion is indicated.

Keywords: clinically relevant blood group antigens, Nigerians, rhesus D negative pregnancies, haemolytic disease of the foetus and newborn, haemolytic transfusion reaction

1. Introduction

1.1 History of Nigeria

Nigeria often referred to the giant of Africa is the largest Black nation in Africa. It is a country located in West Africa bordered by Cameroon in the East, Benin Republic in the West, Niger Republic to the North and Chad Republic to the North East. It is a federation consisting of 36 states with Abuja the Federal Capital territory as the capital. It is located on the Gulf of Guinea with a total area of 923,768 km^2 (356,669 sq. miles). It is the world's 32nd-largest country. Nigeria got her independence from the British on 1st of October 1960. It has an estimated population of over 200 million people. The United Nations estimated the population in 2016 to be 185,989,640 distributed as 51.7% rural and 48.3% urban with a population density of 167.5 persons per square kilometre. Although the official language is English, there are more than 250 ethnic groups with well over 500 different native languages and diverse cultures. There are 3 major ethnic groups in Nigeria (Hausa/Fulani, Igbo and Yoruba). Nigeria is a religiously diverse nation divided into a predominantly Christian South and Muslim North and a minority groups of traditional African religion. Nigeria is a mixed economy dependent and an emerging market. As at 2014 Nigeria was the fastest growing and largest economy in Africa. She is blessed with abundant natural resources and a developing communication, financial, legal and transportation sector. Nigeria is the 12th largest producer of oil in the world, the 8th largest exporter, has the 10th largest proven reserves and supplies a fifth of its oil to the United States of America. Oil plays a significant role in the Nigerian economy and accounts for 40% of GDP and 80% of all government earnings. Healthcare delivery is the responsibility of the 3 tiers of government (federal, state and local government). There is a number of health-related challenges in Nigeria (HIV/AIDS, malaria, polio, poor access to potable and clean water, lack of proper sanitation system, high infant and maternal mortality rates). Although the recurrent expenditure on health in Nigeria has increased over the years, healthcare delivery and infrastructural endowment remains suboptimal with health tourism on the increase [1]. The Nigerian health care system is continuously faced with a number of challenges; shortage of healthcare workers [2] predominantly due to significant emigration of skilled medical personnel to developed economies of the world (brain drain), suboptimal funding, decaying infrastructure, inter-professional conflict, perennial strike actions by healthcare professionals, lack of political will as well as bureaucratic bottlenecks in public health care delivery in Nigeria [3].

2. UHC and the WHO model lists as governmental obligations to implement before 2030

Nigeria is a party to the United Nation (UN) General Assembly adopted 2030 agenda for Sustainable Development and the UN High-Level Meeting (UN HLM) Universal Health Coverage (UHC) UHC2030. In September 2015, the UN General Assembly adopted the 2030 Agenda for Sustainable Development that included 17 Sustainable Development Goals (SDGs) ensuring that all persons are carried along and that no one is left behind [4]. The agenda laid emphasis a holistic approach aimed at achieving sustainable development for all. The 17 sustainable development goals (SDGs) included; no poverty, zero hunger, good health and well-being, quality education, gender equality, clean water and sanitation, affordable and clean energy, decent work and economic growth, industrial innovation and infrastructure, reduced inequality, sustainable cities and communities, responsible consumption and production, climate action, life below water, life on land, peace and justice strong institutions and partnerships to achieve goal. On September 23rd 2019, a high-level meeting on universal health coverage held at the United Nations General Assembly. The meeting focussed on Universal Health Coverage: Moving Together to Build a Healthier World (UHC2030) and brought together heads of state, political and health leaders, policy-makers, and universal health coverage champions to advocate for health for all. The meeting agreed on Key Asks from the UHC Movement aimed at accelerating progress toward Universal Health Coverage (UHC) [4]. Among others, UHC2030 advocates that countries should; ensure political leadership beyond health (that all countries to ensure healthy lives and wellbeing for all at all stages as a social contract), leave no one behind (pursue equity in access to quality health services with financial protection), regulate and legislate (create a strong, enabling regulatory and legal environment responsive to people's needs), uphold the quality of care (build high-quality health systems that people and communities trust), invest more and better (increased domestic investment and allocation of more public financing for health through equitable and mandatory resource) and move together (establishing multi-stakeholder mechanisms for engaging the whole of society for a healthier world). Nigeria is a party to the global commitment ensuring the well-being, universal health coverage and access to quality healthcare when and where they need it, without facing financial hardship [5]. There is general expectation among Nigerians for the government to mix word with action by ensuring that all Nigerians in both rural and urban communities have access and can use the promotive, preventive, curative, rehabilitative and palliative health services they require, that is of sufficient quality and affordable [6].

3. Current situation in Nigeria

3.1 Distribution of ABO and other clinically significant blood groups

The human red blood cell membrane is complex and contains a number of clinically relevant blood group antigens, the most relevant being the ABO and the Rhesus blood group antigens. Apart from the ABO and Rhesus blood group systems, thirty-four other blood group systems have been identified as at November 2014 [7]. In addition to the ABO and Rhesus blood group antigens, 364 other red cell antigens have been identified serologically. The clinical relevance of a blood group system depends on the distribution of antigens of the blood group system in the population, ability of antibodies of the blood group system to cause haemolytic transfusion reaction (HTR) and haemolytic disease of the foetus and newborn (HDFN) [8]. The ABO blood group system is one of the most clinically relevant blood group systems [9]. It was first discovered by Karl Landsteiner in 1901 [10]. The ABO blood group system has three main antigens (A, B and H). Four major ABO groups exist (A, B, AB and O). The ABO blood group system is based on the A and B antigens occurring singly as A or B, doubling as AB or the absence of both as O. Individuals who have lack the A or B antigens on their red cells have the group specific antibody in their serum or plasma. Antibodies of the system are predominantly IgM originally thought to be naturally occurring but are now known to occur in the first years of life as a result of sensitization to ABO-like antigen and environmental substances that occur in nature such as bacteria, viruses and food. Evidence has shown that these antibodies are not present at birth and that animals kept in a sterile room from birth do not produce these antibodies. The ABO blood group system is important in transfusion medicine, HDFN and in organ transplant. Transfusion of ABO incompatible unit can cause severe HTR. Similarly, an immune response can also occur following ABO incompatible organ transplant. ABO blood group incompatibilities between the mother and child does not normally cause HDFN because antibodies of the ABO blood group system are usually of the large molecular weight IgM type, which do not cross the placenta. However, mothers who were previously sensitised (previous incompatible transfusion and pregnancy) can potentially have IgG ABO antibodies that can potentially cause ABO HDFN. The distribution of ABO blood groups varies across the world according to the population. There are also variations in blood type distribution within human subpopulations.

Nigeria is a significantly varied nation in terms of ethnicity. The gene frequency of ABO and Rh blood group varies significantly within the six geopolitical zones in Nigeria [11–18]. Previous studies in most parts of Nigeria indicates that the ABO blood group distribution is in the order O > A > B > AB [19]. Studies from the United States, Mauritania, Morocco, Cameroun, Tunisia, Ethiopia and Iran reported same order (O > A > B > AB) [20–26]. However, study in Madagascar and Guinea reported a contrary trend (O > B > A > AB) [27, 28]. This observation in Nigeria is also at variance with reports from India and Bangladesh where prevalence of B is highest followed by O and the least was AB (B > O > A > AB) [29, 30]. Reports from Turkey and Colombia indicates an order A > O > B > AB [31, 32].

A multi race/ethnic study in the United States reported that blood type O is the most prevalent (46.6%) with White non-Hispanic, Hispanic, Black non-Hispanic, Asian and North American Indian having varying percentage of 45.5, 56.5, 50.2, 39.8 and 54.6 respectively [21]. Other studies in Turkey, Mauritania, Iran, Ethiopia, Colombia, Cameroun, Bangladesh, Madagascar, Morocco, Guinea and Northern India have reported varying percentage in ABO and Rh blood types [20–23, 25–32].

Phenotypic distribution of Rh(D) in Nigeria varies from one part of the country to the other; Kwara (4.5%) [17], Jos Plateau State (4.32) [14], FCT (4.3) [33], Minna (3.3%0) [11], Lagos (3.0, 6, 6.86%) [16, 34, 35], Ogun (6.65 and 2.9%) [36, 37], Osun (6.3%) [38], Oyo (3.3, 6.68, 4.8, 5.89%) [12, 14, 18, 39], Ekiti (4.3%) [40], Akwa Ibom (5.7%) [41], Bayelsa (2%) [42], Delta (1.8%) [43], Benin (6.0%) [13], Rivers (3.2, 7, 8.3%) [44–46], Kano (5.2%) [47], Sokoto (1.55%) [14], Zamfara (1.2%) [48], Enugu (4.49%) [14], Abia (5.3%) [49], Ebonyi (4.2%) [50], Borno (1.92%) [14], Adamawa (4.6%) [51], Yobe (4.6%) [52]. The prevalence of Rhesus negativity varies from one zone to the other; 4.4, 3.1, 6.0, 4.3, 3.9 and 3.1% respectively for the South East, North East, South, South, South West, North Central and North West zone respectively.

The overall average prevalence of Rhesus negativity is 5.1%. The distribution of Rh(D) in Nigeria is in agreement with others parts of the world [20, 23, 25–28, 30, 31]. Blacks have been found to have a lower frequency of Rhesus D negative phenotype (3–5%) [34, 42, 44] compared to the general Caucasian population (15%) [21, 53]. The lower prevalence of Rh(D)− in Nigeria and other developing is important and a blessing in disguise because clinical situations like fetomaternal haemorrhage during the course of pregnancy can give arise through Rh incompatibility and HDFN. In Nigeria and many of these developing countries RAADP and other anti-D HDFN related prevention strategies are not being implemented. **Table 1** shows the prevalence of Rhesus D group among Nigerians based on zones.

The Kell blood group is the third most clinically relevant blood group system after ABO and Rhesus. Individuals without Kell antigens (K_0) who are transfused with Kell positive donor red cells or Kell negative pregnant women exposed to the Kell positive red cells of their baby carry the risk of developing Kell antibody which can cause HDFN [54]. In the developed world all pregnant women and non-pregnant women of child bearing age are transfused with Kell negative blood. Also, patients with other antibodies are transfused with Kell negative and red cells also lacking the antigen to which their alloantibody is specific. This is to prevent them from potentially developing anti-Kell antibody. Kell sensitization is the third

Zone of Nigeria	Percentage of Rhesus negative status	Percentage of Rhesus negative status
South-East	4.4	95.6
South-South	6.0	94
South-West	4.3	95.7
North-East	3.1	96.9
North-West	3.1	96.9
North-Central	3.9	96.1

Table 1.
Prevalence of Rhesus D group among Nigerians based on zones.

most common cause of HDFN after Rh and ABO. Anti-Kell has been shown to cause severe foetal anaemia by suppressing foetal RBC synthesis [55]. HDFN-associated anaemia in Anti-Kell-related HDFN is caused by the ability of anti-K to cause the suppression of foetal production of RBCs [56]. Unlike Rh and ABO, Kell antigens are expressed on the surface of RBC precursors, and anti-K promotes the immune destruction of Kell positive erythroid early progenitor cells by macrophages in the foetal liver rather than only mature foetal RBCs [55]. There are few Kell prevalence studies in Nigeria. Among their cohort of pregnant women in Sokoto, North Western Nigeria, Erhabor and Colleagues [57] obtained a Kell antigen prevalence of 2%. Similarly, Ugboma and Nwauche [58] in Port Harcourt investigated the prevalence of Kell antigen among their patients and reported a Kell antigen prevalence of 2%. The prevalence of Kell antigen among a multi-ethnic cohort of 302 healthy Nigerian individuals indicated a zero prevalence of K antigen [59]. Racial differences seem to exist in Kell blood group antigen distributions [60, 61]. The Nigerian government and governments in other African countries will need to implement this strategy in a bid to reducing Kell-related sensitization and the effect of HDFN.

The prevalence of other clinically significant red cell antigens has been determined among Nigerians. The prevalence of Lewis, Kidd, Duffy, Kell and M blood group antigens among blood donors in Aminu Kano Teaching Hospital, Kano, Nigeria [62] were as follows: Lea: 26.4%, Leb: 15.1%, M: 20.8%, k (cellano): 21.7%. The Duffy (anti Fya, anti Fyb) and Kidd (anti Jka anti Jkb) antigens were not detected among the donors. Out of the 162 pregnant women tested for their Duffy antigens status indicated Fya, Fyb and Fya (a+b+) prevalence of 7 (4.3%), 9 (5.6%) and 1 (0.61%) respectively [63]. Kidd blood group phenotypes were determined among pregnant women in Sokoto, North Western Nigeria [63]. The distribution of Kidd antigens among subjects studied indicated a prevalence of Jka, Jkb and Jk(a+b+) of 8 (4.9%), 13 (8.0%) and 0 (0.0%), respectively. There is need for the phenotyping of donor's blood for clinically significant red cell antigens. There is also the need to routinely screen all pregnant women for alloantibodies to facilitate the selection of antigen negative units for those with clinically significant alloantibodies who require a red cell transfusion. This can potentially optimise the obstetric management of HDFN.

The prevalence of Rh c and e phenotype among 200 pregnant women attending antenatal clinic (ANC) in Usmanu Danfodiyo University Teaching Hospital Sokoto was determined. The prevalence of Rh c was 92% while Rh e was 98.5% [64]. The frequencies of Rh blood group antigens and phenotypes of the Ibibio, Efik, and Ibo ethnic nationalities in Calabar municipality, Nigeria, were determined using standard serologic techniques. Of the 720 Calabar individuals tested, the frequencies of the Rh antigens within the nationalities were c (100%), e (96.38%),

D (96.38%), E (15.22%), and C (3.62%) for the Ibibios; c (100%), e (95.60%), D (96.70%), E (21.98%), and C (0%) for the Efiks; and c (100%), e (94.29%), D (91.43%), E (28.57%), and C (2.86%) for the Ibos. The overall frequencies of the Rh antigens in these 720 individuals were c (100%), e (95.56%), D (94.44%), E (18.89%), and C (2.78%). Forty (5.56%) were found to be D−, while all were found to possess the c antigen. The most frequently occurring Rh phenotype was Dccee, with a frequency of 73.61%. The alternative allele, C, did not appear in homozygous form (CC) in the population tested [65]. Of the 374 pregnant women studied in Port Harcourt, Nigeria, the frequencies of the Rh antigens within the population were D (89.0%), c (82.0%), e (54.0%), C (24.3%), E (20.1%). The frequencies of the Rh antithetical antigens were DD/Dd (91.2%), Cc (19.5%), cc (84.5%), Ee (13.9%), ee (54.3%), CC (25.1%), EE (19.8%) and dd (10.4%). Seven (1.9%) were found to be Rhnull, sixteen (4.3%) were found to be D− or exalted D. Phenotypes without RhD reactivity were -c- (2.9%), -Cc (0.3%), -C- (0.3%), -Ee (0.5%) and -E- (0.3%) [66]. A multi-ethnic cohort of healthy Nigerian individuals were studied. The antigen status of these individuals for Rh was determined. The prevalence of the Rh antigens in the study cohort was found to be: D (92.7%), C (20.5%), c (97.7%), E (19.5%), and e (97.4%). Dce was the most common Rh phenotype (53.3%) [59]. Few countries in sub-Saharan Africa have systematic testing for antigens C, c, E, and e of the Rh and Kell system antigens in the donor and recipient, thereby exposing transfused patients to the risk of developing antibodies that can cause HTR and HDFN. Among 651 blood donors tested in Abidjan for antigens of the Rh blood group system, the antigen frequencies of D, c, e, C, and E were; 92.93, 99.85, 99.85, 21.97, and 13.82% respectively. K antigen is was found in 0.77% of donors [67].

3.2 Universal donor phenomenon: the need to implement a policy of universal haemolysin testing of group O donor units

ABO blood group system is one of the most clinically relevant blood group systems. Individuals above the age of 6 months have clinically significant anti-A and/or anti-B in their serum particularly if they lack the corresponding antigens on their red cells. Whole blood transfusion still thrives in Nigeria despite the advantages of component therapy and challenges associated with whole blood transfusion (development of febrile transfusion reactions, graft-versus-host disease, alloimmunization to leukocyte antigens, immunomodulatory effects, transmission of diseases such as cytomegalovirus, Human T-Lymphotrophic Virus I/II and Epstein Barr (EBV) for which leukocytes may be the vector) [68]. Blood group O donor blood is the most common blood group among Nigerian blood donors [69] and their red cells are commonly used as universal donor units for transfusion to A, B and AB recipient particularly in emergency situations. Blood group O individuals lack the A and B antigens on their red cells and thus are inappropriately called Universal donors. These individuals have anti A and Anti B in the plasma. Due to the absence of A and B on their red cell, their red cells could be given to A, B, and AB individuals. This is quite useful particularly in Nigeria and other developing countries where there is inadequate supply of donor blood. However, some group O individuals have potentially lytic anti-A and lytic anti-B in their plasma that bind to antigens A and B on the surface of erythrocytes in recipients and potentially activate the complement cascade resulting in acute intravascular haemolysis. To avoid this, all blood group O donor units intended for transfusion to non-O patient must be tested for the presence of these anti-A and lytic anti-B haemolysis. Those donors found negative can have their blood given to non-O patients while those that test positive are reserved for group O recipients only. Haemolysin testing to identify the presence of haemolytic anti-A and anti-B antibodies has emerged as a useful screening in most countries to identify high levels of anti-A and/or anti-B antibodies to prevent HTRs. Routine haemolysis testing of blood group O donor units intended for transfusion to A, B or AB recipient is not routinely carried out in most settings in Nigeria despite the high prevalence of haemolysins observed among Nigerians in previous studies [70–75]. The Nigeria government can learn from evidenced-based best practices in most developed settings [76, 77] and implement a policy to routinely test all group O donor units for haemolysins in other to identify group O donors with high titre of IgG anti A and/or anti B whose blood should be reserved only for transfusion to group O recipient while those that test negative can be transfused to A, B or AB individual as a way to maximising the use of our limited allogeneic stock.

3.3 Screening for clinically significant alloantibodies

Alloantibodies are antibodies produced in a patient as a result of exposure to foreign red cell antigen via transfusion, pregnancy or transplantation. In countries such as Nigeria, there are multiple ethnic groups and racial or genetic heterogeneity among the population. This can often be associated with a wide variation of alloantibodies [78]. Other common factors that facilitate alloantibody formation in the recipient include: the immune competence, the dose of the antigen the recipient is exposed to, the route of exposure and how immunogenic the foreign antigen is [79, 80]. Development of alloantibodies can lead to difficulty in finding compatible blood for transfusion or it can result in severe delayed haemolytic transfusion reaction if the antibody titre is low, undetected, missed and if antigen positive units is transfused [81]. Evidenced-based best practice in the developing world requires that alloantibody testing is carried out as part of pre-transfusion testing of patients who require a red cell transfusion as well as pregnant women presenting to antenatal clinic at booking [82, 83]. The aim of this test is to detect the presence of unexpected red cell antibody in the patient's serum [84, 85]. Once these antibodies are detected during the alloantibody screening, every effort must be made to identify the specificity of the alloantibody by doing a panel test. The aim of identifying the specificity of the alloantibody in a patient that requires a red cell transfusion is to enable the Medical Laboratory or Biomedical Scientist to select antigen negative donor unit for appropriate crossmatch (indirect antiglobulin test) for such patient [86]. The aim of a panel test in the case of a pregnant women coming for antenatal booking is to identify the alloantibody, determine whether the antibody can potentially cause HDFN [87] and to allow the monitoring of the titre or quantification of the antibody every 4 weeks from booking until 28 weeks' gestation and every 2 weeks thereafter until delivery [88]. The obstetrician requires this information to determine to what extent the developing foetus is affected by HDFN, decide whether to monitor the baby for anaemia using Doppler ultrasound, determine whether the baby will require intrauterine transfusion and to make an informed decision to possibly deliver the baby earlier. These evidence-based best practices are not being implemented in many settings in Nigeria. Testing of donor units for other clinically relevant red cell antigens other than ABO and Rhesus D is not routinely carried out. Also, donor units particularly those intended for transfusion to pregnant women and neonates are also not routinely screened for CMV and Hepatitis E virus like it is routinely done in more advanced part of the world. This is a complete failure in stewardship by the Nigerian government and can compromise the transfusion service delivery to pregnant women and patients that require red cell transfusion.

4. Challenges for the future

4.1 Absence of universal access to prophylactic anti-D through the routine antenatal anti-D prophylaxis (RAADP) program

RAADP or routine antenatal anti-D prophylaxis is a recommended treatment option for all Rhesus D negative pregnant women who are not known to be sensitised previously to the RhD antigen. The D antigen is the most immunogenic and most clinically relevant of the Rhesus antigens. A mother who is RhD negative and married to a homozygous or heterozygous D positive husband has a 100 and 50% chance respectively of carrying a D positive baby. During such pregnancies as a result of feto maternal haemorrhage (FMH) following potentially sensitising events [abdominal trauma, abortion or termination of pregnancy, antepartum haemorrhage (APH), amniocentesis, chorionic villus sampling, external cephalic version (ECV) and miscarriages] during pregnancy, small amounts of foetal blood can enter into the maternal circulation. The foetal RhD-positive cells can irreversibly sensitise the mother to produce alloantibody D. The risk of sensitisation occurring is dependent on a number of factors; ABO blood group of the developing foetus (there is a higher risk if there is ABO compatibility between mum and baby), dose of foetal cells entering the maternal circulation, immune competence of the mother and type of pregnancy (risk is significantly higher in the first decreasing in the subsequent pregnancies. The antibody produced is immune IgG antibody that is a low molecular weight antibody and can potentially cross the placenta barrier. The maternal immune anti-D are small molecular weight IgG immunoglobulin and can pass through the placenta in subsequent D positive pregnancy and destroy the foetal red cells with increased production of bilirubin a product of red cell breakdown (HDFN). While in womb the mother manages the bilirubin on behalf of the baby by production of glucoronyl transferase enzyme which break down (conjugate) the bilirubin to water soluble forms that can be excreted in the urine. However, after delivery, the excess bilirubin released from the breakdown of the foetal red cells leads to jaundice. With the baby's liver poorly developed and not producing enough glucoronyl transferase enzyme to conjugate the bilirubin to excretable form, the level can potentially rise above the blood brain barrier and cause kernicterus (permanent brain damage) with attendant neurodevelopmental problems (cerebral palsy, deafness neuromotor and speech delay). Routine antenatal anti-D prophylaxis (RAADP) is a program under which Rhesus D negative non-sensitised pregnant women are universally offered anti-D prophylaxis at 28–34 weeks' gestation with the aim of preventing the sensitization of Rh D-negative women and by extension prevent anti-D HDFN in subsequent pregnancy [89]. The aim of the RAADP programme is the reduction in the incidence of anti-D related HDFN; improve the survival of the children delivered by Rhesus D negative women, reduce the incidence of disability and health-related quality of life of children and mortality in children delivered by Rhesus D negative women who would have developed anti-D related-HDFN if mothers were not offered prophylaxis. The RAADP program is based on offering either two doses of at least 500 IU at 28- and 34-weeks' gestation or a single dose of at least 1500 IU at 28 weeks gestation followed by a further dose of at least 1500 IU within 72 h of delivery of a Rh D positive baby. The dose offered post-delivery is dependent on the result of feto maternal haemorrhage testing result (flow cytometry of Kleihauer testing). Both methods quantify in millilitres the amount of foetal red cells that has entered maternal circulation to facilitate the administration of adequate dose of prophylactic anti-D. As a general rule 1 25 IU of anti-D is administered to clear 1 ml of foetal red cells from maternal circulation. The introduction of anti-D prophylaxis using Rhesus D immunoglobulin (given intramuscular or intravenous administration) has led to a significant fall in the number of women becoming sensitised and by extension reduced the incidence and severity of this condition. The anti D immunoglobulin used as prophylaxis is prepared from plasma of male Rhesus D negative donors who have high levels of plasma anti-D due to deliberate or intentional immunisation with D positive red cells. Anti D is also administered to Rhesus D negative women following a potentially sensitising events during pregnancy. The anti-D facilitates the clearance of foetal red cells from the maternal circulation to prevents active immunisation, thus preventing the production of alloantibody D. Prior to the availability and widespread use of anti-D prophylaxis for Rhesus negative pregnant women, the incidence of Rh D sensitization among Rhesus D negative women following two deliveries of D positive and ABO-compatible, infants was approximately 16% and haemolytic disease of the foetus and newborn (HDFN) due to immune anti-D was a significant cause of morbidity and mortality [90]. Following the implementation of anti-D prophylaxis, the rate of sensitization has declined significantly to approximately 2%. With the implementation of RAADP by providing anti-D prophylaxis in the 3rd trimester between 28 and 34 weeks gestation, there has been a further remarkable reduction in the sensitisation rate to 0.17–0.28% [91]. Mortality from D-related HDFN related has also declined significantly from 46/100,000 births to 1.6/100,000 births [89]. Evidence from best practice implementation in England and Wales indicates that RAADP has reduced the incidence of sensitisation and hence of HDFN [92]. Conservative estimate indicates that it cost £2–£3.5 million for England and Wales to provide RAADP to all her Rh D-negative pregnant women. The Nigerian government can learn from this evidence-based best practice by implementing RAADP program for her population of Rhesus D negative pregnant population with the hope of reducing sensitization, incidence and severity of anti-D related HDFN and mortality in Nigeria.

4.2 Absence of facility for foetal genotype testing for D, K and other clinically relevant red cell antigens

Rhesus D grouping is relevant for blood donors, transfusion recipients and for women of child bearing age including pregnant women. This is because the Rh blood group antigens particularly D is significantly immunogenic. Rh D negative individuals often lack the D antigens on their red cells and can potentially be sensitised when exposed to D antigen positive red cells during pregnancy and blood transfusion. Such antibodies are often capable of causing a haemolytic transfusion reaction (HTR) and haemolytic disease of the foetus and newborn (HDFN). Since the introduction of prophylactic anti-D and implementation of evidence based best practice of careful management and monitoring of D negative pregnant women for all the potentially sensitising events that occur during pregnancy, the prevalence of HDFN because of Rh D incompatibility between the mother and baby has declined significantly [90]. In order to prevent Rhesus D negative women who are not previously sensitised from developing alloantibody D, these women are offered prophylactic anti-D during pregnancy under the Routine Antenatal Anti-D Prophylaxis program between 28 and 34 weeks' gestation. The half-life of the administered anti-D is 12 weeks. The anti-D prevents the mother from being sensitised by micro foetal maternal haemorrhage that can occur as a result of potentially sensitising events that occur during pregnancy. These women should have a fetomaternal haemorrhage testing following any potentially sensitising events that occur after from 20 weeks' gestation. This test quantifies the amount of foetal red cells that entered the maternal circulation to allow for the administration of adequate dose of anti-D to clear the fotal cells and prevent them from sensitising the mother. Anti-D (125 IU) is required to remove 1 ml of foetal red cells from maternal circulation. RhD alloimmunisation is still a significant cause of foetal and neonatal morbidity and mortality particularly in Nigeria and other developing countries [93–95] because of absence of evidence-based best practices and non-implementation of Rh D prophylaxis during pregnancy. This often result in a significant number of unfortunate women developing alloantibody D through no fault of theirs but rather as a result of failure in stewardship by the Nigerian government. Also, non-invasive foetal blood group genotyping (DNA) testing of maternal plasma to determine the antigen status of the developing foetus carried by an alloimmunised pregnant women is vital as it provides useful information as to whether a foetus is carrying the group specific antigen and in fact at risk of HDFN. This will help prevent the need for extensive laboratory testing (titration and quantification of antibody every 4 weeks from booking till 28 weeks' gestation and every 2 weeks from 28 weeks to delivery) and clinical monitoring in antigen negative cases. Molecular testing of maternal plasma for foetal DNA can be performed during the second trimester. DNA probes for the most common antigens associated with HDFN are now available [96]. Knowledge of the molecular basis of the blood group systems has facilitated the development of assays for blood group genotyping. Foetal Rhesus D genotyping can potentially tell at 16 weeks' gestation through the analysis of amniotic fluid or through maternal plasma the foetal D genotype of the developing foetus. In previously sensitised alloimmunised pregnant women, knowledge of the foetal D antigen status is beneficial to enable obstetricians optimally manage these women [95]. In non-sensitised Rhesus negative pregnant women, the knowledge of the foetal D antigen status is quite important for several reasons; prevent us from exposing the mother to a prophylactic anti-D (a human blood product that even though significantly virally tested for TTIs) she does not need, allow for the optimal utilisation of the product in patients in whom it is indicated and spare the woman the pain of the product being administered intramuscularly. *RHD* genotyping of foetuses carried by Rh D-negative women using foetal DNA obtained invasively through amniocentesis or chorionic villus sampling used to be critical to the clinical management of these women. Technological advances now allows for accurate determination of foetal *Rh D* genotype using cell-free foetal DNA from maternal blood, thus overcoming the invasive procedures [97]. *Rh D* genotyping are based on polymerase chain reaction using non-invasive blood sample from the mum are quite sensitive with low incidence of false positive result [98, 99]. Although there are cases of D-negative genomes possessing fragments of mutated Rh D genes, the most notable of which is the Rh D pseudogene found in Africans. Rh D genotyping tests have been developed to differentiate these alleles and thus enhance the diagnosis in a multi-ethnic population [100].

Foetal blood group genotype of a developing foetus can also be determined for Rh C, c, E and Kell (K) using cffDNA from maternal plasma [101]. Many European Union countries have suggested the mass application of foetal genotyping for all foetuses carried by D-negative women. This advocacy is based on clear benefit of conserving anti-D stocks and prevention of unnecessary administration of this human-derived blood product that has associated risk [102, 103]. In Denmark and the Netherlands this evidenced-based best practice of foetal *Rh D* testing for all non-sensitised D negative pregnant women have been introduced [104]. Also, non-invasive foetal blood group genotyping (DNA) testing of maternal plasma to determine the antigen status of the developing foetus carried by an already alloimmunised pregnant women is vital as it provides useful information as to whether a foetus is carrying the group specific antigen and in fact at risk of haemolytic disease. This will help prevent the need of extensive laboratory (titration and quantification of antibody every 4 weeks till 28 weeks' gestation and every 2 weeks from 28 weeks to delivery) and clinical monitoring in antigen-negative cases.

4.3 Absence of facility for intrauterine transfusion for children with HDFN that are severely anaemic in utero

The maternal alloantibody D produced as a result of sensitization of the Rh D negative mother to the Rhesus D positive foetal red cells are low molecular weight IgG antibody. This antibody can potentially cross the placenta barrier into the foetal circulation and can destroy the foetal red cells resulting in anaemia, heart failure, hydrops foetalis (fluid retention and swelling) and intrauterine death. In utero the diagnosis of foetal anaemia used to be made by carrying out ultrasound guided foetal blood sampling for analysis of the foetal haemoglobin and haematocrit or amniocentesis-an invasive ultrasound guided procedure with a significant 2% risk of foetal loss associated with entering the amniotic sac and obtaining amniotic fluid which is analysed for product of haemoglobin breakdown. However, non-invasive diagnosis of foetal anaemia can now be made using non-invasive Doppler ultrasound technology by measuring the middle cerebral artery peak systolic velocities (MCA PSV). The foetal anaemia can be managed with intrauterine blood transfusions. Intrauterine transfusion is associated with a number of risks; foetal bradycardia, foetal death, cord haematoma, haemorrhage from the puncture site, miscarriage, preterm labour and vessel spasm. The blood used for such transfusions must meet certain requirements; gamma irradiated red cells to prevent transfusion-associated graft-versus-host disease, haemoglobin S negative, CMV negative and significantly high PCV (0.70–0.85) [105, 106], unit must be C-, D-, E- and K-, leucocyte depleted to less than 1×10^6 leucocytes per unit, less than 5 days old, free from clinically significant irregular blood group antibodies and negative for high-titre anti-A and anti-B haemolysin. If the mother has other alloantibodies apart from D, it is vital that suitable unit negative for the specific antigens to which those maternal alloantibodies are specific are selected. Once the baby is delivered, intensive phototherapy and IV immunoglobulin along with antiglobulin (DAT) test should be carried out. There should also be continuous monitoring of the haemoglobin, haematocrit and bilirubin level. A positive DAT is diagnostic of HDFN and the baby sample should be sent for elution to identify if the antibody coating the foetal red cell is maternal alloantibody. If the bilirubin is not responsive to intensive phototherapy and continues to rise, the associated neonatal anaemia and hyperbilirubinemia can be managed by carrying our exchange blood transfusion (EBT) to prevent bilirubin encephalopathy by removing a significant number of maternal antibodies-coated foetal red cells and excess bilirubin and replacing it with donor red cells. The red cell product used for EBT must meet certain requirements; group O or ABO compatibility (mum and baby), compatible with any maternal antibody, gamma irradiated, collected in saline, adenine, glucose and mannitol (SAGM), fresh less than 5 days old, have high haematocrit (0.5–0.55) to prevent of post-exchange anaemia and polycythaemia and negative for high titre haemolysins. A number of these evidenced-based best practices; facility for intrauterine blood transfusion, facilities for diagnosis of foetal anaemia in utero, maternal alloantibody testing, elution testing, facility for gamma irradiation of blood, CMV testing of donors units, testing of donor units for other clinical significant red cell antigens apart from ABO and Rhesus D, SAGM units and leucodepletion of donor units are often not available in Nigeria and most developing countries. This failure in stewardship by government in these countries limits the delivery of best possible care in the management of HDFN and appropriate transfusion in these patients.

4.4 Absence of facility to monitor the antibody titre and quantification in pregnant women who have developed HDFN causing alloantibody during pregnancy

Haemolytic Disease of the Foetus and Newborn (HDFN) is the destruction of foetal and newborn red cells by maternally derived alloantibody directed against a red cell antigen often inherited from the father and expressed on foetal cells. These maternal IgG antibodies are low molecular weight and can pass through the placenta barrier into the foetal circulation and bind to the corresponding foetal red cell antigen. The resultant maternal IgG-coated cells interact with foetal macrophages in resulting in their removal by the foetal spleen. This often results in anaemia, erthroblastosis with compensatory erythropoiesis resuming in the foetal liver and spleen, resulting in hepatosplenomegaly and portal hypertension. Maternal antibody screening is undertaken to detect clinically significant antibodies, which might affect the foetus and/or newborn, and to detect antibodies that may cause problems with the provision of compatible blood products for the woman and for the foetus/newborn. Approximately 1% of pregnant women are found to have clinically significant red cell antibodies [107–109]. The detection of clinically significant antibodies among antenatal women plays an important role in transfusion safety and preventing HDFN. A previous study among antenatal multiparous women in Jammu region of India indicated that the commonly observed alloantibodies were anti-D, anti-E, anti-C and anti-K [110]. Once an antibody has been detected, it is identified by carrying out a panel test. If the antibody specificity is one that has the potential to cause HDFN, the titre/quantification must be carried out periodically. Antibody quantification and titration is performed on patients' samples, to support the prediction and management of HDFN and ABO mismatched organ transplant. Antibody quantification of anti-D, and anti-c for management of HDFN. Antibody titration in ABO mismatched transplant is carried out to allow clinical assessment of the possibility of carrying out an ABO mismatched transplant, and monitoring of treatment to reduce antibody titre in preparation for ABO mismatched transplant. All clinically significant maternal antibodies detected during antenatal booking or follow up visit must be referred to the reference laboratory for confirmation of specificity, determination of the possibility of the antibody to cause HDFN and for and titre/quantification to allow for the monitoring of antibody. Evidence based best practice in developed countries requires the monitoring of women with red cell antibodies of specificities known to have potential to cause significant HDFN (anti-D, anti-c and anti-K), covering frequency of testing (every 4 weeks from booking until 28 weeks and every 2 weeks there after till delivery), measurement of antibody concentration (by quantification or titration as appropriate), referral to a foetal medicine specialist and follow-up required post-delivery. Antibodies that require quantification include anti-c, anti D, anti c + D, and anti-c + E. The antibodies that require titration include Anti-e, c, E, C+ e, G, CW, Fya, Fyb, K, k, Kpa, Kpb, Jsa, Jsb, M, S, and s. Antibody titration (ABT) is a semi quantitative method used to detect the strength of an alloantibody/antibodies present in the patient's plasma [111]. Antibody titration is used prenatally to screen for risk of HDFN, haemolytic transfusion reactions and assessment in solid organ or haematopoietic stem cell transplant. To assess risk for HDFN, the titre of the clinically significant alloantibody is performed. When the antibody and the titre strength are identified, ABT is periodically performed throughout pregnancy, whereby plasma samples are compared in parallel with the previously frozen samples to determine if the titre or strength of the antibody is static, decreasing or increasing. Obstetricians can use this information in conjunction with middle cerebral artery Doppler assessment to determine the extent to which the developing infant is affected, the presence of foetal anaemia, decision to carry out intrauterine transfusion as well as decision on whether to deliver the baby earlier to allow for a better and less risky physical management rather than ultrasound-guided in utero management [112]. Colour Doppler ultrasonography a non-invasive technique is currently being used to assess cerebral artery blood flow [113]. Increased cerebral artery blood flow is an indicator of foetal anaemia [114]. Invasive procedures such as amniocentesis or cordocentesis, with subsequent analysis of amniotic fluid and foetal blood sampling obtained by ultrasonography guided procedure are invasive and significantly risky with potential attendant negative effect to the foetus. Accepted titration methodologies include the tube and gel column technology method [115]. A difference of 2 dilutions or a score of 10 is usually an indication of significant change in antibody production. The antibody titre/quantification often rises as a result of re-exposure of the maternal immune system to red cell antigen following the initial sensitising events that occur during pregnancy. Every re-exposure to the initial offending antigen from the foetus to the mother's immune system often becomes booster doses. These booster doses often result in more antibody production, attendant increase in the titre and quantification. Antibody titration is also commonly used for screening blood products, particularly platelets and plasma as well as group O donor blood intended for transfusion to blood group A, B and AB patients. This is to decrease the risk of haemolytic transfusion reactions due to passive anti-A/anti-B antibodies. The titre of group O products is determined and those with high titers [51, 114] are labelled and used for group O individuals only while those negative for HT haemolysin can be given to A, B and AB individuals [116]. Also, ABT also has a potential role in preventing graft rejection in ABO-incompatible solid organ transplants (heart, liver, and lung) [117] as well as in erythroid engraftment after haematopoietic progenitor cell transplants [118]. Previous report indicates that the performance of antenatal titrations by column agglutination technology (CAT) is at least as sensitive as the performance by the indirect antiglobulin test (IAT) tube method. CAT was found to show greater sensitivity than IAT tube when dealing with anti-c compared to titrating Anti-K. The CAT method also appears to be more sensitive for detecting samples that require referral to the obstetrician [119]. Evidenced-based best practice requires that all pregnant women are tested for the presence of alloantibodies and its titers/quantification during pregnancy as a way of calculating the risk of developing HDFN [120]. Guidelines of the British Committee for standards in Haematology requires that, all pregnant women should be ABO and D antigen typed and screened for presence of alloantibodies at booking and at the 28th week of gestation [121]. Similarly, in the Netherlands, it has been mandatory to screen all pregnant females for presence of alloantibodies [122]. The aim of periodic antibody titration and quantification (every 4 weeks from detection at booking till 28 weeks and every 2 weeks thereafter until delivery) is to determine whether the titre/quantification is static, decreasing or increasing. A static titre/quantification shows that there is no increase in severity over time, a dropping titre/quantification indicate a low risk for HDFN while a rising titre/quantification is an indication of a potentially severe HDFN. For anti-D quantification a level of 4–15 IU indicates a moderate risk while a level > 15 IU indicates a high risk for HDFN. For anti-c a level > 7.5 IU indicates a high risk of HDFN. For anti-K, a titre of 1:32 or greater is indicative of HDFN risk. Generally, a 4-fold increase in the titre of an HDFN-associated alloantibody is an indication of a significant risk for HDFN [68]. In Nigeria and some other African countries alloantibody testing at booking and at 28 weeks gestation is not available, facilities for alloantibody identification and titration/quantification is not available. A number of pregnant women have alloantibodies without knowing and the risk of mortality from HDFN is high.

Nigerian and most of these countries can afford to provide the best possible antenatal care for their pregnant population like it obtains in the developed world. However, lack of political will, failure in stewardship and endemic corruption and misappropriation of the people's resources remains a major challenge to the effective management of the women. African government must rise to the responsibilities and do what is right by implementing evidence-based practice to allow for the effective management of pregnancies associated with clinically significant alloantibodies and its associated HDFN.

4.5 Challenge associated with use of anti-D immunoglobulin for the prevention of haemolytic disease of the foetus and newborn

Alloantibody-D are produced in a woman of child bearing age either as a result of Rhesus D incompatible transfusion (deliberate or erroneous transfusion of D positive donor red cells to Rhesus D negative women) or as a result of prior Rhesus D incompatibility between the mother and the developing foetus. These sensitizations are often as a result of fetomaternal haemorrhage during pregnancy or during delivery. This is often associated with D positive red cells entering into the maternal circulation to sensitise the mother to produce these immune antibody D. This immune D is an IgG class antibody and can potentially cross the placenta in subsequent D positive pregnancies to cause D HDFN. If a Rhesus D negative woman is married to Rh D positive men who are either homozygous or heterozygous for blood group antigen D, there is a 100 and 50% chance respectively of potentially carrying a Rhesus D positive foetus. In such pregnancies the risk of sensitization of the mother during the first pregnancy as a result of fetomaternal haemorrhage (during pregnancy or delivery) of D positive foetal red cell into maternal circulation is high. The recommend that prophylaxis be provided as soon as possible and always within 72 h of the following potentially sensitising event taking place in Rh D negative pregnant women (Amniocentesis, chorionic villus biopsy and cordocentesis, APH, PV bleed during pregnancy, ECV, Abdo trauma (sharp/blunt, open/closed, ectopic pregnancy, evacuation of molar, pregnancy, IUFD, intrauterine intervention during pregnancy (transfusion, surgery, insertion of shunts and laser), miscarriages, TOP, delivery (normal, instrument or C/S) and intraoperative cell salvage) to prevent sensitization and anti-D-related HDFN in subsequent pregnancy. Evidence-based best practice in most developed countries is to prevent this sensitization from taking place by the implementation of the Routine Antenatal Anti-D Prophylaxis (RAADP) programme. This program is alloimmunization prevention where all Rh D negative women are universally offered anti prophylaxis during pregnancy (28 weeks gestation) and following the delivery of a Rhesus positive baby. The implementation of this program has significantly reduced the number of residual alloimmunization from 16% to less than 0.1% [123]. The justification for this implementation is based of scientific evidence that 92% of women who develop an alloantibody-D during pregnancy do so at or after 28 weeks gestation [124, 125].

This implementation has significantly reduced the number of women who are sensitised and by extension the number of D HDFN. However, in countries like Nigeria and some other developing countries where this policy has not been implemented, a significant 14% of unfortunate foetuses are born dead while 50% of those who are born alive suffer from brain injury and neonatal death [126]. This cases of preventable death of Nigerian and African children is a humanitarian emergency that require urgent attention and good will by the Nigerian, African government and people of good will across to globe. Rh_0(D) immune globulin (RhIG) is a medication that can be given to non-sensitised Rhesus D negative pregnant women to prevent Rh D sensitization. The medication is often administered intramuscularly or intravenously and has a half-life of 12 weeks. Rho(D) immune globulin used for prophylaxis is a human derived fractionated plasma product produced from blood donors who have high levels of anti-D Ig either due to previous sensitization or intentional immunisation of Rh D negative men to produced immune D. This product is significantly virally tested (HBsAg, anti-HIV and HCV RNA) and includes viral inactivation steps in order to further reduce the risk of viral transmission. There is still a small unquantifiable possibility of transmitting prion particularly vCJD or other infectious agents. Product safety data submitted by manufacturers to National Institute of Health and Clinical Excellence technical appraisal guidance 156 (National Institute for Health and Clinical Excellence [127]) indicates a very low rate of adverse event (less than one non-serious per 80,000 doses of anti-D administered) [89]. There is no evidence till date to suggest that prophylactic anti-D administered to Rhesus D negative women during pregnancy is harmful to the foetus. Child birth or delivery is a potential sensitising event that can potentially expose the mother to the Rhesus D positive cells of the baby. Following delivery in these women, the cord blood is tested for ABO, Rh D group and DAT. If the infant is Rhesus D positive, the mother sample taken within 72 h is tested for fetomaternal haemorrhage (flow cytometry of Kleihauer-Betke test). These tests quantify the number of foetal cells that has entered the maternal circulation and thus facilitates the determination of the optimal dosage of prophylactic anti-D to be administered. As a general rule 125iu of anti-D is required to clear 1 ml of foetal cells from maternal circulation. A dose of 300 μg or 1500 IU is often sufficient to prevent alloimmunization after delivery in 99% of cases [128]. If the D-type of a newborn or stillborn is unknown or cannot be determined, a dose of anti-D prophylaxis should be administered. However, if the infant is found Rhesus D negative, prophylaxis will not be required. Evidenced-based best practices in most developed countries as part of their HDFN prevention program recommend the following [92].

In Nigeria and many countries in Africa, these recommendations and best practices are not being implemented. Government in these countries will need to rise up to their responsibilities by implementing these recommendations to prove the sincerity of their resolve to offer their people particularly Rhesus negative women the best possible health care delivery.

4.6 Unaffordability due to high cost of prophylactic anti-D

Anti-D related HDFN often result from the transplacental passage of maternal allo-antibodies directed against foetal red cell antigens inherited from the father affects the foetus or neonate. Majority of the mothers becomes sensitised following small feto-maternal haemorrhages during pregnancy and at delivery of the first Rh D-positive infant. These antibodies can potentially cause HDFN in successive Rh D-positive infants. Implementation of universal access to prophylactic anti-D given during antenatal and post-partum period following the delivery of a Rh D positive baby can help prevent primary Rh D immunisation and risk of HDFN in subsequent pregnancies [129]. It is recommended that routine antenatal anti-D prophylaxis (RAADP) is offered to all non-sensitised pregnant women who are Rh D negative to reduce the risk of sensitization and by extension D-related HDFN [130]. The World Health Organisation (WHO) recommends that antenatal prophylaxis with anti-D immunoglobulin should be given to non-sensitised Rh-negative pregnant women at 28 and 34 weeks of gestation to prevent Rh D alloimmunization. It is estimated that single dose of anti-D can cost around US$ 50 (500 IU) to US$ 87 (1500 IU), depending on the brand and local taxes. Therefore, the cost of antenatal prophylaxis for two 500 IU doses could be as much as US$ 100 per woman. Additional costs will include screening for blood typing in settings where Rh blood tests are not currently performed [131]. However, providing anti-D prophylaxis universally to all Rh D negative non-sensitised pregnant women is not cheap. The cost benefit analysis of preventing sensitization, HDFN and its related physical disabilities, mental retardation and death of affected children supports investing in the implementation of this policy by responsible government who believes that every life count. Routine antenatal anti-D prophylaxis provides a cost effective intervention for preventing HDFN in non-sensitised Rh D-negative pregnant women [132]. Health economic model indicates a significant cost per quality-adjusted life-year (QALY) gained by the implementation of RAADP given to Rh D-negative primigravidae versus no RAADP is between £9000 and £15,000, and for RAADP given to all RhD-negative women rather than to Rh D-negative primigravidae only is between £20,000 and £35,000. It is suggested that a programme of routine prophylaxis would be cost saving if HDFN were eradicated by its implementation [130]. The National Institute for Health and Clinical Excellence reported that when RAADP for all Rh D-negative women was compared with that for primigravidae, the additional cost per incident of sensitisation prevented ranged from £2900 to £8200 depending on the regimen used. The cost per HDFN-associated foetal loss avoided was £42,000–120,000. It does make economic sense for African government to rise to their responsibilities by proving universally anti-D prophylaxis to all non-sensitised Rhesus D negative women. There is also potential to significantly reduce the cost of implementing RAADP by these governments investing on facilities to non-invasive determination of foetal D genotyping for all non-sensitised Rh D negative pregnant women. This will help identify women who are carrying Rhesus D negative mothers who will not require the prophylaxis. Also, because the prevalence of Rh D negative status is significantly lower among Nigerians (6%) [133] compared to the West ≥15% [134], it is likely to cost African countries a lot less to implement universal access to anti-D prophylaxis [135].

4.7 Challenges associated with the provision of antigen negative red cells to patients with clinically significant red cell antibodies

Evidenced based best practice in management of patients including pregnant women requires that patients are transfused with red cells lacking the group specific antigens to which the recipient alloantibody is specific [136]. This aim of this implementation is to prevent immune mediated destruction of the donor red cells containing the offending antigen [137, 138]. For example, pregnant women who have alloantibody Kell should be given K-negative donor units. The provision of antigen negative blood units for these patients is a special challenge particularly in Nigeria and many other countries in Africa [139]. Although these countries have national blood transfusion services, majority of them are often not fit for purpose. Majority of them test blood donors only for their ABO and Rhesus antigen status [139]. Routine testing of blood donors for other clinically significant red sell antigens are not routinely done. This has a significant implication on haemolytic transfusion reaction and HDFN. In the alloimmuned pregnant women who have low molecular weight immune IgG antibodies, IAT crossmatching should ideally be carried out using donor red cells suspended in low ionic strength saline preferably using highly sensitive column agglutination technique instead of the conventional less sensitive tube methods. Many of these technologies are often not available in most settings in Nigeria and other African countries. Transfusion of antigen positive donor red cells to patient with the group specific antibodies like it potentially happens in Nigeria and some other African countries have significant negative consequences [140]. These antibodies can cause clinically significant haemolytic transfusion reactions, difficulty in cross-matching blood and getting compatible blood in future, cause decrease in RBC survival and thus negate the aim of red cell transfusion of managing anaemia, improving the quality of life and improving the oxygen carrying capacity of the recipient's blood [141]. Also, there is also the effect of managing donor red cell clearance and the product of red cell breakdown due to haemolysis which often results in multiple organ failure, electrolyte perturbations, coagulopathy and in some severe cases, death [142]. Nigerians and citizens of other African countries deserve the best quality transfusion service like their counterparts in the West. It is the responsibility of African government to work smartly and effectively by avoiding waste and eradicating corruption to ensure that citizens get the best quality health care they deserve.

4.8 Lack of facilities for feto-maternal haemorrhage testing

The accurate detection and quantification of foetal red blood cells (RBCs) in the maternal circulation are necessary for the prevention of Rhesus D alloimmunization among D-negative women because of FMH. It is critical to the administration of adequate amount of anti-D prophylaxis are necessary for the prevention of Rhesus D alloimmunization. As a result of D incompatibility between mother (Rhesus D negative and foetus (D-positive), foetal red cells can enter into maternal circulation and sensitise the mother to produce anti-D alloantibody. These anti-D alloantibodies (small molecular weight IgG antibodies) can pass through the placenta barrier in subsequent D positive pregnancies cause HDFN (haemolysis, foetal anaemia, hydrops foetalis, kernicterus or even death). FMH testing helps obstetrician to determine that a potential sensitising event has taken place and facilitate the administration of adequate amount of prophylactic anti-D (125 IU per 1 ml bleed of foetal red cells into maternal circulation). The widespread use of FMH testing in the evidenced-based provision of adequate immunoprophylaxis with anti-D immunoglobulin has resulted in a significant reduction in the incidence of anti-D related HDFN mortality. Evidence-based best practice implementation of FMH test and provision of immunoprophylaxis with anti-D immunoglobulin in England and Wales has brought about a significant reduction in the number of infants affected with HDFN from affected in 1.2 per 1000 births in 1970 to 0.02 per 1000 births by 1989. There are several methods available for FMH testing (Quantitative and qualitative). Three qualitative methods (micro Du, rosette test, and PEG Du) and two quantitative methods (acid elution and Flow Cytometry) for assessing FMH were evaluated with particular attention given to PEG Du and FC. Of the qualitative techniques, the micro Du test was the least sensitive with 20% false-negative results occurring at 0.5% foetal cells. The PEG Du test was only slightly more sensitive and offered no clinical advantage. The rosette test was the most sensitive, consistently detecting foetal cells at concentrations of 0.25% or greater. Flow Cytometry and acid elution showed similar results, with good correlation obtained between measured and expected quantities of foetal cells ($r = 0.99$ and 0.96, respectively). One of 26 postpartum samples was positive by all screening techniques; acid elution and FC detected 0.3% concentrations of fetal cells and 0.17% [143, 144]. The rosette screen is a highly sensitive in qualitatively detecting 10 mL of foetal whole blood in the maternal circulation. As the screen is reliant on the presence of the D antigen to distinguish foetal from maternal cells, it cannot be used to detect FMH in D-positive mothers or in D-negative mothers carrying a D-negative fetus. The Kleihauer-Betke acid-elution test, the most widely used confirmatory test for quantifying FMH, relies on the principle that foetal RBCs contain mostly foetal haemoglobin (HbF), which is resistant to acid-elution whereas adult haemoglobin is acid-sensitive. Although the Kleihauer-Betke test is inexpensive and requires no special equipment, it lacks standardisation and precision, and may not be accurate in conditions with elevated F-cells. Flow cytometry is a promising alternative, although its use is limited by equipment and staffing costs. The two well-established confirmatory tests are the Kleihauer-Betke acid-elution assay and flow cytometry. The rosette screen is a highly sensitive FDA approved method to qualitatively detect 10 mL or more of foetal whole blood, or 0.2% foetal cells (volume/volume) in the maternal circulation [143]. The principle is based upon the formation of microscopic foetal D+ aggregates upon incubation of foetal cells with enzyme0-treated group O D-positive indicator RBCs and reagent anti-D serum. The foetal cells must be D-positive and the maternal cells D-negative for the test to be valid. In summary the maternal blood sample is first incubated with anti-D and then washed. The indicator D-positive RBCs are added and the sample is examined under a light microscope. In the presence of anti-D coated foetal D-positive cells, the indicator cells will form aggregates (or rosettes) around the foetal cells. The main limitation of this method is that falsely positive result may occur is the mum has a variant of the D antigen and falsely negative if the foetus or neonate is weak D. Also, mothers that have a positive direct antiglobulin test (DAT) or an autoantibody can produce a false positive result due to the agglutination of the mother's antibody coated red cells.

A positive rosette test is indicative of FMH > 10 mL. In a negative rosette test administration of is 300 μg (1500 IU) of Rh Ig is sufficient to prevent immunisation in 99% of patients. If the rosette test is positive quantification of the FMH by either the Kleihauer-Betke acid elution test or flow cytometry is indicated to determine the optimal dose of prophylactic anti-D immunoglobulin to be administered. The Kleihauer-Betke acid-elution test is an inexpensive method and requires no special equipment and thus can possibly be implemented in developing country like Nigeria and other resource-limited settings. The method is based on the principle that foetal RBCs containing foetal haemoglobin (HbF) to resist acid elution whereas adult haemoglobin does not. When a peripheral smear prepared from a EDTA anticoagulated maternal blood sample is exposed to an acid buffer such as Shepherds stain, haemoglobin in the cytoplasm of maternal red cells are eluted while HbF in the foetal red cells resist acid elution. Subsequent counterstaining with haematoxylin results in red cell containing foetal haemoglobin staining pink while the maternal adult haemoglobin containing red cells appear as ghost. **Figure 1** shows a positive Kleihauer-Betke test. To calculate the number of foetal cells in maternal circulation using Kleihauer-Betke test, get a stained thin film on a microscope and replace one of the objectives of the microscope with a graticule (Miller square) (**Figure 2**). Focus the microscope making sure the graticule is on the top left-hand corner. Select the ×40 lens and count at least 50 fields of the area of the film where the red cells are just touching each other. For each field count all the foetal cells in the large and small square. Count all the maternal cells in the small square. Count fields with at least 25–30 maternal cells. To calculate the total number of maternal cells, add the total number of maternal cells together and multiply by 9. Also add the total number of foetal cells from the 50 fields. The calculation of FMH is done using Mollison's rule.

Mollison's rule = 2400 × number of foetal cells ÷ number of maternal cells

For example, if the number of foetal red cells is 20 and the maternal cells is 2000, the FMH = number of maternal cells = 2000 × 9 = 18,000

25 × 2400/18,000 = 3.3 mls bleed.

Calculation of dose of anti-D. Anti-D administered is calculated by giving 125 IU per ml of FMH. For a 3.3 ml bleed you will have to administer 3.3 × 125 IU = 413 IU of anti-D.

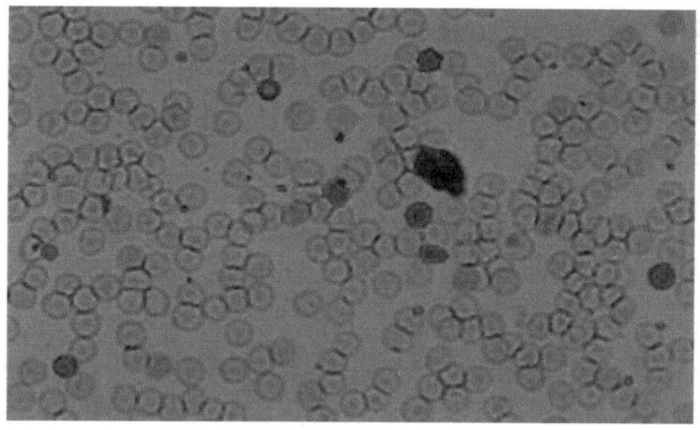

Figure 1.
Positive Kleihauer-Betke test.

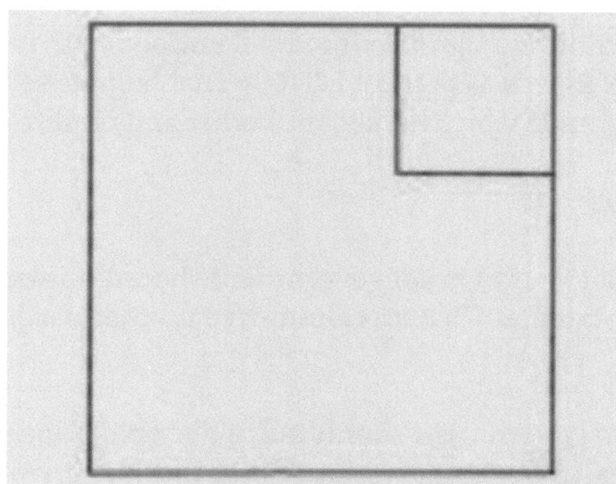

Figure 2.
Diagram of Miller square (graticule).

The Kleihauer-Betke method is a labour intensive and subjective method. The accuracy and precision of this method is hampered by lack of standardisation which can potentially lead to slight variations in result (thickness of blood smear, pipetting skill of analyst, pH variations in the buffer used, inter analyst variations). Over- and underestimation of FMH using the Kleihauer-Betke test has been reported [145, 146]. The disadvantages of this method include; laborious to perform, lacks standardisation, is imprecise and may not be accurate in conditions associated with elevated haemoglobin F containing red cells. However, standardisation of the Kleihauer-Betke test can make the result potentially comparable to result from flow cytometry [147]. Haemoglobin F containing red cells are increased in haemoglobinopathies including sickle cell disease and β-thalassemia and hereditary persistence of foetal haemoglobin (HPFH). In 25% of pregnant women, HbF tend to be increased and can cause false positive results [148, 149]. In pregnant women with conditions such as sickle cell disease, thalassaemia and HPFH an alternative method for FMH testing such as flow cytometry should be employed. Despite its limitations, a good correlation has been reported between the Kleihauer-Betke test and flow cytometry for both small and large FMH [150, 151].

Flow cytometry involves using a flow cytometer using monoclonal antibodies directed against. Flow cytometric determination of FMH is superior to Kleihauer-Betke test for a number of reasons; cytometric methods can accurately distinguish adult foetal haemoglobin containing red cells from foetal RBCs, flow cytometers rapidly analyses a significantly higher number of cells (≥50,000), thus improving its quantitative accuracy and flow cytometry is automated non-subjective and has greater reproducibility. The only disadvantage is that it requires trained staff to perform test coupled with the fact that it is it is expensive and may not be affordable in low-resource settings.

5. Conclusions

There is paucity of data on the distribution of clinically significant blood group antigens apart from ABO and Rhesus D among Nigerians. Management of Rhesus D negative pregnancies and pregnancies associated with clinically significant alloantibody is suboptimal. This failure in stewardship by the Nigerian government has a significant implication for Haemolytic Disease of the Foetus and Newborn and haemolytic transfusion reaction. There is need to introduce routine screening of pregnant women in Nigeria for clinically significant red cell antibodies to facilitate the effective management of HDFN as well as prevent HTR by enabling the selection of antigen negative red cells for women who have alloantibodies and require a red cell transfusion.

5.1 Recommendations

We recommend that the Nigerian government should implement the following evidence-based best practices (British Committee for Standards in Haematology [152–155].

1. That the Nigerian government should fulfil her obligations under goal 3.8 of the Universal Health Coverage initiative and the Sustainable Development goal 3.b which emphasises the need for access to safe, effective, quality and affordable essential medicines for all by implementing universal access to anti-D prophylaxis for previously unsensitized Rhesus D negative pregnant women.

2. Screen donor units for clinically significant antigen status to facilitate the selection of antigen negative donor units for transfusion to patients with a clinically significant alloantibody.

3. Routinely screening all blood group O donors whose units are intended for transfusion to non-O recipients for high titre haemolysin.

4. Anti-D immunoglobulin should be available in cases of potentially sensitising events such as amniocentesis, cordocentesis, antepartum haemorrhage, vaginal bleeding during pregnancy, external cephalic version, abdominal trauma, intrauterine death and stillbirth, in utero therapeutic interventions, miscarriage, and therapeutic termination of pregnancy.

5. All Rhesus D negative women having a termination of pregnancy (abortion) must be tested for Rhesus D group and those found to be Rhesus D negative must be offered prophylaxis following the procedure.

6. Routine foetal genotyping using non-invasive testing of maternal sample to identify Rhesus negative pregnant women who are carrying Rhesus negative infants for whom prophylaxis is not indicated.

7. Facilities for intrauterine transfusion of infants who become anaemic in utero as a result of HDFN and require a red cell transfusion. Facilities to test donor

red cells to ensure that they meet the requirements for intrauterine, exchange and top up transfusion.

8. Facilities for the implementation of alloantibody titration and quantification should be provided for pregnant women with a clinically significant, HDFN causing alloantibody.

9. There is need for the provision of facilities for fetomaternal haemorrhage testing to facilitate the administration of optimal amount of anti-D prophylaxis following a sensitising event to prevent HDFN.

10. Knowledge of anti-D prophylaxis and management of women with clinically significant antibodies among Obstetricians, Laboratory of Biomedical Scientist, Midwives, Traditional Birth Attendants, Pharmacists and Nurses in Nigeria and other countries in Africa needs to be improved. This will facilitate quality antenatal and postnatal care offered particularly to Rh-negative pregnant women and those with clinically significant alloantibodies.

11. That anti-D prophylaxis be provided in Rhesus D negative pregnant pregnancies <12 weeks gestation, following ectopic pregnancy, molar pregnancy, therapeutic termination of pregnancy. FMH haemorrhage (FMH) testing is often not required for sensitising events at <12 weeks gestation.

12. That for all potentially sensitising events occurring between 12- and 20-weeks' gestation, prophylaxis should be administered within 72 h of the event without need for FMH testing.

13. That for potentially sensitising events after 20 weeks gestation, prophylaxis should be administered within 72 h of the event along with testing for FMH. This is to determine if additional dose of anti-D Ig is required for a significant bleed.

14. That in the event of an intrauterine foetal death (IUFD), where no sample can be obtained from the baby or foetus, an appropriate dose of prophylactic anti-D should be administered to Rhesus D negative, previously non-sensitised women within 72 h of the *diagnosis of IUFD*, irrespective of the time of subsequent delivery.

15. That following intra-operative cell salvage (ICS) during Caesarean section in D negative, previously non-sensitised women, and where cord blood group is confirmed as D positive (or unknown), a minimum dose of 1500 IU prophylactic anti-D should be administered following the re-infusion of salvaged red cells. Also, the maternal sample should be taken for estimation of FMH 30–45 min after reinfusion to confirm if a further dose of anti-D Ig is required.

16. That in cases of therapeutic termination of pregnancy (abortion), whether by surgical or medical methods, and regardless of gestational age, all previously non-sensitised D negative women should receive a dose of prophylactic anti-D within 72 h of having the procedures.

17. That anti-D prophylaxis should be administered to all cases of ectopic pregnancy in previously non-sensitised, D negative women regardless of the mode of management.

18. That there is significant potential for sensitisation in cases of molar pregnancy. Anti-D prophylaxis should be administered to all cases of molar pregnancy in previously non-sensitised, D negative women.

19. That D negative women presenting with continual uterine bleeding between 12- and 20-weeks' gestation should be offered anti-D prophylaxis at a minimum of 6 weekly intervals.

20. That under normal circumstances, D negative platelets should be transfused to D negative females or women of child bearing age, who need a platelet transfusion. Occasionally, if the appropriate product is not available or its availability is likely to cause unacceptable delay and harm, it may be necessary to transfuse D positive platelets. In these situations, prophylaxis against possible sensitisation by the D positive red cells contaminating the platelet product should be given. A dose of 250 IU anti-D immunoglobulin is sufficient to cover up to five adult therapeutic doses of D positive platelets given over a 6-weeks period.

Author details

Osaro Erhabor*, Tosan Erhabor, Teddy Charles Adias and Iwueke Ikechukwu Polycarp
Department of Haematology, School of Medical Laboratory Science, Usmanu Danfodiyo University, Sokoto, Nigeria

*Address all correspondence to: n_osaro@yahoo.com

References

[1] Bakare AS, Olubokun S. Health care expenditure and economic growth in Nigeria: An empirical study. Journal of Emerging Trends in Economics and Management Sciences. 2011;**2**(2):83-87

[2] Uneke C, Ogbonna A, Ezeoha A, Oyibo P, Onwe F, Ngwu B, et al. The Nigeria health sector and human resource challenges. International Journal of Health. 2007;**8**(1):1-5

[3] Duru EJ, Nwagbos CI. The problems and prospects of public health care development in Nigeria's local government system. Global Journal of Social Sciences. 2007;**6**(1):51-56

[4] United Nations. Moving Together to Build a Healthier World Key Asks from the UHC Movement UN High-Level Meeting on Universal Health Coverage. UHC2030. Available from: https://www.uhc2030.org/fileadmin/uploads/uhc2030/Documents/UN_HLM/UHC_Key_Asks_final.pdf [Accessed: October 10, 2019]

[5] Wagner AK, Graves AJ, Reiss SK, Lecates R, Zhang F, Ross-Degnan D. Access to care and medicines, burden of health care expenditures, and risk protection: Results from the World Health Survey. Health Policy. 2011;**100**:151-158

[6] WHO. The World Health Report—Health Systems Financing: The Path to Universal Coverage. Geneva: World Health Organization; 2010

[7] ISBT. Table of Blood Group Systems. International Society of Blood Transfusion. 2014. Retrieved 19 February 2016

[8] Marcela C, Antole L. Antigens in human blood. In: Postgraduate Haematology. 4th ed. Boston, Mass, USA: Butterworth-Heinemann; 1999. pp. 186-189 (chapter 10)

[9] Giangrande PL. The history of blood transfusion. British Journal of Haematology. 2000;**110**(4):758-767

[10] Landsteiner K. On agglutination of normal human blood. Transfusion. 1901;**1**(1):5-8

[11] Anifowoshe AT, Oyeyemi BF, Iyiola OA, Ahmed IO, Akinseye KM. Gene frequencies of ABO and Rh (D) blood group alleles in Minna, North-Central, Nigeria. Nigerian Journal of Pure and Applied Sciences. 2015;**28**:2644-2657

[12] Bakare AA, Azeez MA, Agbolade JO. Gene frequencies of ABO and rhesus blood groups and haemo globin variants in Ogbomosho, South-West Nigeria. African Journal of Biotechnology. 2006;**5**:224-229

[13] Enosolease ME. Distribution of ABO and Rh_D blood groups in the Benin area of implication for regional blood transfusion. Asian Journal of Transfusion Science. 2008;**2**(1):3-5

[14] Falusi AG, Ademowo OG, Latunji AC, Okeke C, Olatunji PO, Onyekwere TO, et al. Distribution of ABO and Rh genes in Nigeria. African Journal of Medicine and Medical Sciences. 2000;**29**:23-26

[15] Hassan A, Babadoko AA, Ahmed AJ, Isa HA, Suleiman AM. The pattern of distribution of ABO blood groups in North Western Nigeria. Annals of Nigerian Medicine. 2005;**1**(2):17-18

[16] Iyiola OA, Igunnugbemi OO, Bello OG. Gene frequencies of ABO and Rh(D) blood group alleles in Lagos, South-West Nigeria. Egyptian Journal of Medical Human Genetics. 2012;**13**:147-153

[17] Iyiola OA, Igunnugbemi OO, Raheem UA, Anifowoshe AT. Gene

frequencies of ABO and Rh(D) blood group alleles in Ilorin, North-Central Nigeria. World Journal of Biological Research. 2011;**4**(1):6-14

[18] Omotade OO, Adeyemo AA, Kayode CM, Falade SL, Ikpeme S. Gene frequencies of ABO and Rh (D) blood group alleles in a healthy infant population in Ibadan, Nigeria. West African Journal of Medicine. 1991;**18**(4):294-297

[19] Anifowoshe AT, Owolodun OA, Akinseye KM, Iyiola OA, Oyeyemi BF. Gene frequencies of ABO and Rh blood groups in Nigeria: A review. Egyptian Journal of Medical Human Genetics. 2017;**18**(3):205-210

[20] Benahadi A, Alami R, Boulahdid S, Adouani B, Laouina A, Mokhtari A, et al. Distribution of ABO and Rhesus D blood antigens in Morocco. Internet Journal of Biological Anthropology. 2013;**6**(1):1-6

[21] Garratty G, Glynn SA, McEntire R. ABO and Rh (D) phenotype frequencies of different racial/ethnic groups in the United States. Transfusion. 2004;**44**(5):703-706

[22] Hamed CT, Bollahi MA, Abdelhamid I, Mahmoud M, Ba B, Ghaber S, et al. Frequencies and ethnic distribution of ABO and Rh (D) blood groups in Mauritania: Results of first nationwide study. International Journal of Immunogenetics. 2012;**39**(2):151-154

[23] Ndoula ST, Noubiap JJN, Nansseu JRN, Wonkam A. Phenotypic and allelic distribution of the ABO and Rhesus (D) blood groups in the Cameroonian population. International Journal of Immunogenetics. 2014;**41**(3):206-210

[24] Said N, BenAhmed F, Doghri A, Ghazouani E, Layouni S, Gritli V, et al. The ABO system polymorphism in Tunisian blood. Transfusion Clinique et Biologique. 2003;**10**:331

[25] Tesfaye K, Petros Y, Andargie M. Frequency distribution of ABO and Rh (D) blood group alleles in Silte Zone, Ethiopia. Egyptian Journal of Medical Human Genetics. 2015;**16**(1):71-76

[26] Torabizade Maatoghi J, Paridar M, Mahmodian Shoushtari M, Kiani B, Nori B, Shahjahani M, et al. Distribution of ABO blood groups and rhesus factor in a large-scale study of different cities and ethnicities in Khuzestan province, Iran. Egyptian Journal of Medical Human Genetics. 2016;**17**(1):105-109

[27] Loua A, Lamah MR, Haba NY, Camara M. Frequency of blood groups ABO and Rhesus D in the Guinean population. Transfusion Clinique et Biologique. 2007;**14**:435

[28] Randriamanantany ZA, Rajaonatahina DH, Razafimanantsoa FE, Rasamindrakotroka MT, Andriamahenina R, Rasoarilalamanarivo FB, et al. Phenotypic and allelic profile of ABO and Rhésus D blood group system among blood donor in Antananarivo. International Journal of Immunogenetics. 2012;**39**(6):477-479

[29] Chandra T, Gupta A. Frequency of ABO and Rhesus blood groups in blood donors. Asian Journal of Transfusion Science. 2012;**6**(1):52-53

[30] Dewan G. Comparative frequency and allelic distribution of ABO and Rh (D) blood groups of major tribal communities of southern Bangladesh with general population and their determinants. Egyptian Journal of Medical Human Genetics. 2015;**16**(2):141-147

[31] Causil-Vargas L, Gómez-Mercado L, Otero-Díaz D, Moscote-Blanco L, Monterrosa-Mestra L, Burgos-Flórez D, et al. Frecuencia de grupos sanguíneos

(sistema ABO) entre estudiantes de la universidad de córdoba sede berástegui. Ciencia e Investigación Medico Estudiantil Latinoamericana. 2016;**21**(1):24-26

[32] Kayiran SM, Oktem O, Kayiran PG, Paloglu E, Gurakan B. Frequency of ABO and Rhesus blood groups among neonates born at a private hospital in Istanbul. The Southeast Asian Journal of Tropical Medicine and Public Health. 2012;**43**(2):467-470

[33] Olaniyan TO, Ajibola BM, Rasong H, Dare BJ, Shafe MO. Blood group and rhesus factor pattern among indigenes of FCT, Abuja, Nigeria. Journal of Community Medicine and Health Education. 2013;**3**(3):208

[34] Adeyemo OA, Soboyejo OB. Frequency distribution of ABO, RH blood groups and blood genotypes among the cell biology and genetics students of University of Lagos, Nigeria. African Journal of Biotechnology. 2006;**5**(22):2062-2065

[35] Alimba CG, Adekoya KO, Oboh BO. Prevalence and gene frequencies of phenylthiocarbamide (PTC) taste sensitivity, ABO and Rhesus factor (Rh) blood groups, and haemoglobin variants among a Nigerian Population. Egyptian Journal of Medical Human Genetics. 2010;**11**(2):153-158

[36] Oluwadare I, Shonekan S. ABO and Rhesus 'D' blood type distribution in students admitted into MoshoodAbiola Polytechnic, Abeokuta, Nigeria in 2006. African Journal of Biotechnology. 2008;**7**(11):1641-1643

[37] Temitayo OI, Timothy SO. Frequency distribution of haemoglobin variants and rhesus blood groups among pregnant. American Medical Journal. 2013;**4**(1):78-81

[38] Olubayode B, Dennis SA, Abiola OA. Distribution of ABO and rhesus blood groups among medical students in Bowen University, Iwo, Nigeria. Annals of Biological Research. 2013;**4**(11):1-6

[39] Akhigbe RE, Ige SF, Adegunlola GJ, Adewumi MO, Azeez MO. Malaria, haemoglobin genotypes abd ABO blood group genotypes in Ogbomoso, Nigeria. International Journal of Tropical Medicine. 2011;**6**(4):73-76

[40] Famoni PO, Adekoya-Benson T, Ajala O, Agbaje A, Olatimehin O, Adeosun OC, et al. Frequencies of ABO blood groups among blood donors in Ado-Ekiti and its metropolis, South-West, Nigeria. International Journal of Healthcare Sciences. 2015;2(2):126-129

[41] Akpan EB, Iwah-Udo IS. Studies of the distribution of ABO blood groups and Rhesus factors in Uyo, Akwa Ibom State, Nigeria. African Journal of Applied Zoology and Environmental Biology. 2006;**8**:159-161

[42] Egesie UG, Egesie OJ, Usar I, Johnbull TO. Distribution of ABO, Rhesus blood groups and haemoglobin electrophoresis among the undergraduate students of Niger Delta University Nigeria. Nigerian Journal of Physiological Sciences. 2008;**23**:5-8

[43] Odokuma EI, Okolo AC, Aloamaka PC. Distribution of Abo and Rhesus blood groups in Abraka, Delta State, Nigeria. Nigerian Journal of Physiological Sciences. 2007;**22**(1-2):89-91

[44] Erhabor O, Adias TC, Jeremiah ZA, Hart ML. Abnormal hemoglobin variants, ABO, and Rhesus blood group distribution among students in the Niger Delta of Nigeria. Pathology and Laboratory Medicine International. 2010;**2**:41-46

[45] Akinnuga AM, Bamidele O, Amosu AM, Ugwah GU. Distribution of ABO and Rh blood groups among major

ethnic groups of medical students of Madonna University Teaching Hospital, Elele, Nigeria. Asian Journal of Medical Sciences. 2011;**3**(3):106-109

[46] Jeremiah ZA. Abnormal haemoglobin variants, ABO and Rh blood groups among students of African descent in Port-Harcourt, Nigeria. African Health Sciences. 2006;**6**(3):177-181

[47] Chima OK, Mohammed TB, Aisha K, Alhaji SA, Muhammad BM, Kwaru AH. ABO and rhesus blood groups among blood donors in Kano, North-Western Nigeria. Nigerian Journal of Basic and Clinical Sciences. 2012;**9**(1):11-13

[48] Erhabor O, Isaac IZ, Saidu A, Ahmed HM, Abdulrahaman Y, et al. The distribution of ABO and rhesus blood groups among residents of Gusau, Zamfara State, North Western Nigeria. Research and Reviews: Journal of Medical and Health Sciences. 2013;**2**(4):58-63

[49] Obeagu EI, Ogbodo OR, Onyenweaku F, Emelike CU, Udochukwu AI. Frequency distribution of ABO, Rh blood groups and blood genotypes among the students and staff of Michael Okpara University of Agriculture, Umudike Abia State, Nigeria. International Journal of Research and Reviews in Pharmacy and Applied Science. 2013;**3**(4):561-565

[50] Ugwu ZI. Pattern of ABO and Rhesus blood group distribution among students of Ebonyi State University, Abakaliki, South Eastern Nigeria. Asian Journal of Medical Sciences. 2016;**7**(1):101-104

[51] Abdulazeez AA, Alo EB, Rebecca SN. Carriage rate of human immunodeficiency virus (HIV) infection among different ABO and rhesus blood groups in Adamawa state, Nigeria. Biomedical Research. 2008;**19**(1):41-44

[52] Babadoko AA, Takai IU, Kawuwa MB. Distribution of ABO, Rh d blood groups and haemoglobin phenotypes among antenatal clinic attendees in Federal Medical Centre Nguru, Nigeria. Borno Medical Journal. 2014;**11**(2):86-91

[53] Cerny T, Fey M, Oppliger R, Castiglione M, Nachbur B, Gertsch M, et al. Prevalence of the rhesus-negative phenotype in Caucasian patients with small-cell lung cancer (SCLC). International Journal of Cancer. 1992;**52**:504-506

[54] Lin M, Wang CL, Chen FS, Ho LH. Fatal haemolytic transfusion reaction due to anti-Ku in a K null patient. Immunohematology. 2003;**19**(1):19-21

[55] Vaughan JI, Manning M, Warwick RM, Letsky EA, Murray NA, Roberts IA. Inhibition of erythroid progenitor cells by anti-Kell antibodies in foetal alloimmune anaemia. New England Journal of Medicine. 1998;**338**(12):798-803

[56] Vaughan JI, Warwick R, Letsky E, Nicolini U, Rodeck CH, Fisk NM. Erythropoietic suppression in fetal anemia because of Kell alloimmunization. American Journal of Obstetrics and Gynecology. 1994;**171**(1):247-252

[57] Erhabor O, Ladan MA, Zama I, Ahmed Y, Mairo H. Distribution of Kell phenotype among pregnant women in Sokoto, North Western Nigeria. The Pan African Medical Journal. 2015;**21**:301

[58] Ugboma HA, Nwauche CA. Kell blood group antigen in Port Harcourt, Nigeria—A pilot study. Port Harcourt Medical Journal. 2009;**4**(2). ISSN 0795-3038

[59] Adewoyin AS, Lee GM, Adeyemo TA, Awodu OA. Rh and

Kell blood group antigen prevalence in a multi-ethnic cohort in Nigeria: Implications for local transfusion service. Immunohematology. 2018;**34**(2):61-65

[60] Lamba DS, Kaur R, Basu S. Clinically significant minor blood group antigens amongst north Indian donor population. Advances in Hematology. 2013;**2013**:215454

[61] Redman CM, Russo D, Lee S. Kell, Kx and the McLeod syndrome. Baillière's Clinical Haematology. 1999;**12**(4):621-635

[62] Yusuf Jamoh B, Gwaram BA, Abdullahi S, Tasiu M. 12th World Hematologists Congress; March 15-16, 2018; London, UK. 2018

[63] Erhabor O, Shehu CE, Alhaji YB, Yakubu A. Duffy red cell phenotypes among pregnant women in Sokoto, North Western Nigeria. Journal of Blood Disorders & Transfusion. 2014;**5**:223

[64] Okwesili A, Sani AB, Onuigwe F, Hauwa B, Bagudo A, Ibrahim K, et al. Prevalence of rhesus C and E phenotype among pregnant women attending antenatal clinic in Usmanu Danfodiyo University Teaching Hospital, Sokoto. Journal of Gynecology and Neonatal Biology. 2016;**2**(1):13-16

[65] Jeremiah ZA, Odumody C. Rh antigens and phenotype frequencies of the Ibibio, Efik, and Ibo ethnic nationalities in Calabar, Nigeria. Immunohematology. 2005;**21**(1):21-24

[66] Jeremiah ZA, Biribo AA, Adias TC, Uko EK. Uncommon Rh phenotypes in a cross section of Nigerian antenatal women: Implications for molecular genotyping of blood groups. Journal of Blood Disorders & Transfusion. 2012;**S10**:001

[67] Siransy BL, Dembele B, Sekongo Y, Abisse S, Konaté S, Sombo M. Phenotypic Profile of Rh and Kell Blood Group Systems among Blood Donors in Cote d'Ivoire, West Africa. Journal of Blood Transfusion. 2014;**2014**:4

[68] Erhabor O, Adias TC. From whole blood to component therapy: The economic, supply/demand need for implementation of component therapy in sub-Saharan Africa. Transfusion Clinique et Biologique. 2011;**18**(5-6):516-526

[69] Ahmed OA, Agomo PU, Olukoya DK, Esan GJ. The prevalence of ABO blood group antigens and antibodies in Lagos State, Nigeria. African Journal of Medicine and Medical Sciences. 1993;**22**:49-53

[70] Emeribe AO. The status of alpha and beta haemolysins in Nigerian blood donors. East African Medical Journal. 1990;**67**(3):205-208

[71] Obisesan OA, Ogundeko TO, Iheanacho CU, Abdulrazak T, Idyu VC, Idyu II, et al. Evaluation of alpha (α) and beta (β) haemolysin antibodies incidence among blood group 'O' donors in ATBUTH Bauchi-Nigeria. American Journal of Clinical Medicine Research. 2015;**3**(3):42-44

[72] Okafor LA, Enebe S. Anti-A and anti-B haemolysins, dangerous universal blood donors and the risk of ABO antagonism in a Nigerian community. Tropical and Geographical Medicine. 1985;**37**:270-272

[73] Olawumi HO, Olatunji PO. Prevalence and titre of alpha and beta haemolysins in blood group 'O' donors in Ilorin. African Journal of Medicine and Medical Sciences. 2001;**30**(4):319-321

[74] Oyedeji OA, Adeyemo TA, Ogbenna AA, Akanmu AS. Prevalence of anti-A and anti-B hemolysis among blood group O donors in Lagos.

Nigerian Journal of Clinical Practice. 2015;**18**:328-332

[75] Uko EK, Erhabor O, Ahmed HM, Isaac IZ, Abdulrahaman Y, Wase A, et al. Prevalence of high titre alpha and beta haemolysins among blood donors in Sokoto, North Western Nigeria. International Journal of Medical Sciences and Health Care. 2013;**1**(11):1-7

[76] Castilho L. ABO isohemagglutinin titration or hemolysin test: What should we do to reduce the risk of passive hemolysis? Revista Brasileira de Hematologia e Hemoterapia. 2015;**37**(4):215-216

[77] Mathai J, Sindhu PN, Sulochana PV, Sathyabhama S. Haemolysin test for characterization of immune ABO antibodies. The Indian Journal of Medical Research. 2003;**118**:125-128

[78] Nadarajan SN, Hlaing AA, Maung TH, Jeyajoti I, Kyu TN, Ranjana KJ, et al. Incidence of red cell alloantibodies in a multi-ethnic hospital patient population. Vox Sanguinis. 2007;**93**:63-64

[79] Schonewille H, van de Watering LMG, Loomans DSE, Brand A. Red blood cell alloantibodies after transfusion: Factors influencing incidence and specificity. Transfusion. 2006;**46**:250-256

[80] Singer ST, Wu V, Mignacca R, Kuypers FA, Morel P, Vichinsky EP. Alloimmunization and erythrocyte autoimmunization in transfusion dependent thalassemia patients of predominantly Asian descent. Blood. 2000;**96**:3369-3373

[81] Jan RH, Yu LC, Wen SH, Tsai SS, Lin TY. Incidence of alloantibodies in transfused patients in Eastern Taiwan. Tzu Chi Medical Journal. 2009;**21**:66-69

[82] Ameen R, Al-Eyaadi O, Al-Shemmari S, Chowdhury R, Al-Bashir A. Frequency of red blood cell alloantibody in Kuwaiti population. Medical Principles and Practice. 2005;**14**:230-234

[83] Makarovsk-Bojadzieva T. Blood group antibodies that cause problems in pretransfusion testing. Blood Banking and Transfusion Medicine. 2004;**2**:89-93

[84] Al-Joudi F, Ali AB, Ramli MB, Ahmed S, Ismail M. Prevalence and specificities of red cell alloantibodies among blood recipients in the Malaysian state of Kelantan. Asian Journal of Transfusion Science. 2011;**5**(1):42-45

[85] Yousuf R, Abdul Aziz S, Yusof N, Leong CF. Incidence of red cell alloantibody among the transfusion recipients of Universiti Kebangsaan Malaysia Medical Centre. Indian Journal of Hematology and Blood Transfusion. 2013;**29**(2):65-70

[86] Poole J, Daniels G. Blood group antibodies and their significance in transfusion medicine. Transfusion Medicine Reviews. 2007;**21**:58-71

[87] Illanes S, Soothill P. Management of red cell alloimmunisation in pregnancy: The non-invasive monitoring of the disease. Prenatal Diagnosis. 2010;**30**(7):668-673

[88] Tong KF, Tse KT, Lee AW, Mak CS, So CC. Is antenatal antibody screening worthwhile in Chinese. British Journal of Haematology. 1997;**97**:917-919

[89] Pilgrim H, Lloyd-Jones M, Rees A. Routine antenatal anti-D prophylaxis for Rh D negative women: A systematic review and economic evaluation. Health Technology Assessment. 2009;**13**:1-126

[90] Urbaniak SJ, Greiss MA. Rh D haemolytic disease of the fetus and the newborn. Blood Reviews. 2000;**14**:44-61

[91] MacKenzie IZ, Bowell P, Gregory H, Pratt G, Guest C, Entwistle CC. Routine antenatal rhesus D immunoglobulin prophylaxis: The results of a prospective 10-year study. British Journal of Obstetrics and Gynaecology. 1999;**106**:492-497

[92] Qureshi H, Massey E, Kirwan D, Davies T, Robson S, White J, et al. BCSH guideline for the use of anti-D immunoglobulin for the prevention of haemolytic disease of the foetus and newborn. Transfusion Medicine. 2014;**24**(1):8-20

[93] Koelewijn JM, de Haas M, Vrijkotte TGM, van der Schoot CE, Bonsel GJ. Risk factors for RhD immunisation despite antenatal and postnatal anti-D prophylaxis. BJOG. 2009;**116**:1307-1314

[94] Koelewijn JM, Koelewijn JM, Vrijkotte TG, de Haas M, van der Schoot CE, Bonsel GJ. Risk factors for the presence of non-rhesus D red blood cell antibodies in pregnancy. BJOG. 2009;**116**(5):655-664

[95] Moise KJJ. Management of rhesus alloimmunization in pregnancy. Obstetrics and Gynecology. 2008;**112**:164-176

[96] Reid ME. Application of DNA-based assays in blood group antigen and antibody identification. Transfusion. 2003;**43**:1748-1757

[97] Avent ND. RHD genotyping from maternal plasma: Guidelines and technical challenges. Methods in Molecular Biology. 2008;**444**:185-201

[98] Scheffer PG, van der Schoot CE, Page-Christiaens GC, de Haas M. Noninvasive fetal blood group genotyping of rhesus D, c, E and of K in alloimmunised pregnant women: Evaluation of a 7-year clinical experience. BJOG. 2011;**118**(11):1340-1308

[99] Tóth T, Papp C, Tóth-Pál E, Nagy B, Papp Z. Fetal RhD genotyping by analysis of maternal blood. A case report. Journal of Reproductive Medicine. 1998;**43**(3):219-222

[100] Singleton BK, Green CA, Avent ND, Martin PG, Smart E, Daka A, et al. The presence of an RHD pseudogene containing a 37 base pair duplication and a nonsense mutation in Africans with the Rh D-negative blood group phenotype. Blood. 2000;**95**:12-18

[101] van der Schoot CE, Tax GH, Rijnders RJ, de Haas M, Christiaens GC. Prenatal typing of Rh and Kell blood group system antigens: The edge of a watershed. Transfusion Medicine Reviews. 2003;**17**(1):31-44

[102] Chan FY, Cowley NM, Wolter L, Stone M, Carmody F, Saul A, et al. Prenatal RHD gene determination and dosage analysis by PCR: Clinical evaluation. Prenatal Diagnosis. 2001;**21**(4):321-326

[103] Hromadnikova I, Vesela K, Benesova B, Nekovarova K, Duskova D, Vlk R, et al. Non-invasive fetal RHD and RHCE genotyping from maternal plasma in alloimmunized pregnancies. Prenatal Diagnosis. 2005;**25**(12):1079-1083

[104] Clausen FB, Christiansen M, Steffensen R, et al. Report of the first nationally implemented clinical routine screening for fetal RHD in D− pregnant women to ascertain the requirement for antenatal RhD prophylaxis. Transfusion. 2012;**52**:752-758

[105] Lindemburg ITM, van Kamp IL, van Zwet EW, et al. Increased perinatal loss after intrauterine transfusion for alloimmune anaemia before 20 weeks of gestation. BJOG: An International Journal of Obstetrics and Gynaecology. 2013;**120**:847-852

[106] Rodeck CH, Deans A. Red cell alloimmunisation. In: Rodeck CH, Whittle MJ, editors. Fetal Medicine: Basic Science and Clinical Practice.

2nd ed. London: Churchill Livingstone; 2008. pp. P559-P577

[107] Howard H, Martlew V, McFaden I, Clarke C, Duguid J, Bromilow I, et al. Consequences for fetus and neonate of maternal red cell Allo-immunisation. Archives of Disease in Childhood—Fetal and Neonatal Edition. 1998;**78**:F62-F66

[108] Koelewijn JM, Vrijkotte TG, van der Schoot CE, Bonsel GJ, de Haas M. Effect of screening for red cell antibodies, other than anti-D, to detect hemolytic disease of the fetus and newborn: A population study in the Netherlands. Transfusion. 2008;**48**(5):941-952

[109] Smith HM, Shirey RS, Thoman SK, Jackson JB. Prevalence of clinically significant red blood cell alloantibodies in pregnant women at a large tertiary-care facility. Immunohematology. 2013;**29**:127-130

[110] Meena S, Renu B, Naveen A, Vijay S. Prevalence, specificity and titration of red cell alloantibodies in multiparous antenatal females at a tertiary care Centre from North India. Indian Journal of Hematology and Blood Transfusion. 2016;**32**(3):307-311

[111] Finck R, Lui-Deguzman C, Teng SM, Davis R, Yuan S. Comparison of a gel microcolumn assay with the conventional tube test for red blood cell alloantibody titration. Transfusion. 2013;**53**(4):811-815

[112] Ebbing C, Rasmussen S, Kiserud T. Middle cerebral artery blood flow velocities and pulsatility index and the cerebroplacental pulsatility ratio: Longitudinal reference ranges and terms for serial measurements. Ultrasound in Obstetrics & Gynecology. 2007;**30**(3):287-296

[113] Steiner EA, Judd WJ, Combs M, Watkins K, Weissman P, Mann N, et al. Prenatal antibody titers by the gel test. In: Scientific Abstract, Ortho Clinical Diagnostics. 2002 AABB Annual Meeting Presentation. 2002

[114] Mari G, Deter RL. Non-invasive diagnosis by doppler ultrasonography of foetal anaemia due to maternal red-cell alloimmunization. New England Journal of Medicine. 2000;**342**:9-14

[115] Kumlien G. Comparing the tube and gel techniques for ABO antibody titration, as performed in three European centers. Transplantation. 2007;**84**:S17-S19

[116] Hill EA, Bryant BJ. Comparison of antibody titers in donor specimens and associated AS-1 leukoreduced donor units. Transfusion. 2014;**54**(6):1580-1584

[117] Schwartz J, Winters JL, Padmanabhan A, et al. Guidelines on the use of therapeutic apheresis in clinical practice-evidence-based approach from the Writing Committee of the American Society for Apheresis: The sixth special issue. Journal of Clinical Apheresis. 2013;**28**(3):145-284

[118] Booth GS, Gehrie EA, Bolan CD, Savani BN. Clinical guide to ABO incompatible allogeneic stem cell transplantation. Biology of Blood and Marrow Transplantation. 2013;**19**(8):1152-1158

[119] Adriaansen MJ, Perry HE. Validation of column agglutination technology for blood group alloantibody titration. New Zealand Institute of Medical Laboratory Science. 2013;**67**:92-96

[120] Judd WJ, Luban NLC, Ness PM, Silberstein LE, Stroup M, Widmann FK. Prenatal and perinatal immunohematology: Recommendations for serological management of the fetus, newborn, infant and obstetric patients. Transfusion. 1990;**30**(2):175-183

[121] British Committee for Standards in Haematology. Guidelines for blood grouping and red cell antibody testing during pregnancy. 2008

[122] Semmekrot BA, de Man AJ, Boekkooi PF. Irregular blood group antibodies during pregnancy: Screening is mandatory. Nederlands Tijdschrift voor Geneeskunde. 1999;**143**:449-452

[123] Bowman JM. Controversies in Rh prophylaxis. Who needs Rh immune globulin and when should it be given? American Journal of Obstetrics and Gynecology. 1985;**151**(3):289-294

[124] ACOG. Prevention of Rh D Alloimmunization. ACOG Practice Bulletin Number 4. Washington, DC: American College of Obstetricians and Gynaecologists; 1999

[125] Bowman JM. The prevention of Rh immunization. Transfusion Medicine Reviews. 1988;**2**(3):129-150

[126] Provan D, Stasi R, Newland AC, et al. International consensus report on the investigation and management of primary immune thrombocytopenia. Blood. 2010;**115**(2):168-186

[127] National Institute for Health and Clinical Excellence (NICE). Routine antenatal anti-D prophylaxis for women who are rhesus D negative) (National Institute for Health and Clinical Excellence (NICE CG156)). 2008

[128] Klein HG, Anstee DJ. Haemolytic disease of the fetus and newborn. In: Mollison's Blood Transfusion in Clinical Medicine. 11th ed. Oxford: Blackwell; 2005. pp. 496-545

[129] Chilcott J, Lloyd Jones M, Wight J, Forman K, Wray J, Beverley C, et al. A Review of the Clinical Effectiveness and Cost-Effectiveness of Routine Anti-D Prophylaxis for Pregnant Women Who Are Rhesus-Negative. NIHR Health Technology Assessment Programme: Executive Summaries. Southampton (UK): NIHR Journals Library; 2003

[130] National Institute for Health and Clinical Excellence. Overview—Routine antenatal anti-D prophylaxis for Rh D-negative women. 2008

[131] WHO Reproductive Health Library. WHO Recommendation on Antenatal Anti-D Immunoglobulin Prophylaxis. (December 2016). The WHO Reproductive Health Library. Geneva: World Health Organization; 2016

[132] Jim C, Paul T, Myfanwy LJ, Jeremy W, Katie F, Julie W, et al. The economics of routine antenatal anti-D prophylaxis for pregnant women who are rhesus negative. BJOG: An International Journal of Obstetrics and Gynaecology. 2004;**111**(9):903-907

[133] Udomah FP, Isaac IZ, Aliyu N, Erhabor O, Ahmed MH, et al. Haemoglobin electrophoretic patterns, ABO and rhesus D blood groups distribution among antenatal women in Sokoto, Nigeria. Obstetrics and Gynaecology Cases—Reviews. 2015;**2**:034-037

[134] Golassa L, Tsegaye A, Erko B, Mamo H. High Rhesus (Rh (D)) negative frequency and ethnic-group based ABO blood group distribution in Ethiopia. BMC Research Notes. 2017;**10**(1):330

[135] Downe S, Finlayson K, Tunçalp Ö, Gülmezoglu AM. Factors that influence the provision of good quality routine antenatal care services by health staff: A qualitative evidence synthesis. Cochrane Database of Systematic Reviews. 2016;**2016**

[136] Thakral B, Saluja K, Sharma RR, Marwaha N. Red cell alloimmunization in a transfused patient population: A study from a tertiary care hospital in North India. Hematology. 2008;**13**(5):313-318

[137] Bujandrić NB, Grujić JN, Krga-Milanović MM. Transfusion management of patients with red blood cell antibodies. Medicinski Pregled. 2013;**66**(11-12):491-496

[138] Pandey H, Das SS, Chaudhary R. Red cell alloimmunization in transfused patients: A silent epidemic revisited. Asian Journal of Transfusion Science. 2014;**8**(2):75-77

[139] Natukunda B, Schonewille H, van de Watering L, Brand A. Prevalence and specificities of red blood cell alloantibodies in transfused Ugandans with different diseases. Vox Sanguinis. 2010;**98**(2):167-171

[140] Pahuja S, Pujani M, Gupta SK, Chandra J, Jain M. Alloimmunization and red cell autoimmunization in multi transfused thalassaemic of Indian origin. Haematology. 2010;**15**:174-177

[141] Zimring JC, Welniak L, Semple JW, Ness PM, Slichter SJ, Spitalnik SL, et al. Current problems and future directions of transfusion-induced alloimmunization: Summary of an NHLBI working group. Transfusion. 2011;**51**:435-441

[142] Daniels G, Poole J, de Silva M, Callaghan T, MacLennan S, Smith N. The clinical significance of blood group antibodies. Transfusion Medicine. 2002;**12**:287-295

[143] Bayliss KM, Kueck BD, Johnson ST, Fueger JT, McFadden PW, Mikulski D, et al. Detecting fetomaternal hemorrhage: A comparison of five methods. Transfusion. 1991;**31**(4):303-307

[144] Kim YA, Makar RS. Detection of fetomaternal hemorrhage. American Journal of Hematology. 2012;**87**(4):417-423

[145] Pelikan DM, Mesker WE, Scherjon SA, Kanhai HH, Tanke HJ. Improvement of the Kleihauer-Betke test by automated detection of fetal erythrocytes in maternal blood. Cytometry. Part B, Clinical Cytometry. 2003;**54**(1):1-9

[146] Renshaw AA. An accurate and precise methodology for routine determination of the false-negative rate of Papanicolaou smears screening. Cancer. 2001;**93**(2):86-92

[147] Raafat A, Fraser N, Main R, Urbaniak SJ. A quality assurance scheme for the Kleihauer test: The Scottish experience 1988-1996. Transfusion Medicine. 1997;**7**:221-226

[148] Duguid JK, Bromilow IM. Laboratory measurement of fetomaternal hemorrhage and its clinical relevance. Transfusion Medicine Reviews. 1999;**13**:43-48

[149] Iyer R, McElhinney B, Heasley N. False positive Kleihauer tests and unnecessary administration of anti-D immunoglobulin. Clinical and Laboratory Haematology. 2003;**25**:405-408

[150] Chen JC, Bigelow N, Davis BH. Proposed flow cytometric reference method for the determination of erythroid F-cell counts. Cytometry. 2000;**42**:239-246

[151] Davis BH, Olsen S, Bigelow NC, Chen JC. Detection of foetal red cells in fetomaternal haemorrhage using a foetal haemoglobin monoclonal antibody by flow cytometry. Transfusion. 1998;**38**:749-756

[152] British Committee for Standards in Haematology (BCSH—b). Guidelines for the use of platelet transfusions. British Journal of Haematology. 2003;**122**:10-23

[153] Menitove JE. Immunoprophylaxis for D negative patients receiving platelet

transfusion from D negative donors. Transfusion. 2002;**42**:136-138

[154] Royal College of Obstetrics and Gynaecologists. The management of gestational trophoblastic disease. 2010

[155] Royal College of Obstetrics and Gynaecologists. The Use of Anti-D Immunoglobulin for Rhesus D Prophylaxis. 2011

Section 3

Treatments

Chapter 7

Alternative Immune-Mediated-Based Methods in the Aplastic Anemia Treatment

Vivian Gonzaga, Bruna Policiquio, Cristiane Wenceslau and Irina Kerkis

Abstract

Acquired aplastic anemia (AA) is characterized by partial or total bone marrow (BM) destruction resulting in pancytopenia. Most of the acquired AA is the result of autoimmune condition the imbalance between T-regulatory cells (Treg), abnormal cytokines production and cytotoxic T cells activation, leading to the hematopoietic stem cells (HSCs) death. The first-line treatment is given by HSC transplant, but some patients did not respond to the treatment. Therefore, new technologies need to treat AA nonresponder patients. Studies are in progress to test the efficacy of stem cell-based therapeutic as mesenchymal stem cells (MSCs), which confer low immunogenicity and are reliable allogeneic transplants in refractory severe AA cases. Furthermore, MSCs comprise the BM stromal niche and have an important role in supporting hematopoiesis by secreting regulatory cytokines, providing stimulus to natural BM microenvironment. In addition, MSCs have immunomodulatory property and are candidates for efficient supporting AA therapy.

Keywords: allogeneic transplant, mesenchymal stem cell, immune-mediated aplastic anemia, paracrine effects, immunomodulation

1. Introduction

Aplastic anemia (AA) is a rare disease, caused by bone marrow (BM) aggression resulting in hypo or aplastic BM with precocious fat replacement and consequently to peripheral blood pancytopenia [1, 2]. The autoimmunity process in AA occurs due to the activation of the oligoclonal cytotoxic T cells that will lead the hematopoietic cells to apoptosis. Its triggering occurs by the imbalance between CD8 +, CD4 +, T-Helper (Th), Th type 1 (Th1), Th type 2 (Th2), Th17 type (Th17), Natural Killer (NK) and T-regulatory cells (Treg). Besides, there is also an abnormal production of proinflammatory cytokines, such as tumor necrosis factor-alpha (TNF-α), interferon-gamma (IFN-γ) and transformed growth factor (TGF) [3–7].

For severe cases, immunosuppressive therapy is accepted as the first-line treatment option and the allogeneic transplantation of BM and hematopoietic stem cells (HSCs). However, 30–40% of patients with severe aplastic anemia (SAA) remain pancytopenia following the treatment. The transplant option still has a restricted number of compatibility between suitable donors. Additionally, patients aged >50 years are not eligible for transplant [8].

A new viable alternative for the treatment of AA has been sought and the use of mesenchymal stem (MSCs) therapy may be a promising therapeutic candidate mainly because of their hypoimmunogenicity and the lack of rejection after transplants and immunomodulatory effects, which may promote decreasing the symptoms of the disease [9, 10]. These benefits are attributed to the paracrine effects, above all by its ability to regulate the immune system [11].

Actually, is known that MSCs have wide therapeutically potential attributed by paracrine effects and the past decades have seen explosion research directed to understand better these MSCs mechanism and function [12]. One of the main and most important features of MSCs is the low expression of human leukocyte antigen (HLA) class I, with no expression of HLA class II. This feature allows the cell to be characterized as hypoimmunogenic, since it does not stimulate the patient's immune system and can be used safely in transplants [13]. More recently, the studies showed that the main cause of AA is autoimmunity. Through the secretion of bioactive molecules, MSCs have the capacity of regulating immune responses. The mechanism of MSCs may decrease secretion of proinflammatory cytokines such as transforming growth factor (TGF), IFN-γ TNF-α, interleukin (IL)-17 and increase secretion of many soluble mediators, including anti-inflammatory cytokines stimulation that inhibit antigen-presenting cells (APCs) functions, which are capable to decrease proliferation of dendritic cells (DCs) and regulate macrophage activity by polarizing proinflammatory phenotype (M1) to anti-inflammatory phenotype (M2) [14, 15]. Therefore, the decrease of B cells proliferation and antibodies production and adjustment of T cells activities as well as inhibit the proliferation of cytotoxic T cells and stimulate Treg activity [16].

MSCs therapy has gained space due to its vast therapeutic potentials such as immunomodulation mechanisms and main safety as bioproduct. Thus, this chapter will discuss the challenges of allogeneic MSCs as an alternative for an efficient therapeutic in AA immune-mediated treatment.

2. Aplastic anemia: general features

AA is a disorder characterized by BM hypocellularity, and peripheral blood pancytopenia due to a deficit of HSCs. It affects mostly children, young adults, and adults, over 60 years of age [17]. This condition can be similar to other hematologic disorders, however, in most cases, the AA is caused by reduced HSCs function, an increase in HSCs apoptosis level, consequently, the decreased of HSCs and hematopoietic progenitors and lastly, microenvironment fat replacement [18, 19].

Following the patient diagnosis, AA can be considered as moderate or severe. The patients with pancytopenia may present symptoms of anemia purpura or skin hemorrhage, and in most of the cases there is an infection association, that may worsen the symptoms [20]. Three main criteria are used for the diagnostic: neutrophil count lower than 0.5×10^9 cells/L, reticulocyte count lower than 1% and platelet count lower than 20×10^9 cells/L [21]. To confirm acquired AA, the clinical case must be differentiated from other hematological diseases, as well as from the signs of malignant cell transformation or myelodysplasia [22].

Normally the first AA etiology is uncertain and for this reason, the disorder is considered heterogeneous in origin and characterized as idiopathic [23]. AA is associated with exposures to chemical agents (pesticides and benzene), cytotoxic drugs (antineoplastics, antibiotics, non-steroidal anti-inflammatory drugs), active viral infections exposure (Epstein Barr, hepatitis virus, human immunodeficiency virus parvovirus) and radiation exposure [18, 24, 25]. However, these causes considered secondary etiologies, since the studies are directed to the primary etiology of AA to autoimmunity [26, 27]. AA pathogenesis involves an immunity dysfunction, initially provoked by the activated T cells [23], which leads to an abnormal hematopoietic microenvironment, destruction of hematopoietic stem/progenitor cell and differentiation deficiency. These findings suggest that the immune system plays an important role in the pathogenesis of AA.

2.1 AA pathophysiology

Currently, the studies of AA etiology are focused on the immune mechanism of hematopoietic cells destruction. Many researchers [28, 29–31] have demonstrated that the dysfunction of T cells might be a key factor in recent characterization as an autoimmune disease [28]. Most of the acquired AA is the result of an immune-mediated process as an imbalance between CD8+ and CD4+ T cells, including Th1, Th2, Treg and Th17 cells, NK, and natural killer T cells (NK T) that leads to apoptosis of BM cells triggered by cytotoxic T cells activation [6, 17].

The abnormal immunoregulatory cell functions observed in AA can be attributable to abnormal antigen stimulation and some inappropriate T cells activation [28]. Studies demonstrated that patients with AA have a significantly increased proportion of Th1 cells, and showed a reduced fraction of natural killer T cells and regulatory T cells, together with an increased level of TNF-α, a consequent elevation of IL-6, IL-8, and IL17 productions [18]. Additionally, there is also an abnormal production of proinflammatory cytokines including IFN-γ and TGF [4, 5, 28, 32]. The new T cells subset was characterized as Th17 and currently is known that both Th17 cells and the cytokine IL-17, which is secreted by Th17 cells, also is in an association with AA pathogenesis [31]. Studies showed that AA patients who presented an increase in the frequency of Th17 cells had a positive correlation with an increase in the IFN- γ and IL-17 expression. Autoimmunity promotes inflammatory Th17 immune responses that contributed to disease pathophysiology [29].

Otherwise, AA is attributed to inappropriate antigen stimulation and abnormal APCs activation [28], resulting in the priming of T cells specific for hematopoietic cells [33, 34]. APCs exhibit a significant increase in the expression of major histocompatibility class 2 (MHCII), increasing the recognition of CD4+ T cells. In AA, T cells are also stimulated by unknown antigens or abnormal APC activation as DCs and macrophages, which trigger a series of immune responses. Studies have shown that immunoregulatory cell dysfunction leads to a corresponding immune tolerance disorder and renders the body unable to recognize autologous hematopoietic cells [28].

Although the definitive mechanism has not been identified, some genetic factors are the targets of ongoing research, such as the molecular basis of the aberrant immune response and hematopoietic cell deficiency, telomere repair gene mutations in the target cells and unregulated T cell activation pathways and cytokine genes polymorphisms [9, 26, 28]. These changes in the nucleotide sequence and gene regulation are associated with an increased immune response and suggest a genetic basis for aberrant T cells activation in BM failure [35].

2.2 AA treatment

The treatment depends on the severity of the disease, once for moderate cases are based on red blood cell (RBC) transfusions, on platelet transfusions to prevent bleeding, and on supportive care in association with antibiotic aiming to reestablish blood cell volume and prevent secondary infections [17]. However, the pancytopenia of many moderate cases may progress to severe [21]. For severe cases, immunosuppressive therapy is accepted as a first-line treatment option. However, 30–40% of patients with SAA remain pancytopenia following the treatment. Patients with SAA, which are refractory or have a relapse after immunosuppressive treatment, may undergo allogeneic hematopoietic stem cells transplantation (HSCT). However, about one-third of patients do not have a suitable donor for HSCT. Additionally, patients aged >50 years are not eligible for transplant [8].

Furthermore, the immunosuppressive drug treatment has several side effects on patients. On the other hand, the patients often do not respond adequately to the therapies and are not suitable for life treatment (refractory patients) [24]. Therefore, immunosuppressive drugs are considered supporting AA treatment, once it does not promote the cure [20].

2.3 Allogeneic transplantation and alternative methods for AA treatment

Generally, patients are treated with allogeneic HSCs or whole BM transplantations, which replace since HSCs, hematopoietic precursors, until differentiated bloodstream cells and immune system cells. However, in all types of transplants, the treatment involves a combination of immunosuppressive agents or radiation therapy to prevent and to eliminate residual host BM [24]. The transplantation success varies according to risk factors, such as age and mainly histocompatibility allogeneic HLA-matched sibling donors, which are rare for the majority of patients. Despite being well established for many years, the transplanted patients can trigger late complications, such as the development of graft versus host disease (GVHD) and infections, especially in patients who have received hematopoietic grafts from HLA antigen matched donor [36, 37]. Studies show that the incidence of GVHD after unrelated donor transplantation can achieve ~14%, and overall survival index was 57% for all 8 HLA-loci matched transplants and 39% for 1-loci mismatched transplant [38]. Thus, for BM and HSCT, the immediate challenge is the extension of stem cell therapies to all patients, regardless of age, with a histocompatible sibling [24].

Since then a new viable alternative for the treatment of AA has been sought and the use of MSCs transplantation becomes of choice. The MSCs therapy may be a promising therapeutic candidate mainly because of their hypoimmunogenicity, the lack of rejection after transplants and immunomodulatory effects, which may promote decreasing the symptoms of the disease [39]. These benefits are attributed to MSCs paracrine effects, above all to their ability to regulate the immune system. MSCs may help for AA treatment, especially for autoimmune type [11].

3. Mesenchymal stem cell: general features

MSCs are multipotent progenitors, which were first isolated from an adult organism by Friedenstein and colleagues in 1968, and described years later by Caplan and colleagues [40, 41]. These cells include firstly an inherent autocrine effect, as self-renewal and differentiation potential for a variety of cell types, as main adipocytes, osteoclasts, and chondrocytes [42], depending on the surrounding microenvironment conditions [43]. Currently, such cells have shown to be isolated from many postnatal and adult tissues, such as adipose tissue, umbilical cord, placenta, dental pulp, and others [44, 45].

Initially, the mechanism therapeutic potential of the MSCs was based only on the potential for regeneration through cellular self-renewal and its plasticity.

Further studies have shown low engraft of MSCs in injured areas that questioned the hypothesis that MSCs repair tissue damage by replacing cell loss with newly differentiated cells [46, 47].

3.1 MSC: paracrine effects

It is known that MSCs have wide therapeutically potential attributed to paracrine effects and the past decades explosion research was directed to understand better these MSCs mechanism and function [12]. Although the therapeutic mechanisms of MSCs are not yet well characterized, it is possible to say that their paracrine effects consist in the secretion of bioactive molecules such as a variety of cytokines and growth factors as like anti-inflammatory, anti-apoptotic and angiogenic [46–51].

MSCs can to migrate to the lesion site through signals from specific chemokines. This process called homing consists of the steps of activating adhesion molecules, rolling to the endothelium, adhesion, and migration to the tissue that is the source of chemokine inflammation production [52, 53]. The current hypothesis is that paracrine factors secreted by MSCs promote protective microenvironment and repair by local tissue-resident progenitor populations, favoring the hypothesis of detecting favorable effects even in the absence of the cells at lesion sites [54].

3.2 MSC: immunogenic effect and safety for transplantation

One of the main and most important features of MSC is the low expression of HLA class I, with no expression of HLA class II. Also, MSCs do not appear to express the co-stimulatory molecules CD80 or CD86 required for effector T cell induction [55]. The absence of co-stimulatory molecules implies that any residual engagement of the T cell receptor on Th cells would result in absence of the normal immune response to a particular antigen and contribute to tolerance rather than allogeneic responses. This feature allows the cell to be characterized as hypoimmunogenic, since it does not stimulate the patient's immune system and can be used safely in transplants [113]. As well, MSCs have properties attributed to immune functions, indicating their ability to immunomodulatory activity. Studies indicated that MSCs can regulate immune responses during chronic inflammation through the innate and adaptive immune system, regulating the recruitment and their function [56, 57].

3.3 MSC: immunomodulatory potential

The paracrine effects of MSCs may have great importance in the treatment of autoimmune diseases. Through the secretion of bioactive molecules, MSCs have the capacity of regulating immune responses. These cells can regulate adaptive immune responses through multiple redundant pathways, interacting with various immune cells and secreting soluble mediators such as IL-6, IL-10, prostaglandin E2 (PGE2), nitric oxide (NO), transforming growth factor-β1 (TGF-β1), and hepatocyte growth factor (HGF), indoleamine-pyrrole 2, 3-dioxygenase (IDO) [58, 59]. They can regulate APCs activity, decreasing maturation and proliferation of DCs [14]. MSC also may regulate macrophage activity by polarizing its pro-inflammatory phenotype (M1) to its anti-inflammatory phenotype (M2) [15]. Therefore, suppress T cell proliferation and activation and regulate the differentiation of Th cells and act on the humoral response by inhibiting of B cell activation and antibody production [60]. MSCs may also reduce pro-inflammatory cytokines proliferation, such TNF-α, which has an important role of the pathogenesis of autoimmune diseases and chronic inflammation (**Figure 1**) [14, 16, 61].

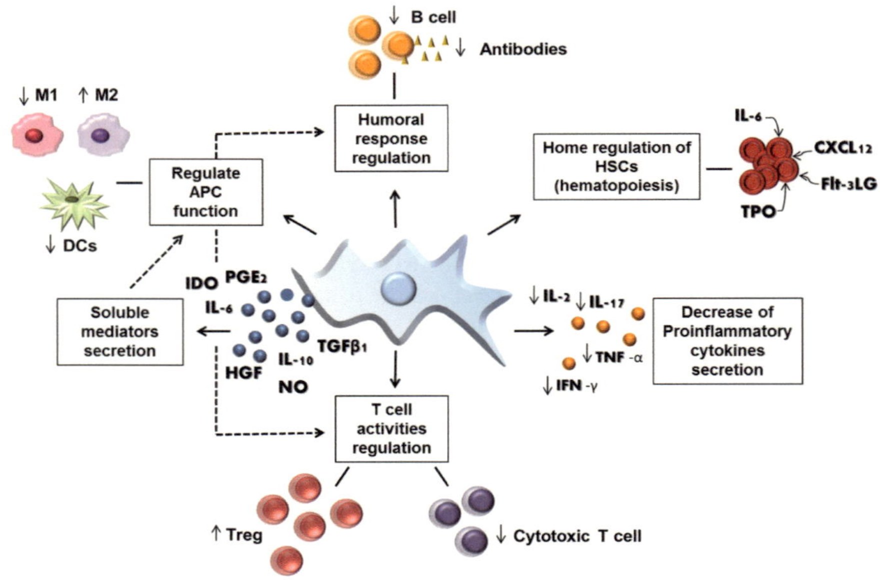

Figure 1.
Benefits of MSCs paracrine effect (immunomodulatory) on immune cells imbalance. MSCs secrete many soluble mediators, including anti-inflammatory cytokines stimulation that regulates APCs functions capable to decrease proliferation of DCs and regulate macrophage activity by polarizing proinflammatory phenotype (M1) to anti-inflammatory phenotype (M2). Therefore, they are responsible for humoral response regulation by the decrease of B cells proliferation and antibodies production. The APCs are also capable to regulate the T cell activities as well as inhibit cytotoxic T cell proliferation and upregulation and increase of Treg cells. MSCs may also promote the decrease of proinflammatory cytokines secretion. And act on the homing regulation of HSCs mechanism on stages of adhesion, expansion, and migration through chemokine and other factors secretion.

4. MSC mechanism in AA treatment

The first paracrine effect, showed for MSCs, was the capacity to support HSCs growth *in vitro*. Afterward, adipose tissue (AT) – derived MSCs also supported HSCs growth *in vitro* [62, 63]. Therefore, the most successful clinical application of MSCs is involved in the hematological disease.

At BM microenvironment, MSCs niche supports hematopoietic cells and produce factors recruiting HSCs and supporting hematopoiesis [64]. This mechanism occurs through chemokine secretion of C-X-C motif chemokine ligand 12 (CXCL12), which acts on the homing regulation of HSCs, regulating the stages of adhesion, expansion and migration [65, 66]. The secretion of other factors is also important in the proliferation of HSCs mechanisms such as Flt-3 ligand (FLT3LG) [67], thrombopoietin (TPO) [68] and IL-6 [17]. That despite being a proinflammatory cytokine in general, when IL-6 is secreted in BM microenvironment, is capable to stimulate hematopoiesis [69, 70].

More recently, the studies showed that the main cause of AA is autoimmunity. This process occurs in the result of an imbalance between CD8 + and CD4 + T cells, including Th1, Th2, Th17, NK, leading to the death of hematopoietic cells and their precursors [28]. Many studies have hypothesized that the onset of the immune imbalance in AA begins by stimulating APCs through an unknown antigen resulting in the T cells activation [71]. Another important mechanism of MSCs is the immunomodulation mechanism. MSCs can act directly on AA imbalance by T cells suppression, inhibiting activation and proliferation of T cells [72]. MSCs also inhibit the secretion of two important cytokines present in the pathology of AA, the

AA disorders x MSC benefits	
Aberrant secretion of pro-inflammatory cytokines ↑IFN-γ ↑TNF-α ↑IL-17 ↑IL-2;	Immunomodulatory effect: Decreased secretion of proinflammatory cytokines, ↓IFN-γ ↓TNF-α ↓IL-17 ↓IL-2;
Imbalance between CD8+ and CD4+ T cells; ↑ Cytotoxic T cell ↓Treg	Regulation of T cell activity and Treg cell proliferation ↓ Cytotoxic T cell ↑Treg
Apoptosis of HSC and progenitor cells ↑ Apoptosis	Protect BM by antiapoptotic properties ↓ Apoptosis
BM hypoplasia	Recovery of BM ↑ Hematopoiesis improvements ↑ CXCL12 ↑FLT3LG ↑TPO ↑IL-6
Abnormal APC activation ↑ DCs ↑ Macrophage	Regulate APCs functions ↓ DCs maturation and proliferation and ↓ Macrophages M1 activation ↑ Macrophages M2 activation
Abnormal humoral response ↑ B cells ↑ Antibodies production	Regulate humoral response ↓ B cells ↓ Antibodies production
Irregular activity of NK cells ↑ Cytotoxicity of NK cells	↓ Cytotoxicity of NK cells

MSC can decrease secretion of pro-inflammatory cytokines such as TGF, IFN-γ TNF-α, IL-17, regulate T cell activity, inhibit proliferation of cytotoxic T cells and stimulate Treg activity. MSC has anti-apoptotic properties, protects BM environment and recovery BM through cytoprotective effect and stimulates macrophages M2 activation and hematopoiesis improvements. MSCs may also regulate APCs functions, humoral response, and cytotoxicity of NK cells.

Table 1.
Table shows disorders characterized in AA and the mechanism of action of MSCs in AA pathology.

INF-γ and TNF-α and stimulate the proliferation of Treg, promoting the production of the anti-inflammatory cytokine IL-10 **Table 1** [73, 74]. In addition, some studies also show that MSCs also acts through its anti-apoptotic effects [75].

5. Biodistribution and engraftment of allogeneic MSC in BM

In the last years, several studies have been exploring intravenous administrations (IV) due to being safe and do not present morbidity risk for patients. However, still lack the data about the biodistribution mechanism of MSCs and about how these cells engraftment on the target organ, which is essential for the success of clinical studies. It is known that the biodistribution is influenced in vivo and in vitro conditions. Stromal cell-derived factor 1 (SDF-1) (also known as CXCL12) is upregulated at sites of injury and acts as a chemoattractant to recruit circulating or residing MSCs expressing its cognate receptor CXC chemokine receptor 4 (CXCR4). It has been demonstrated that the CXCR4-SDF-1 axis is critical for BM homing [76]. Diverse studies demonstrate that some in vitro conditions may influence the expression of adhesion molecules [77, 78]. For instance, long expansion periods [79] and cells culturing at high density may reduce CXCR4 cell expression; the cells cultured at higher confluence secrete more metalloproteinase inhibitor 3, which decreases migration of MSCs when compared to those cultured at the low confluence [80]. Hypoxia condition may increase CXCR4 expression; on the other hand, hypoxia may decrease matrix metalloproteinase-2 secretion and an increase in membrane-type 1 matrix metalloproteinase [81].

In vivo engraftment is influenced by interactions of MSCs with different types of immune cells that depend on their ability to respond to signals from the immune system. On the other hands, the MSCs biodistribution and homing depend on the host niche. Interesting the MSCs migration and homing to target tissue can be influenced positively by irradiation. It has been demonstrated an increased absolute number of human MSCs in the brain, heart, bone marrow, and muscles after total body irradiation and MSCs IV administrations in mice, when compared to the untreated control [82].

Some animal studies evidence that MSCs can engraftment in BM after systemic administration [83]. Studies in patients showed MSCs engraftment into BM 30 days after the second MSCs IV administration. Although, after MSCs infusion was observed no recovery of hematopoietic tissue, interstitial hemorrhage, edema, and all adipocytic necrosis disappeared in BM [84]. Other studies indicate the engraftment due to myeloid and plated recovery after HSCs and MSCs transplantation [85, 86].

6. MSC use in clinical studies

6.1 Clinical potential and market of MSC in hematopoietic disorders

MSCs have been implicated in immunomodulatory therapy, in particular, in GVHD treatment and as an adjunct to hematopoietic stem cell transplantation (HSCT) to help enhance engraftment [87, 88]. The first major clinical trial of MSCs (Prochymal) was for the treatment of steroid-refractory of GVHD (NCT00366145) [89, 90]. The primary endpoint of the study was complete remission at day 28 after allogeneic BM-MSCs infusion but was not significantly increased compared to placebo [89, 91]. In 2012, MSCs have bens conditional approval to treat children GVHD in Canada, based on subset analysis that suggested children with GVHD were responsive to MSCs [89, 92, 93]. Many new studies have been developed in recent years; however, a few of them have attempted to look at biological correlates of response to therapy. Isolated studies reported serum biomarkers of GVHD severity including IL-2, *tumor necrosis factor receptor 1* (TNFR1), regenerating islet-derived protein 3 alpha (Reg3a), and levels of inflammatory cytokines, which not clearly correlate with the response in humans. More studies are needed to obtain correlative research data [94, 95]. This outcome results in the first Food and Drug Administration (FDA) approved MSCs product in the United States [96, 97].

6.2 Clinical studies with MSC in combination to HSCT transplantation for treat AA

Cotransplantation of HSCs with (umbilical cord) UC-MSCs has been performed to study whether the last will be able to support hematopoiesis, enhance the engraftment of HSCs, and reduce the incidence of GVHD following HSCT [98–100]. These studies include adult and children in AA patients [101, 102]. Stem cells application was mainly intravenous. In some of the studies multiple (five) infusions were used. All clinical protocols have been developed in the presence of traditional immunosuppressive protocol to prevent GVHD manifestation [98–102].

One pioneer study, where the conditioning of patients was myeloablative or reduced, followed BM-MSCs treatment together with allogeneic HSCT. This study showed that co-transplantation of MSCs resulted in fast engraftment of absolute neutrophil count and platelets and 100% donor chimerism [87]. In turn, Yamei and co-workers (2014) demonstrate prolonged survival (follow up of 78 months) in 80.9% patients after cotransplantation of the culture-expanded third party donor-derived UC-MSCs in 21 young people with SAA undergoing haplo-HSCT [103]. Even so, the patients did not show infusion toxicity. This study showed that MSCs support *in vivo* normal hematopoiesis and display potent immunosuppressive effects. The other metacentric study shows that cotransplantation of BM-MSCs and haplo-HSCT could reduce the risk of graft failure and severe GVHD in SAA [104]. Similar data were obtained in a study that used cotransplantation of haploidentical HSCs and BM-MSCs into children with SAA without an HLA-identical sibling donor. It was shown that such cotransplantation seems to be safe and may improve survival rates and reduce the risk of graft failure [105]. Another multicenter study, which explored cotransplantation of BM-MSCs with allo-HSCT, reported that such treatment could ameliorate clinical outcomes of a GVHD, viremia, and survival in allo-HSCT for AA patients [106].

6.3 Clinical studies with MSC for treat AA

Nowadays there a few clinical studies using only MSCs single to treat AA. All studies used MSCs isolated from BM s and adult patients with severe or non-severe AA and refractory. The via of MSCs administration used was IV and the number of administrations was 2 until 5 depending on study in combination with conventional immunosuppressive therapy.

The study development by Pang et al. showed, six of 18 patients (33.3%) achieved a complete response or a partial response to MSCs treatment [107]. In six patients, two achieved a complete response including recovery of three hematopoietic cell lines after MSCs therapy. Similar results was achieved by Cle et al. 2015 using MSCs being 22% of all patients (18 patients) presents hematologic response at 6 months after MSCs transplantation [108]. One clinical trial phase II conducted in China evaluated the MSC overall response rate and safety using a significant number of refractory AA younger patients (n = 72). The study performed full quality control of BM-MSCs production, which includes counts, viability, morphology, endotoxin, aseptic culture, immunophenotype. It was the first clinical study that showed significant results in BM functional recovery. The rate response of patients was 28.4% being that 6.8% complete response and 21.6% partial response after MSCs transplantation. Among patients with hematologic response, ten patients had normalization of cellularity BM followed for more than 1 year MSCs transplantation. Seven patients got adverse events such as fever and headaches. No other adverse events were observed in the study. At the follow-up endpoint, nine patients died. One patient with RAEB-II died of disease progression, two patients died of intracranial hemorrhages, and six patients died of serious infection [107]. In other two studies were reported adverse events such as, fever, hypoxemia, mild dyspnea and diarrhea during MSCs administration or some hours after MSCs injection, this phenomenon occurs in 2 of 16 patients [107] and 7 of the 18 patients [108]. None major adverse effects were reported in all studies during months of follow-up of each respective study. Fuillard et al., 2003 reported one death due to fungal infection and Cle et al. 2015 four patients died in consequence result of heart failure and bacterial or invasive fungal infections and none of the deaths in both studies were directly attributable to MSCs infusions [84, 108].

These preliminary studies support the concept that MSCs replacement can improve BM stroma and may alleviate symptoms severe and non-severe AA patients. However, larger studies with a significant number of patients are needed to evaluate the utility of MSCs further.

7. Conclusion and future perspectives

The progress in dissecting the underlying and complex pathophysiology of AA has been gain space over the past years in the hematology research community [26]. In addition to that, the need for an optimal alternative of a targeted treatment for this disorder. It is too soon to place the conventional AA treatment methods, but MSCs have gained space for demonstrating positive results in several AA clinical studies and other hematological diseases. The hypoimmunogenicity advantages, ensuring the absence of rejection in patients due to no expression of MHC class II, prevention and treatment of GVHD traditional transplants, and mainly immunomodulatory action presented [109]. Essential in the environment imbalance provoked by own immune system in people committed by the AA disorder. The MSCs are able in a modulating way to relieve the BM self-attack [110].

Contemporary, personalized therapies are famous in the whole scientific world. The MSCs may fit into this class due to their paracrine effects. These cells can assist in diverse situations such as: migration, injury recovery, stimulates cells renewal, death cell prevention, anti-inflammatory and modulation of the immune system to control the autoimmune environment [111]. Thus, MSCs have the heterogeneous capacity in varied therapies field. And the patient may have alternative use according to their needs.

In that event, the current way is providing the MSCs safety and acceptance by regulatory agencies as new biological product [112], which has already been proven to be more efficient than synthetic industries products [113]. And finally, implement the MSCs as ideal allogeneic transplant model, even for adequacy periods used as support for other established therapies.

Acknowledgements

Thanks to everyone on the Cellavita team who helped us so much. Special thanks to the company Cellavita Ltda., for financial and professional supporting. And to Butantan Institute, to providing us space and the research opportunity.

Conflict of interest

The authors declare no conflict of interest.

Author details

Vivian Gonzaga[1,2*], Bruna Policiquio[1], Cristiane Wenceslau[2] and Irina Kerkis[1*]

1 Laboratory of Genetics, Butantan Institute, São Paulo, SP, Brazil

2 CellAvita Ltd, Valinhos, SP, Brazil

*Address all correspondence to: vivia_gonzaga@hotmail.com and irina.kerkis@butantan.gov.br

References

[1] Medinger M, Drexler B, Lengerke C, Passweg J. Pathogenesis of acquired aplastic anemia and the role of the bone marrow microenvironment. Frontiers in Oncology. 2018;**8**:587. DOI: 10.3389/fonc.2018.00587

[2] Marsh JCW, Ball SE, Cavenagh J, Darbyshire P, Dokal I, Gordon-Smith EC, et al. Guidelines for the diagnosis and management of aplastic anaemia. British Journal of Haematology. 2009;**147**:43-70. DOI: 10.1111/j.1365-2141.2009.07842.x

[3] Zoumbos NC, Gascon P, Djeu JY, Young NS. Interferon is a mediator of hematopoietic suppression in aplastic anemia in vitro and possibly in vivo. Proceedings of the National Academy of Sciences. 1985;**82**(1):188-192. DOI: 10.1073/pnas.82.1.188

[4] Dubey S, Shukla P, Nityanand S. Expression of interferon-γ and tumor necrosis factor-α in bone marrow T cells and their levels in bone marrow plasma in patients with aplastic anemia. Annals of Hematology. 2005;**84**(9):572-577. DOI: 10.1007/s00277-005-1022-8

[5] Zeng W, Miyazato A, Chen G, Kajigaya S, Young NS, Maciejewski JP. Interferon-induced gene expression in CD34 cells: Identification of pathologic cytokine-specific signature profiles. Blood. 2006;**107**:167-175. DOI: 10.1182/blood-2005-05-1884

[6] Li JP, Zheng CL, Han ZC. Abnormal immunity and stem/progenitor cells in acquired aplastic anemia. Critical Reviews in Oncology/Hematology. 2010;**75**:79-93. DOI: 10.1016/j.critrevonc.2009.12.001

[7] Sloand E, Kim S, Maciejewski JP, Tisdale J, Follmann D, Young NS. Intracellular interferon-γ in circulating and marrow T cells detected by flow cytometry and the response to immunosuppressive therapy in patients with aplastic anemia. Blood. 2002;**100**(4):1185-1191. DOI: 10.1182/blood-2002-01-0035

[8] Bacigalupo A. How I treat acquired aplastic anemia. Blood. 2017;**129**(11):1428-1436. DOI: 10.1182/blood-2016-08-693481

[9] Ogawa S. Clonal hematopoiesis in acquired aplastic anemia. Blood. 2016;**128**:337-347. DOI: 10.1182/blood-2016-01-636381

[10] Broglie L, Margolis D, Medin JA. Yin and Yang of mesenchymal stem cells and aplastic anemia. World Journal of Stem Cells. 2017;**9**(12):219-226. DOI: 10.4252/wjsc.v9.i12.219

[11] Rad F, Ghorbani M, Mohammadi Roushandeh A, Habibi RM. Mesenchymal stem cell-based therapy for autoimmune diseases: Emerging roles of extracellular vesicles. Molecular Biology Reports. 2019;**46**:1533-1549. DOI: 10.1007/s11033-019-04588-y

[12] Marquez-Curtis LA, Janowska-Wieczorek A. Enhancing the migration ability of mesenchymal stromal cells by targeting the SDF-1/CXCR4 axis. BioMed Research International. 2013;**2013**. DOI: 10.1155/2013/561098

[13] Oliveira RL, Chagastelles PC, Sesterheim P, Pranke P. In vivo immunogenic response to allogeneic mesenchymal stem cells and the role of Preactivated mesenchymal stem cells Cotransplanted with allogeneic islets. Stem Cells International. 2017;**2017**. DOI: 10.1155/2017/9824698

[14] Zhao Q, Ren H, Han Z. Mesenchymal stem cells: Immunomodulatory capability and clinical potential in immune diseases. Journal of Cellular Immunotherapy. 2016;**2**:3-20. DOI: 10.1016/j.jocit.2014.12.001

[15] Nakajima H, Uchida K, Guerrero AR, Watanabe S, Sugita D, Takeura N, et al. Transplantation of mesenchymal stem cells promotes an alternative pathway of macrophage activation and functional recovery after spinal cord injury. Journal of Neurotrauma. 2012;**29**(8):1614-1625. DOI: 10.1089/neu.2011.2109

[16] Kaundal U, Bagai U, Rakha A. Immunomodulatory plasticity of mesenchymal stem cells: A potential key to successful solid organ transplantation. Journal of Translational Medicine. 2018;**16**(1):31. DOI: 10.1186/s12967-018-1403-0

[17] Gonzaga VF, Wenceslau CV, Lisboa GS, Frare EO, Kerkis I. Mesenchymal stem cell benefits observed in bone marrow failure and acquired aplastic Anemia. Stem Cells International. 2017;**2017**. DOI: 10.1155/2017/8076529

[18] Shipounova IN, Petrova TV, Svinareva DA, Momotuk KS, Mikhailova EA, Drize NI. Alterations in hematopoietic microenvironment in patients with aplastic anemia. Clinical and Translational Science. 2009;**2**(1):67-74. DOI: 10.1111/j.1752-8062.2008.00074.x

[19] Leguit RJ, Van Den Tweel JG. The pathology of bone marrow failure. Histopathology. 2010;**57**:655-670. DOI: 10.1111/j.1365-2559.2010.03612.x

[20] Scheinberg P. Aplastic anemia: Therapeutic updates in immunosuppression and transplantation. Hematology. American Society of Hematology. Education Program. 2012;**2012**:292-300. DOI: 10.1182/asheducation-2012.1.292

[21] Young NS. Introduction: Acquired aplastic anemia. Seminars in Hematology. 2000;**37**(1):2-2

[22] Rovó A, Dufour C, Tichelli A. Diagnosis of Acquired Aplastic Anemia. Congenital and Acquired Bone Marrow Failure. Elsevier Inc.; 2017. pp. 35-50. DOI: 10.1038/bmt.2012.230

[23] Dolberg OJ, Levy Y. Idiopathic aplastic anemia: Diagnosis and classification. Autoimmunity Reviews. 2014;**13**:569-573. DOI: 10.1016/j.autrev.2014.01.014

[24] Young NS. Current concepts in the pathophysiology and treatment of aplastic anemia. Hematology/the Education Program of the American Society of Hematology. 2013;**2013**:76-81. DOI: 10.1182/asheducation-2013.1.76

[25] Găman A, Găman G, Bold A. Acquired aplastic anemia: Correlation between etiology, pathophysiology, bone marrow histology and prognosis factors. Romanian Journal of Morphology and Embryology. 2009;**50**(4):669-674

[26] Shallis RM, Ahmad R, Zeidan AM. Aplastic anemia: Etiology, molecular pathogenesis, and emerging concepts. European Journal of Haematology. 2018;**101**:711-720. DOI: 10.1111/ejh.13153

[27] Baranski BGYN. Autoimmune aspects of aplastic anemia. In Vivo (Brooklyn). 1988;**2**(1):91-94

[28] Liu C, Sun Y, Shao Z. Current concepts of the pathogenesis of aplastic Anemia. Current Pharmaceutical Design. 2019;**25**(3):236-241. DOI: 10.2174/1381612825666190313113601

[29] De Latour RP, Visconte V, Takaku T, Wu C, Erie AJ, Sarcon AK, et al. Th17 immune responses contribute to the pathophysiology of aplastic anemia. Blood. 2010;**116**(20):4175-4184. DOI: 10.1182/blood-2010-01-266098

[30] Russell TB, Kurre P. Double-negative T cells are non-ALPS-specific markers of immune dysregulation found in patients with aplastic anemia. Blood.

2010;**116**:5072-5073. DOI: 10.1182/blood-2010-09-306910

[31] Du HZ, Wang Q, Ji J, Shen BM, Wei SC, Liu LJ, et al. Expression of IL-27, Th1 and Th17 in patients with aplastic anemia. Journal of Clinical Immunology. 2013;**33**(2):436-445. DOI: 10.1007/s10875-012-9810-0

[32] Hara T, Ando K, Tsurumi H, Moriwaki H. Excessive production of tumor necrosis factor-alpha by bone marrow T lymphocytes is essential in causing bone marrow failure in patients with aplastic anemia. European Journal of Haematology. 2004;**73**(1):10-16. DOI: 10.1111/j.1600-0609.2004.00259.x

[33] Stauder R, Valent P, Theurl I. Anemia at older age: Etiologies, clinical implications, and management. Blood. 2018;**131**(5):505-514. DOI: 10.1182/blood-2017-07-746446

[34] Feng X, Chuhjo T, Sugimori C, Kotani T, Lu X, Takami A, et al. Diazepam-binding inhibitor-related protein 1: A candidate autoantigen in acquired aplastic anemia patients harboring a minor population of paroxysmal nocturnal hemoglobinuria-type cells. Blood. 2004;**104**(8):2425-2431. DOI: 10.1182/blood-2004-05-1839

[35] Gupta S. Aplastic anemia. In: Pathobiology of Human Disease: A Dynamic Encyclopedia of Disease Mechanisms. Elsevier Inc; 2014. pp. 1446-1461

[36] Miano M, Dufour C. The diagnosis and treatment of aplastic anemia: A review. International Journal of Hematology. 2015;**101**(6):527-535. DOI: 10.1007/s12185-015-1787-z

[37] Eapen M, Horowitz MM. Alternative donor transplantation for aplastic anemia. Hematology. American Society of Hematology. Education Program. 2010;**2010**:43-46. DOI: 10.1182/asheducation-2010.1.43

[38] Perez-Albuerne ED, Eapen M, Klein J, Gross TJ, Lipton JM, Baker KS, et al. Outcome of unrelated donor stem cell transplantation for children with severe aplastic anemia. British Journal of Haematology. 2008;**141**(2):216-223. DOI: 10.1111/j.1365-2141.2008.07030.x

[39] Frank P, Carmen B, Ulrich G. First-line allogeneic hematopoietic stem cell transplantation of HLA-matched sibling donors compared with first-line ciclosporin and/or antithymocyte or antilymphocyte globulin for acquired severe aplastic anemia. Cochrane Database of Systematic Reviews. 2013;7. DOI: 10.1002/14651858.CD006407.pub2

[40] Caplan AI. Mesenchymal stem cells*. Journal of Orthopaedic Research. 1991;**9**(5):641-650. DOI: 10.1002/jor.1100090504

[41] Friedenstein AJ, Petrakova KV, Kurolesova AIFG. Heterotopic of bone marrow. Analysis of precursor cells for osteogenic and hematopoietic tissues. Transplantation. 1968;**6**(2):230-247

[42] Chamberlain G, Fox J, Ashton B, Middleton J. Concise review: Mesenchymal stem cells: Their phenotype, differentiation capacity, immunological features, and potential for homing. Stem Cells. 2007;**25**(11):2739-2749. DOI: 10.1634/stemcells.2007-0197

[43] Ra JC, Kang SK, Shin IS, Park HG, Joo SA, Kim JG, et al. Stem cell treatment for patients with autoimmune disease by systemic infusion of culture-expanded autologous adipose tissue derived mesenchymal stem cells. Journal of Translational Medicine. 2011;**9**:(1):181. DOI: 10.1186/1479-5876-9-181

[44] Potdar PD. Human dental pulp stem cells: Applications in future regenerative medicine. World Journal of Stem Cells. 2015;7(5):839. DOI: 10.4252/wjsc.v7.i5.839

[45] Narang S, Sehgal N. Stem cells: A potential regenerative future in dentistry. Indian Journal of Human Genetics. 2012;**18**(2):150. DOI: 10.4103/0971-6866.100749

[46] Caplan AI, Correa D. The MSC: An injury drugstore. Cell Stem Cell. 2011;**9**: 11-15. DOI: 10.1016/j.stem.2011.06.008

[47] Caplan AI. Mesenchymal stem cells: Time to change the name! Stem Cells Translational Medicine. 2017;**6**(6): 1445-1451. DOI: 10.1002/sctm.17-0051

[48] Caplan AI, Dennis JE. Mesenchymal stem cells as trophic mediators. Journal of Cellular Biochemistry. 2006;**98**: 1076-1084. DOI: 10.1002/jcb.20886

[49] Gnecchi M, Zhang Z, Ni A, Dzau VJ. Paracrine mechanisms in adult stem cell signaling and therapy. Circulation Research. 2008;**103**:1204-1219. DOI: 10.1161/CIRCRESAHA.108.176826

[50] da Silva ML, Fontes AM, Covas DT, Caplan AI. Mechanisms involved in the therapeutic properties of mesenchymal stem cells. Cytokine and Growth Factor Reviews. 2009;**20**:419-427. DOI: 10.1016/j.cytogfr.2009.10.002

[51] Caplan AI. Adult mesenchymal stem cells: When, where, and how. Stem Cells International. 2015;**2015**. DOI: 10.1155/2015/628767

[52] Yagi H, Soto-Gutierrez A, Parekkadan B, Kitagawa Y, Tompkins RG, Kobayashi N, et al. Mesenchymal stem cells: Mechanisms of immunomodulation and homing. Cell Transplantation. 2010;**19**:667-679. DOI: 10.3727/096368910X508762

[53] Leibacher J, Henschler R. Biodistribution, migration and homing of systemically applied mesenchymal stem/stromal cells mesenchymal stem/ stromal cells - an update. Stem Cell Research & Therapy. 2016;7(1):7. DOI: 10.1186/s13287-015-0271-2

[54] Nombela-Arrieta C, Ritz J, Silberstein LE. The elusive nature and function of mesenchymal stem cells. Nature Reviews Molecular Cell Biology. 2011;**12**:126-131. DOI: 10.1038/nrm3049

[55] Tse WT, Pendleton JD, Beyer WM, Egalka MC, Guinan EC. Suppression of allogeneic T-cell proliferation by human marrow stromal cells: Implications in transplantation. Transplantation. 2003;**75**(3):389-397. DOI: 10.1097/01.TP.0000045055.63901.A9

[56] Munir H, McGettrick HM. Mesenchymal stem cell therapy for autoimmune disease: Risks and rewards. Stem Cells and Development. 2015;**24**(18):2091-2100. DOI: 10.1089/scd.2015.0008

[57] Marigo I, Dazzi F. The immunomodulatory properties of mesenchymal stem cells. Seminars in Immunopathology. 2011;**33**:593-602. DOI: 10.1007/s00281-011-0267-7

[58] Zhao S, Wehner R, Bornhäuser M, Wassmuth R, Bachmann M, Schmitz M. Immunomodulatory properties of mesenchymal stromal cells and their therapeutic consequences for immune-mediated disorders. Stem Cells and Development. 2009;**19**(5):607-614. DOI: 10.1089/scd.2009.0345

[59] Gao F, Chiu SM, Motan DAL, Zhang Z, Chen L, Ji HL, et al. Mesenchymal stem cells and immunomodulation: Current status and future prospects. Cell Death & Disease. 2016;**7**:e2062. DOI: 10.1038/cddis.2015.327

[60] Herrero C, Pérez-Simón JA. Immunomodulatory effect of mesenchymal stem cells. Brazilian Journal of Medical and Biological Research. 2010;**43**:425-430. DOI: 10.1590/S0100-879X2010007500033

[61] Castro-Manrreza ME, Montesinos JJ. Immunoregulation by mesenchymal

stem cells: Biological aspects and clinical applications. Journal of Immunology Research. 2015;**2015**. DOI: 10.1155/2015/394917

[62] Nakao N, Nakayama T, Yahata T, Muguruma Y, Saito S, Miyata Y, et al. Adipose tissue-derived mesenchymal stem cells facilitate hematopoiesis in vitro and in vivo: Advantages over bone marrow-derived mesenchymal stem cells. The American Journal of Pathology. 2010;**177**(2):547-554. DOI: 10.2353/ajpath.2010.091042

[63] Dexter TM. Stromal cell associated Haemopoiesis. Journal of Cellular Physiology. Supplement. 1982;**1**:87-94

[64] Hamzic E, Whiting K, Gordon Smith E, Pettengell R. Characterization of bone marrow mesenchymal stromal cells in aplastic anaemia. British Journal of Haematology. 2015;**169**(6):804-813. DOI: 10.1111/bjh.13364

[65] Sugiyama T, Kohara H, Noda M, Nagasawa T. Maintenance of the hematopoietic stem cell pool by CXCL12-CXCR4 chemokine signaling in bone marrow stromal cell niches. Immunity. 2006;**25**(6):977-988. DOI: 10.1016/j.immuni.2006.10.016

[66] Asri A, Sabour J, Atashi A, Soleimani M. Homing in hematopoietic stem cells: Focus on regulatory role of CXCR7 on SDF1A/CXCR4 axis. EXCLI Journal. 2016;**15**:134-143. DOI: 10.17179/excli2014-585

[67] Oubari F, Amirizade N, Mohammadpour H, Nakhlestani M, Zarif MN. The important role of FLT3-L in ex vivo expansion of hematopoietic stem cells following co-culture with mesenchymal stem cells. *Cell Journal*. 2015;**17**(2):201-210. DOI: 10.22074/cellj.2016.3715

[68] Anthony BA, Link DC. Regulation of hematopoietic stem cells by bone marrow stromal cells. Trends in Immunology. 2014;**35**:32-37. DOI: 10.1016/j.it.2013.10.002

[69] Tvedt THA, Ersvaer E, Tveita AA, Bruserud Ø. Interleukin-6 in allogeneic stem cell transplantation: Its possible importance for immunoregulation and as a therapeutic target. Frontiers in Immunology. 2017;**8**:667. DOI: 10.3389/fimmu.2017.00667

[70] Patchen ML, Macvittie TJ, Williams JL, Schwartz GN, Souza LM. Administration of Interleukin-6 stimulates multilineage Hematopoiesis and accelerates recovery from radiation-induced hematopoietic depression. Blood. 1991;**77**(3):472-480

[71] Young NS. Current concepts in the pathophysiology and treatment of aplastic anemia. Blood. 2006;**108**(8):2509-2519. DOI: 10.1182/blood-2006-03-010777

[72] Bacigalupo A, Valle M, Podestà M, Pitto A, Zocchi E, De Flora A, et al. T-cell suppression mediated by mesenchymal stem cells is deficient in patients with severe aplastic anemia. Experimental Hematology. 2005;**33**(7):819-827. DOI: 10.1016/j.exphem.2005.05.006

[73] Li J, Lu S, Yang S, Xing W, Feng J, Li W, et al. Impaired immunomodulatory ability of bone marrow mesenchymal stem cells on CD4 + T cells in aplastic anemia. Results in Immunology. 2012;**2**:142-147. DOI: 10.1016/j.rinim.2012.07.002

[74] Kyurkchiev D. Secretion of immunoregulatory cytokines by mesenchymal stem cells. World Journal of Stem Cells. 2014;**6**(5):552. DOI: 10.4252/wjsc.v6.i5.552

[75] Qiao SK, Ren HY, Shi YJ, Liu W. Allogeneic compact bone-derived mesenchymal stem cell transplantation increases survival of mice exposed to lethal total body irradiation:

A potential immunological mechanism. Chinese Medical Journal. 2014;**127**(3):475-482. DOI: 10.3760/cma.j.issn.0366-6999.20132001

[76] Moll NM, Ransohoff RM. CXCL12 and CXCR4 in bone marrow physiology. Expert Review of Hematology. 2010;**3**:315-322. DOI: 10.1586/ehm.10.16

[77] Dar A, Goichberg P, Shinder V, Kalinkovich A, Kollet O, Netzer N, et al. Chemokine receptor CXCR4-dependent internalization and resecretion of functional chemokine SDF-1 by bone marrow endothelial and stromal cells. Nature Immunology. 2005;**6**(10):1038-1046. DOI: 10.1038/ni1251

[78] Yang JX, Zhang N, Wang HW, Gao P, Yang QP, Wen QP. CXCR4 receptor overexpression in mesenchymal stem cells facilitates treatment of acute lung injury in rats. The Journal of Biological Chemistry. 2015;**290**(4):1994-2006. DOI: 10.1074/jbc.M114.605063

[79] Honczarenko M, Le Y, Swierkowski M, Ghiran I, Glodek AM, Silberstein LE. Human bone marrow stromal cells express a distinct set of biologically functional chemokine receptors. Stem Cells. 2006;**24**(4):1030-1041. DOI: 10.1634/stemcells.2005-0319

[80] De Becker A, Van Hummelen P, Bakkus M, Vande BI, De Wever J, De Waele M, et al. Migration of culture-expanded human mesenchymal stem cells through bone marrow endothelium is regulated by matrix metalloproteinase-2 and tissue inhibitor of metalloproteinase-3. Haematologica. 2007;**92**(4):440-449. DOI: 10.3324/haematol.10475

[81] Annabi B, Lee Y-T, Turcotte S, Naud E, Desrosiers RR, Champagne M, et al. Hypoxia promotes murine bone-marrow-derived stromal cell migration and tube formation. Stem Cells. 2003;**21**(3):337-347. DOI: 10.1634/stemcells.21-3-337

[82] François M, Romieu-Mourez R, Li M, Galipeau J. Human MSC suppression correlates with cytokine induction of indoleamine 2,3-dioxygenase and bystander M2 macrophage differentiation. Molecular Therapy. 2012;**20**(1):187-195. DOI: 10.1038/mt.2011.189

[83] Gan J, En G FM, O U XZ, I CL, E YH, Zen XG, et al. Cross mark. Cytotherapy 2015;17:403-417. DOI: 10.1016/j.jcyt.2014.ll.011

[84] Fouillard L, Bensidhoum M, Bories D, Bonte H, Lopez M, Moseley AM, et al. Engraftment of allogeneic mesenchymal stem cells in the bone marrow of a patient with severe idiopathic aplastic anemia improves stroma. Leukemia. 2003;**17**:474-476. DOI: 10.1038/sj.leu.2402786

[85] Hematti P, Kim J, Battiwalla M. Mesenchymal stem cells in hematopoietic stem cell transplantation. In: Stem Cells and Human Diseases. Springer Netherlands; 2014. pp. 101-115. DOI: 10.1007/978-94-007-2801-1_5

[86] Liu FD, Tam K, Pishesha N, Poon Z, Van Vliet KJ. Improving hematopoietic recovery through modeling and modulation of the mesenchymal stromal cell secretome. Stem Cell Research & Therapy. 2018;**9**(1):268. DOI: 10.1186/s13287-018-0982-2

[87] Le Blanc K, Samuelsson H, Gustafsson B, Remberger M, Sundberg B, Arvidson J, et al. Transplantation of mesenchymal stem cells to enhance engraftment of hematopoietic stem cells. Leukemia. 2007;**21**(8):1733-1738. DOI: 10.1038/sj.leu.2404777

[88] Fang B, Li N, Song Y, Li J, Zhao RC, Ma Y. Cotransplantation of haploidentical mesenchymal stem cells to enhance engraftment of

hematopoietic stem cells and to reduce the risk of graft failure in two children with severe aplastic anemia. Pediatric Transplantation. 2009;**13**(4):499-502. DOI: 10.1111/j.1399-3046.2008.01002.x

[89] Kurtzberg J, Prockop S, Teira P, Bittencourt H, Lewis V, Chan KW, et al. Allogeneic human mesenchymal stem cell therapy (Remestemcel-L, Prochymal) as a rescue agent for severe refractory acute graft-versus-host disease in pediatric patients. Biology of Blood and Marrow Transplantation. 2014;**20**(2):229-235. DOI: 10.1016/j.bbmt.2013.11.001

[90] Česen Mazič M, Girandon L, Kneževič M, Avčin SL, Jazbec J. Treatment of severe steroid-refractory acute-graft-vs.-host disease with mesenchymal stem cells–single center experience. Frontiers in Bioengineering and Biotechnology. 2018;**6**. DOI: 10.3389/fbioe.2018.00093

[91] Baron F, Storb R. Mesenchymal stromal cells: A new tool against graft-versus-host disease? Biology of Blood and Marrow Transplantation. 2012;**18**:822-840. DOI: 10.1016/j.bbmt.2011.09.003

[92] Van Pham P. Mesenchymal stem cells in clinical applications. In: Stem Cell Processing. Cham: Springer; 2016. pp. 37-69. DOI: 10.1007/978-3-319-40073-0_2

[93] Keto J, Kaartinen T, Salmenniemi U, Castrén J, Partanen J, Hänninen A, et al. Immunomonitoring of MSC-treated GvHD patients reveals only moderate potential for response prediction but indicates treatment safety. Molecular Therapy. Methods & Clinical Development. 2018;**9**:109-118. DOI: 10.1016/j.omtm.2018.02.001

[94] Galleu A, Milojkovic D, Deplano S, Szydlo R, Loaiza S, Wynn R, et al. Mesenchymal stromal cells for acute graft-versus-host disease: Response at 1 week predicts probability of survival. British Journal of Haematology. 2019;**185**(1):89-92. DOI: 10.1111/bjh.15749

[95] Elgaz S, Kuçi Z, Kuçi S, Bönig H, Bader P. Clinical use of mesenchymal stromal cells in the treatment of acute graft-versus-host disease. Transfusion Medicine and Hemotherapy. 2019;**46**:27-34. DOI: 10.1159/000496809

[96] Galipeau J, Sensébé L. Mesenchymal stromal cells: Clinical challenges and therapeutic opportunities. Cell Stem Cell. 2018;**22**:824-833. DOI: 10.1016/j.stem.2018.05.004

[97] Seng A, Dunavin N. Mesenchymal stromal cell infusions for acute graft-versus-host disease: Rationale, data, and unanswered questions. Advances in Cell and Gene Therapy. 2018;**1**(2):e14. DOI: 10.1002/acg2.14

[98] Tipnis S, Viswanathan C. Umbilical cord matrix derived mesenchymal stem cells can change the cord blood transplant scenario. Int J Stem Cells. 2010;**3**(2):103-118. DOI: 10.15283/ijsc.2010.3.2.103

[99] Rizvanov AA, Persson J, Şahin F, Bellusci S, Oliveira PJ. Hematopoietic and mesenchymal stem cells in biomedical and clinical applications. Stem Cells International. 2016;**2016**. DOI: 10.1155/2016/3157365

[100] Fernández-García M, Yañez RM, Sánchez-Domínguez R, Hernando-Rodriguez M, Peces-Barba M, Herrera G, et al. Mesenchymal stromal cells enhance the engraftment of hematopoietic stem cells in an autologous mouse transplantation model. Stem Cell Research & Therapy. 2015;**6**(1):165. DOI: 10.1186/s13287-015-0155-5

[101] Li H, Wang L, Pang Y, Jiang Z, Liu Z, Xiao H, et al. In patients with chronic aplastic anemia, bone marrow-derived MSCs regulate the Treg/Th17 balance by influencing the notch/RBP-J/

FOXP3/RORγt pathway. Scientific Reports. 2017;7:42488. DOI: 10.1038/srep42488

[102] Jaganathan BG, Tisato V, Vulliamy T, Dokal I, Marsh J, Dazzi F, et al. Effects of MSC co-injection on the reconstitution of aplastic anemia patient following hematopoietic stem cell transplantation. Leukemia. 2010;**24**:1791-1795. DOI: 10.1038/leu.2010.164

[103] Yamei W, Rongmu L, Yongbin C, Yingjian S, Xiaohong L, Xiaomei Z, et al. Improved outcome of haploidentical transplantation in severe aplastic anemia using reduced-intensity fludarabine-based conditioning. Oncotarget. 2017;**8**(48):83817. DOI: 10.18632/oncotarget.19745

[104] Liu Z, Zhang Y, Xiao H, Yao Z, Zhang H, Liu Q, et al. Cotransplantation of bone marrow-derived mesenchymal stem cells in haploidentical hematopoietic stem cell transplantation in patients with severe aplastic anemia: An interim summary for a multicenter phase II trial results. Bone Marrow Transplantation. 2017;**52**(5):704-710. DOI: 10.1038/bmt.2016.347

[105] Wang ZK, Yu HJ, Cao FL, Liu ZH, Liu ZY, Feng WJ, et al. Donor-derived marrow mesenchymal stromal cell co-transplantation following a haploidentical hematopoietic stem cell transplantation trail to treat severe aplastic anemia in children. Annals of Hematology. 2019;**98**(2):473-479. DOI: 10.1007/s00277-018-3523-2

[106] Chen M, Zheng Z, He G, Lin S, Zhang D, Hu H, et al. Co-transplantation of mesenchymal stem cells can ameliorates acute Gvhd and viremia after allogeneic hematopoietic stem cell transplantation for severe aplastic Anemia: A multi-Center retrospective study of 119 patients. Blood. 2018;**132**(1):4653-4653. DOI: 10.1182/blood-2018-99-118758

[107] Pang Y, Xiao HW, Zhang H, Liu ZH, Li L, Gao Y, et al. Allogeneic bone marrow-derived mesenchymal stromal cells expanded In vitro for treatment of aplastic Anemia: A Multicenter phase II trial. Stem Cells Translational Medicine. 2017;**6**(7):1569-1575. DOI: 10.1002/sctm.16-0227

[108] Clé DV, Santana-Lemos B, Tellechea MF, Prata KL, Orellana MD, Covas DT, et al. Intravenous infusion of allogeneic mesenchymal stromal cells in refractory or relapsed aplastic anemia. Cytotherapy. 2015;**17**(12):1696-1705. DOI: 10.1016/j.jcyt.2015.09.006

[109] Kim HJ, Park J-S. Usage of human mesenchymal stem cells in cell-based therapy: Advantages and disadvantages. Development & Reproduction. 2017;**21**(1):1-10. DOI: 10.12717/dr.2017.21.1.001

[110] Figueroa FE, Carrión F, Villanueva S, Khoury M. Mesenchymal stem cell treatment for autoimmune diseases: A critical review. Biological Research. 2012;**45**(3):269-277. DOI: 10.4067/S0716-97602012000300008

[111] Parekkadan B, Milwid JM. Mesenchymal stem cells as therapeutics. Annual Review of Biomedical Engineering. 2010;**12**(1):87-117. DOI: 10.1146/annurev-bioeng-070909-105309

[112] Fagioli F, Ferrero I. Mesenchymal stem cell manufacturing for clinical use. In: Progress in Stem Cell Transplantation. Rijeka: InTechOpen; 2015. DOI: 10.5772/61370

[113] Erickson B, Nelson WP. Perspective on opportunities in industrial biotechnology in renewable chemicals. Biotechnology Journal. 2012;7:176-185. DOI: 10.1002/biot.201100069

Chapter 8

Harmonized and Quality Sample Handling in Biobank-Supported Multicenter Prospective Studies

Verónica Valdivieso-Gómez, Javier Garrancho-Pérez, Inés Aroca-Siendones and Rocío Aguilar-Quesada

Abstract

In the frame of multicenter research studies, biobanks ensure the harmonization and traceability of the prospective collection of quality samples. This is significant because pre-analytical variables must be carefully considered to guarantee the integrity of biomarkers to be tested and to avoid bias affecting the validity of the analytical results. According to a quality management system, biobanks contribute with documents and records; consumable preparation for collection, processing, and conservation; sample quality controls; and centralized management of sample handling, storage, and distribution. Traceability of samples is based on unique standard codes and the use of pre-assigned, pre-coded, and pre-labeled materials for sample collection, processing, and conservation. By using these supporting tools, quality derivatives are obtained based on common and evidence-based standard operating procedures (SOPs), with associated traceability information in relation with their collection, processing, conservation, and distribution. The biobank-supported workflow, specifically designed and implemented for each project, allows obtaining harmonized quality samples contributing to the quality of large and complex research projects and the corresponding validity of the analyses.

Keywords: multicenter prospective project, sample handling, traceability, workflow harmonization, quality-assured biobanking

1. Introduction

Professionalism is the current hallmark of biobanks [1], which are driven by standards and best practices. A biobank is "an entity that receives, stores, processes, and/or distributes specimens, as needed. It encompasses the physical location as well as the full range of activities associated with its operation [2]." Different types of biobanks have been proposed [3], although the definitive model will be the result of the activities performed in support of the particular needs of attended projects, including real or virtual collection, processing, conservation, and distribution.

Biobanks have been involved in large quality-assured prospective studies based on validated and standardized sample handling and storage protocols [4, 5]. When a prospective multicenter research project is designed, multiple variables must be considered such as the number and type of donations, recruitment sites and analytical laboratory locations, pre-analytical requirements of samples and derivatives obtained, and processing and storage facilities. Attending to the complexity of the project, a specific workflow is implemented after process definition identifying every factor involved in (site, staff, equipment, method, materials, samples and transferences) and their corresponding checkpoints.

2. Harmonization of sample collection and derivative preservation

To guarantee the integrity of biomarkers to be tested and to avoid bias, pre-analytical variables must be carefully considered [6]. In fact, many studies are being conducted to elucidate the effects of pre-analytical variables on analytical profiles. In this sense, a study has been recently published to determine acceptable delays to fixation for formalin-fixed paraffin-embedded (FFPE) tissue samples [7]. In order to mitigate their impact in the complex frame of multicenter projects, biobanks contribute through supervised materials and sample handling and continuous and overlapped checkpoints.

2.1 Centralized preparation of consumables for sample collection, processing and preservation

With the objective to ensure the consistency in sample collection, stabilization, and preservation, specific kits with the consumables necessary for only a donation are defined in function of pre-analytical requirements of obtaining samples and derivatives (**Figure 1**). A careful selection of collection devices is critical here since differences in biomarker testing have been reported [8, 9]. Consumables such as modified cards (IsoCode cards or FTA cards) for blood spot collection, in addition to multibarrier pouches with desiccant packs for room-temperature transportation and future conservation, could be also included for traceability purposes [10]. For

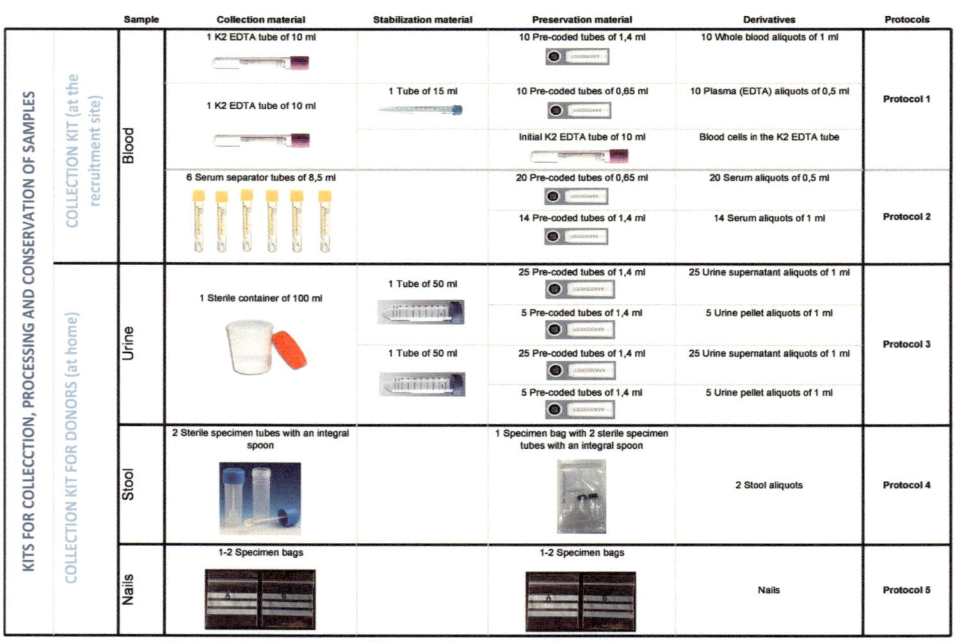

Figure 1.
Consumables included for sample collection, stabilization, and preservation in representative kits, classified by the corresponding protocol and derivatives obtained.

noninvasive samples (nails, stool, etc.), kits targeted to donors may be designed for a more accessible collection at home, with the appropriate consumables to guarantee the integrity of samples until they are receipted by the biobank or analytical laboratory. When processing is performed by a different center from the recruitment site, two kits are prepared in independent boxes for collection and processing, especially when the sample collection is made by the donor on his own.

Materials included in the kits are classified in several bags according with the downstream protocol. Expiration date and batch numbers for consumables must be considered during the purchasing process in relation with the recruitment rates and the validity of the results, respectively. Additionally, expiration date is identified for each kit according to the most recent expiration date from the consumables, and it is used as a reference to track and replace expired consumables by the biobank when the recruitment rate is not the expected.

2.2 Sample processing and quality controls

Evidence-based standard operating procedures (SOPs) are elaborated for sample processing taking the sample requirements provided by the testing laboratories into consideration. The number and volume of samples necessary for analytical assays and the type of derivative, anticoagulant or preservative must be identified in order to choose the most appropriate and approachable option of prospective collection of samples providing high-quality biomarkers useful for downstream applications [11]. Additional requirements from guides [12] or previous scientific publications [13] are also taken into account in relation with specific sample collection and derivative stabilization. Preservation delay and resources available for long-term storage will influence the selection of the collection device as well. In fact, room-temperature storage alternatives have been proposed [14]. When the same sample allows obtaining different derivatives (i.e., blood for plasma, buffy coat, and RBCs), protocols will adjust the number and type of collection tubes or devices to minimize the quantity of sample collected from the donor. On the other hand, the number of aliquots of liquid samples must be set in function of the different analyses to be performed avoiding unnecessary freeze-thaw cycles.

These pre-analytical conditions of samples and derivatives will determine where each process (collection, initial sample processing, provisional cryopreservation of derivatives, long-term storage, testing) will be performed depending on the recruitment site, the biobank, and the analytical laboratory locations and facilities. Accordingly, transportation of samples at the corresponding temperature should be organized [15] following the international recommendations.

Obtaining of specific derivatives such as nucleic acid isolation may be centralized in the biobank or testing laboratories in order to avoid bias. In the same sense, reactive batches must be controlled. When possible, automation of processes must be implemented to avoid traceability errors and decreasing hands on time. Samples should be handled following validation of standard operating protocols by using samples not belonging to the particular project, specifically collected and approved for this purpose by an ethical committee.

The quality of samples must be evaluated after processing by means of a comprehensive analysis of quality indicators [16]. Because of the current lack of qualification tools for each type of derivative and pre-analytical variable, numerous studies are trying to identify new markers to assess the fitness-for-purpose of samples. Thus, new scores and indicators have been proposed for the quality of samples in relation with the impact derived from the pre-analytical phase [17–23]. In the same way, participation in external quality assurance (EQA) schemes like the EQA program developed by the International Society for Biological and Environmental

Repositories (ISBER) focused on sample processing and testing evaluation [24]; it is a highly recommended complementary tool for the internal quality control (IQC). Biobank collaboration through international working groups focused on standardization of sample processing, and biological sample quality control will contribute to the implementation of the last innovations in the field as well.

2.3 Monitored storage of biological samples and distribution

In relation with sample conservation, derivatives are long-term stored in the most appropriate conditions to maintain their original characteristics, being very important for the sample stability the selection of the temperature storage [15]. When samples are receipted in the storage facilities, aliquots are immediately revised to check the shipment temperature; the number, integrity, and volume of each aliquot regarding the expected; and incidents reported, maintaining the cold chain. Racks and boxes are previously prepared to directly store the derivatives in a reduced and optimized space within the conservation equipment classified by the type of container. In addition, derivatives are preferably stored separately in different equipment and preservation rooms as a safety measure.

So, long-term storage facilities may be located in one or more rooms or buildings and may even be assumed by several institutions when transportation of samples and temperature variations are minimized. In any case, sample handling and positions must be under control and restricted access. Both the preservation rooms and storage equipment are constantly controlled through a monitoring system that records critical parameters such as temperature, humidity, CO_2, and O_2 levels (where necessary) and the proper functioning of equipment (compressors, battery power, display) (**Figure 2**). The system triggers an alarm when any parameter is out of the established range, thus activating an emergency plan. Briefly, warnings are received by specifically dedicated staff available for 24 h who analyze and classify the failure to initiate the defined corrective actions. In case it could not be repaired, samples are evacuated to backup equipment.

If previous instructions are followed, samples could be preserved in good conditions for a long time. However, the specific period of time will depend on the type of sample but, most importantly, on the biomarker to be detected by a particular methodology, with a range from minutes to years [15]. In this sense, fitness-for-purpose procedures should be validated and established when a prospective workflow is designed, taking into consideration the general good practices that do allow the most use of samples [2, 12]. Independently, other approaches have been reviewed for the conservation of samples at room temperature by biobanks [25].

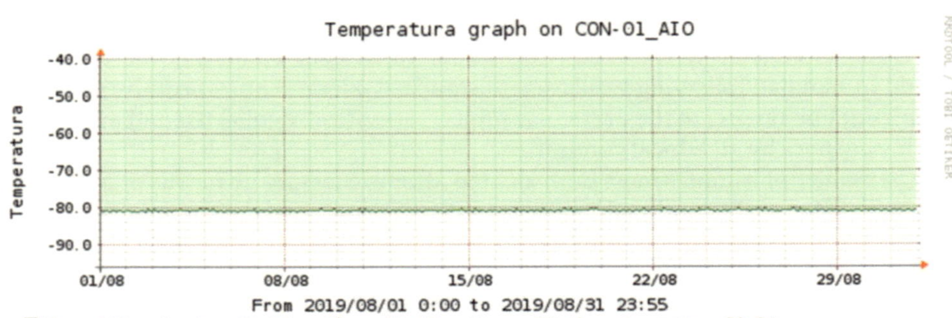

Figure 2.
Representative graph of a monitoring system showing a temperature of an ultra-freezer at −80°C.

Before sending of samples to analytical laboratories from the storage facilities, a checkpoint is introduced to guarantee that each aliquot is compliant with the corresponding study or with the necessary volume of sample to thus supplement with additional aliquots. Additional quality controls should be performed when incidents during the sample conservation occur or after a non-validated long-term storage. The remaining precious samples may be again received for long-term storage from the testing laboratories followed by a new quality control.

3. Traceability of biological samples

3.1 Electronic database

The electronic database used by biobanks allows the integral management of multicenter prospective projects with a maximum level of security through restricted access. Donors, biological samples, and associated information, as well as the ethical-legal documentation associated to the project, are recorded. In detail, the system allows an exhaustive control of collaborating centers and researchers, preparation of sample collection kits maintaining the traceability of all materials used, donor and clinical information, informed consent forms, ethical and scientific committees' approvals, agreements, sample handling by different sites (reception, processing, storage and shipments), quality incidents, and even the project monitoring by using any recorded information, for example, the recruitment rates from each clinical site. The electronic database may be also connected to external databases incorporating additional information such as temperature information from storage equipment. So, traceability is achieved from all the processes.

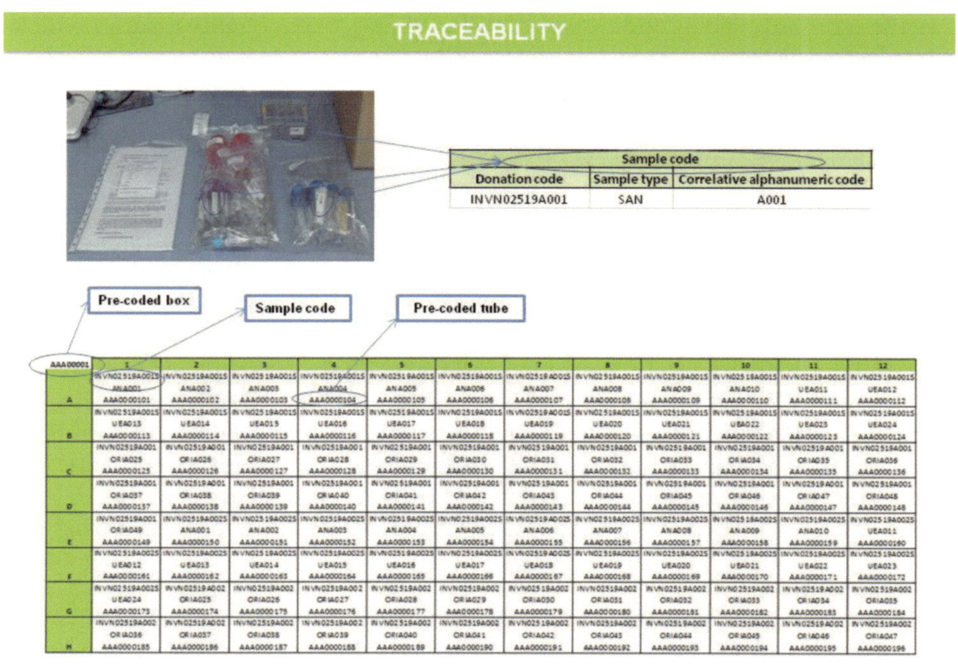

Figure 3.
Identification of samples and materials with structured codes and representative box map with pre-coded tubes.

3.2 Identification of materials and samples

Unique standardized codes are generated by the electronic database to identify each donation, sample, and material included in its corresponding collection kit, thanks to label printing (**Figure 3**). Therefore, samples (and associated information) are de-identified in compliance with applicable laws. Records included in the kit are also identified in relation with donations.

Commercially available pre-coded tubes are selected to prepare derivative aliquots so that specific pre-coded tubes are pre-assigned to each type of sample for a donation during the kit preparation by using the electronic database, supporting the traceability of samples (**Figure 3**). Similarly, racks for the pre-coded tubes included in the kits are identified as well. The process of generation of a new donation code to the positions of aliquots within the storage equipment is recorded in the electronic database. Code generation and identification also accompany manual or automated sample processing to identify the samples by using code readers.

4. Quality management system

A variety of quality standards can be implemented by laboratories, being requirements from ISO 9001 for the quality management system (QMS) the most widely used [26]. Briefly, ISO 9001 is characterized by a process-based approach following the plan-do-check-act cycle, not only focused on the quality of a product or service or the satisfaction of its users but on the way to obtain them. This QMS involves the definition and systematic management of the processes and the interactions between them in order to meet the legal, regulatory, and users' requirements and to achieve the expected results by continuously improving efficiency. Specifically for biobank activities, the ISO 20387:2018 Biotechnology-Biobanking-General Requirements for Biobanking has been launched under which other more specific standards will be additionally developed [27]. Next, quality assurance tools related with the harmonization and traceability of samples in multicenter prospective studies are shown.

4.1 Protocols, records, and other documents

The definition of processes (strategic, key, and support) involves identifying every factor involved (staff, equipment, method) with the objective of describing them through procedures and keeping them well controlled. Strict adherence to procedures by each stakeholder involved in the multicenter projects is mandatory to avoid pre-analytical deviations. A scheme summarizing the project workflow may be useful to clearly represent the responsibilities of all the stakeholders (**Figure 4**).

Clear and schematic protocols are developed for each type of collection device included in the kits in order to make easier the procedure interpretation (**Figure 5**). This action is especially critical when kits are targeted to donors for collection at home. The protocols include associated records to be filled with pre-analytical information of donations or samples, to report any incident that occurred during collection and preservation, even rack maps as guide for derivatives aliquoting into the specific tubes.

After centralized derivatives are obtained, a technical report specifying the sample processing features is accompanied in the shipments to analytical laboratories. Once all the samples for a study are sent from storage facilities to analytical laboratories, a final report is prepared with the missing samples, because of insufficient quantity of aliquots or any incident reported, and with the remaining

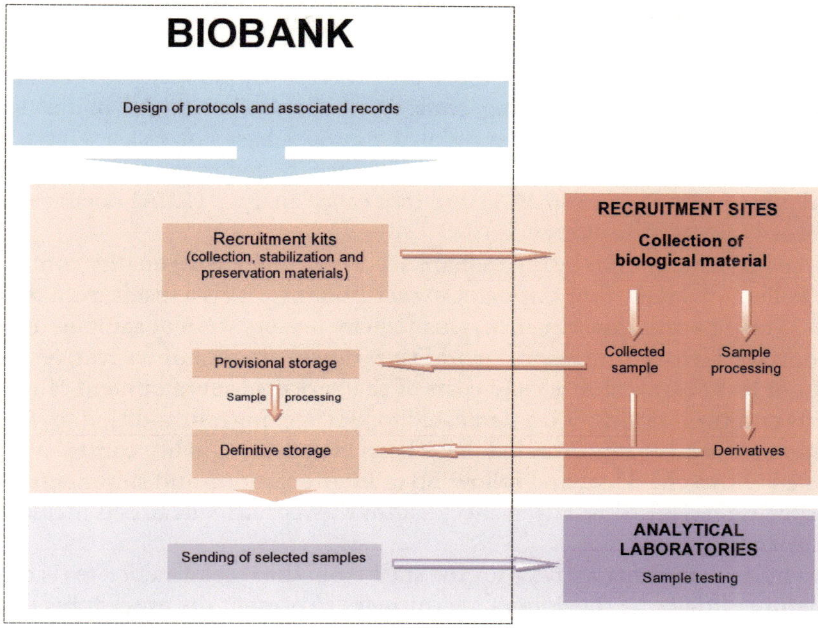

Figure 4.
Biobank-supported workflow for sample handling.

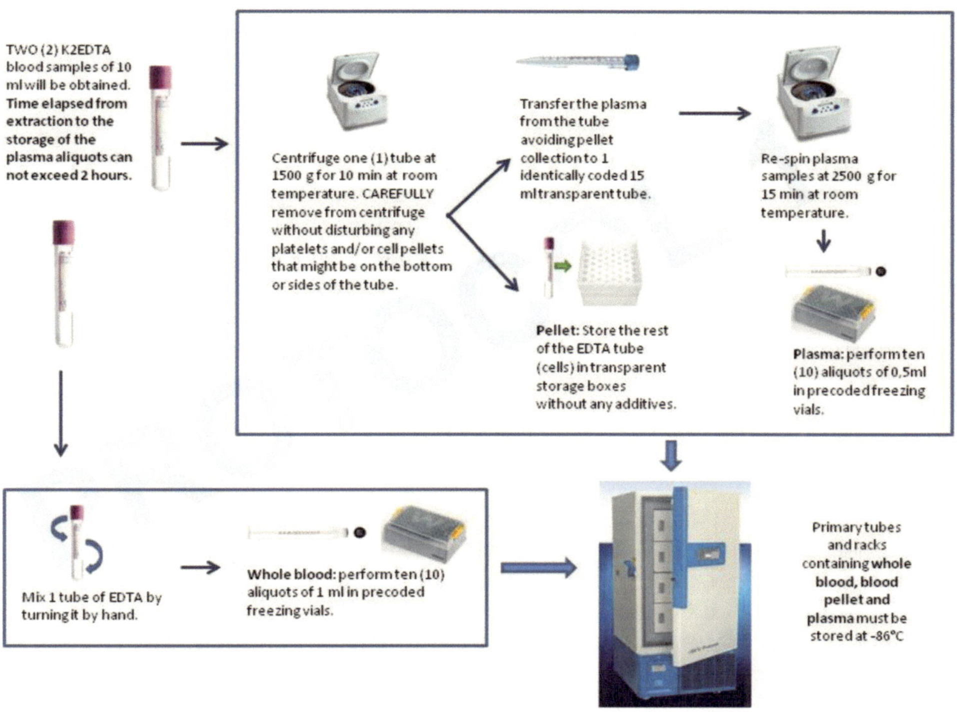

Figure 5.
Representative schematic protocol for derivative stabilization and preservation.

material for the study. Transaction forms specifying the samples included are necessary to declare the derivative shipment to the next facility involved in the project workflow.

4.2 Risk management tool

As part of the quality assurance tools, the processes of prospective sample collection, stabilization and processing, conservation, and distribution in multicenter research studies are managed under a global approach based on risk analysis, aimed at preventing undesired results. Since incidents are treated in the format of corrective and preventative action (CAPA) and root cause analysis (RCA) documentation, these records are used as reference.

So, the implementation by the biobanks of a comprehensive quality control for sample collection kits before shipment to recruitment sites is a result from this risk analysis. The potential consequences (inadequate preservation of samples due to inappropriate devices, containers, or additives, lower amount of derivatives for analysis, or loss of traceability) and costs of this process (new shipment of replacement kits and time of technician dedicated to kit checking), in addition to the number of nonconforming kits detected, have been evaluated. Quality control of kits is performed with a checklist, and follow-up of kit preparation and shipments is made with a specific record. Similarly, a checklist for the recruitment sites is included to track the reception of kits.

In addition, a training activity for the staff from the recruitment sites is organized before initializing the donors' recruitment to present the procedures for sample handling and the kit composition and usage. On the other hand, a pilot in a recruitment site is necessary to validate the model designed and to propose improvement measures.

5. Conclusions

The biobank-supported workflow, specifically designed and implemented for each research study, allows obtaining prospective, harmonized, and quality samples avoiding pre-analytical bias and contributing to the validity of the analytical results. Through biobanking processes and continuous and overlapped checkpoints, quality derivatives are obtained based on common and evidence-based standard operating procedures and supervised materials, with associated traceability information in relation with their collection, processing, conservation, and distribution. The effective workflow established is valid for large and complex multicenter projects.

Acknowledgements

This work was supported by Consejería de Salud y Familias-Junta de Andalucía, Ministerio de Economía y Competitividad-Gobierno de España, and Instituto de Salud Carlos III (grant number PT17/0019/0004 co-financed by FEDER). Thanks go to the staff from the Andalusian Public Health System Biobank for their continuous effort and improvements that make these supporting activities possible. Several projects have been satisfactorily attended following the previous premises.

Conflict of interest

The authors have declared no conflict of interest.

Author details

Verónica Valdivieso-Gómez, Javier Garrancho-Pérez, Inés Aroca-Siendones and Rocío Aguilar-Quesada*
Andalusian Public Health System Biobank, Coordinating Node, Granada, Spain

*Address all correspondence to: rocio.aguilar.quesada@juntadeandalucia.es

References

[1] Simeon-Dubach D, Kozlakidis Z. New standards and updated best practices will give modern biobanking a boost in professionalism. Biopreservation and Biobanking. 2018;**16**(1):1-2. [Epub 2018/02/03]

[2] International Society for Biological and Environmental Repositories (ISBER). Best Practices: Recommendations for Repositories [Internet]. 4th ed. 2018. Available from: https://www.isber.org/page/BPR. [Accessed: September 26, 2019]

[3] Riegman PH, Morente MM, Betsou F, Blasio P, Geary P. Marble arch international working group on biobanking for biomedical research. Biobanking for better healthcare. Molecular Oncology. 2008;**2**(3):213-222. DOI: 10.1016/j.molonc.2008.07.004. Epub 2008/07/30

[4] Elliott P, Peakman TC. The UK biobank sample handling and storage protocol for the collection, processing and archiving of human blood and urine. International Journal of Epidemiology. 2008;**37**(2):234-244. Epub 2008/04/03

[5] Haumann R, Verspaget HW. Quality-assured biobanking: The Leiden University Medical Center model. Methods in Molecular Biology. 1730;**2018**:361-370. [Epub 2018/01/25]

[6] Ellervik C, Vaught J. Preanalytical variables affecting the integrity of human biospecimens in biobanking. Clinical Chemistry. 2015;**61**(7):914-934. Epub 2015/05/17

[7] Jones W, Greytak S, Odeh H, Guan P, Powers J, Bavarva J, et al. Deleterious effects of formalin-fixation and delays to fixation on RNA and miRNA-Seq profiles. Scientific Reports. 2019;**9**(1):6980. DOI: 10.1038/s41598-019-43282-8

[8] Kozaki T, Lee S, Nishimura T, Katsuura T, Yasukouchi A. Effects of saliva collection using cotton swabs on melatonin enzyme immunoassay. Journal of Circadian Rhythms. 2011;**9**(1):1. DOI: 10.1186/1740-3391-9-1

[9] Häntzsch M, Tolios A, Beutner F, Nagel D, Thiery J, Teupser D, et al. Comparison of whole blood RNA preservation tubes and novel generation RNA extraction kits for analysis of mRNA and MiRNA profiles. PLoS One. 2014;**9**(12):e113298. DOI: 10.1371/journal.pone.0113298. eCollection 2014

[10] Parrish RS, Garafalo AV, Ndifor V, Goetz KE, Reeves MJ, Yim A, et al. Sample confirmation testing: A short tandem repeat-based quality assurance and quality control procedure for the eyeGENE biorepository. Biopreservation and Biobanking. 2016;**14**(2):149-155. DOI: 10.1089/bio.2015.0098. [Epub 2016 Feb 18]

[11] Lucena-Aguilar G, Sanchez-Lopez AM, Barberan-Aceituno C, Carrillo-Avila JA, Lopez-Guerrero JA, Aguilar-Quesada R. DNA source selection for downstream applications based on DNA quality indicators analysis. Biopreservation and Biobanking. 2016;**14**(4):264-270. [Epub 2016/05/10]

[12] International Agency for Research on Cancer (IARC). Common Minimum Technical Standards and Protocols for Biobanks Dedicated to Cancer Research. IARC Technical Publication No. 44 [Internet]. 2017. Available from: https://www.google.es/search?source=hp&ei=uWaMXciFNIu-aM33lJAN&q=Common+Minimum+Technical+Standards+and+Protocols+for+Biobanks+Dedicated+to+Cancer+Research&oq=Common+Minimum+Technical+Standards+and+Protocols+for+Biobanks+Dedicated+to+Cancer+Research&gs_l=psy-ab.3..0i19.595.595..1380...

0.0..0.150.150.0j1......0....2j1..gws-wiz. mQHl2WGrdAg&ved=0ahUK EwiIxuXT-e3kAhULHxo KHc07BdIQ4dUDCAk&uact=5 #spf=1569482428652. [Accessed: September 26, 2019]

[13] Bernini P, Bertini I, Luchinat C, Nincheri P, Staderini S, Turano P. Standard operating procedures for pre-analytical handling of blood and urine for metabolomic studies and biobanks. Journal of Biomolecular NMR. 2011;**49**(3-4):231-243. [Epub 2011/03/08]

[14] Lou JJ, Mirsadraei L, Sanchez DE, Wilson RW, Shabihkhani M, Lucey GM, et al. A review of room temperature storage of biospecimen tissue and nucleic acids for anatomic pathology laboratories and biorepositories. Clinical Biochemistry. 2014;**47**(4-5):267-273. DOI: 10.1016/j.clinbiochem.2013.12.011. Epub 2013 Dec 18

[15] Hubel A, Spindler R, Skubitz AP. Storage of human biospecimens: Selection of the optimal storage temperature. Biopreservation and Biobanking. 2014;**12**(3):165-175. DOI: 10.1089/bio.2013.0084. [Epub 2014 Jun 11]

[16] Betsou F, Bulla A, Cho SY, Clements J, Chuaqui R, Coppola D, et al. Assays for qualification and quality stratification of clinical biospecimens used in research: A technical report from the ISBER biospecimen science working group. Biopreservation and Biobanking. 2016;**14**(5):398-409. [Epub 2016 Apr 5]

[17] Ammerlaan W, Trouet J, Sachs MC, Guan P, Carithers L, Lambert P, et al. Small nucleolar RNA score: An assay to detect formalin-overfixed tissue. Biopreservation and Biobanking. 2018;**16**(6):467-476. DOI: 10.1089/bio.2018.0042

[18] Kofanova O, Bellora C, Quesada RA, Bulla A, Panadero-Fajardo S, Keipes M, et al. IL8 and EDEM3 gene expression ratio indicates peripheral blood mononuclear cell (PBMC) quality. Journal of Immunological Methods. 2019;**465**:13-19. DOI: 10.1016/j.jim.2018.11.012. [Epub 2018 Nov 26]

[19] Schwarz N, Knutti N, Rose M, Neugebauer S, Geiger J, Jahns R, et al. Quality assessment of the preanalytical workflow in liquid biobanking: Taurine as a serum-specific quality Indicator for preanalytical process variations. Biopreservation and Biobanking. 2019;**17**(5):458-467. DOI: 10.1089/bio.2019.0004

[20] Mathieson W, Mommaerts K, Trouet JM, Mathay C, Guan P, Carithers LJ, et al. Cold ischemia score: An mRNA assay for the detection of extended cold ischemia in formalin-fixed, paraffin-embedded tissue. Journal of Histochemistry and Cytochemistry. 2019;**67**(3):159-168. DOI: 10.1369/0022155418819967. [Epub 2018 Dec 18]

[21] Neumeister VM, Parisi F, England AM, Siddiqui S, Anagnostou V, Zarrella E, et al. A tissue quality index: An intrinsic control for measurement of effects of preanalytical variables on FFPE tissue. Laboratory Investigation. 2014;**94**(4):467-474. DOI: 10.1038/labinvest.2014.7. Epub 2014 Feb 17

[22] Trezzi JP, Bulla A, Bellora C, Rose M, Lescuyer P, Kiehntopf M, et al. LacaScore: A novel plasma sample quality control tool based on ascorbic acid and lactic acid levels. Metabolomics. 2016;**12**:96. [Epub 2016 Apr 27]

[23] Kofanova O, Henry E, Aguilar Quesada R, Bulla A, Navarro Linares H, Lescuyer P, et al. IL8 and IL16 levels indicate serum and plasma quality. Clinical Chemistry and Laboratory Medicine. 2018;**56**(7):1054-1062. DOI: 10.1515/cclm-2017-1047

[24] Shea K, Betsou F. Development of external quality assurance programs for biorepositories. Biopreservation and Biobanking. 2012;**10**(4):403-404. DOI: 10.1089/bio.2012.1044

[25] Muller R, Betsou F, Barnes MG, Harding K, Bonnet J, Kofanova O, et al. Preservation of biospecimens at ambient temperature: Special focus on nucleic acids and opportunities for the biobanking community. Biopreservation and Biobanking. 2016;**14**(2):89-98. DOI: 10.1089/bio.2015.0022. [Epub 2016 Feb 17]

[26] Valdivieso-Gomez V, Aguilar-Quesada R. Quality management systems for laboratories and external quality assurance programs. In: Zaman GS, editor. Quality Control in Laboratory. London: IntechOpen; 2018. DOI: 10.5772/intechopen.73052

[27] Furuta K, Allocca CM, Schacter B, Bledsoe MJ, Ramirez NC. Standardization and innovation in paving a path to a better future: An update of activities in ISO/TC276/WG2 biobanks and bioresources. Biopreservation and Biobanking. 2018;**16**(1):23-27. DOI: 10.1089/bio.2017.0117. [Epub 2018 Feb 2]

Chapter 9

Contribution of Biomedical Equipment Management to Better Management of Sickle Cell Disease in Africa

Vincent Mulunda-a-Mulunda, Pierre Kouam and Taty Oke Ingwen

Abstract

Sickle cell anemia is a serious disease with manifestations and complications that directly affect the patient's quality of life and his entourage. This is not a shameful disease on the contrary; it is linked to a mutation that arose for us to defend against severe forms of malaria. It is due to the so-called selective pressure that has enabled AS carriers to resist severe forms of malaria. This advantage explains among other things why, although cosmopolitan, sickle cell disease predominates in Africa and its geographical distribution is superimposed on the malaria one. In the Democratic Republic of the Congo (DRC), it is estimated that there are 25–30% heterozygous healthy carriers (AS) and about 50,000 homozygous newborns (SS) each year, equating to 2% of newborns. Therefore, an effective medical care is very indispensable. The management of any pathology implies the appropriate choice of techniques and technologies. Unfortunately, very often in sub-Saharan countries, there is a lack of global strategy to providing effective solution. The choice of equipment performed after an objective needs analysis enables to optimize the acquiring process, to ensure the quality of reported results, and to provide more accessible costs to target populations that are generally poor. Biomedical engineers may enhance health by assessing and managing health technologies.

Keywords: sickle cell anemia, project management, biomedical equipment, planning

1. Introduction

By way of introduction, the quotation below significantly translates the problem of sickle cell disease both in the Democratic Republic of the Congo and in most countries of sub-Saharan Africa:

> *"Sickle cell disease is a genetic inherited disorder where hemoglobin (Hb) normal A (HbA) is replaced by another abnormal, HbS."*

Sickle cell anemia is a *serious disease* with manifestations and complications that directly affect the patient quality of life and his entourage. *This is not a shameful disease* contrary; it is linked to a mutation that arose for us to defend against severe forms of malaria. It is due to the so-called *selective pressure* that has enabled AS carriers to resist severe forms of malaria. This advantage explains among other things why, although cosmopolitan, sickle cell disease predominates in Africa and its geographical distribution is superimposed on the malaria one.

There are *four major outbreaks of sickle cell disease* based on genetic markers called haplotypes: Arabo-Indian, Beninese, Senegalese, and Central African or Bantu. Among Bantu haplotype carriers, the clinical expression of the sickle cell disease is more severe because of, among other things, the relatively low rate of the fetal hemoglobin (HbF) and other genetic factors.

According to WHO estimates, approximately 300–500,000 children are born each year with hemoglobinopathy; 80% of them are born in developing countries, particularly in Africa. The sickle cell anemia is a hemoglobin disorder most common in Africa, where every year about *200,000 newborns with sickle cell disease* are diagnosed and 80% will not reach the age of 5 years.

In the Democratic Republic of the Congo (DRC), it is estimated that there are 25–30% heterozygous healthy carriers (AS) and about *50,000 homozygous newborns (SS) each year*, equating to 2% of newborns [1].

Sickle cell disease is particularly common among people from sub-Saharan Africa, India, Saudi Arabia, and Mediterranean countries. Migration has increased the frequency of the offending gene in the Americas. In parts of sub-Saharan Africa, sickle cell disease affects up to 2% of newborns. More broadly, the prevalence of sickle cell disease (healthy carriers that inherited the mutant gene from only one parent) in equatorial Africa is 10–40%, compared to only 1–2% on the coast of North Africa and less than 1% in South Africa. This distribution reflects the fact that the sickle cell trait confers an advantage in terms of survival against malaria and that the selection pressure due to malaria has made the mutant gene more frequent, especially in areas with high malaria transmission. In West African countries such as Ghana and Nigeria, the rate of trafficking is 15–30%, while in Uganda, where marked tribal variations are observed, it is 45% among the Bahamas of west of the country [2].

2. Problems of financing of health systems and their corollary in the DR Congo

2.1 Deficit in sources of health-care funding

A country's problem of access to health care depends on its ability to finance the required health systems. This presupposes that the country concerned can offer structures, viable infrastructures, and competent personnel. However, low-income countries are struggling to find adequate budget balances to effectively meet the ever-growing health needs of their populations [3], and this is the case of the DR Congo and many other countries in sub-Saharan Africa.

Indeed, the current sources of financing useful for universal health coverage are essentially public expenditure, donor funding, and compulsory contributions to social health insurance [4]. Since under current conditions household contributions to health care remain relatively low, with a few exceptions when community initiatives are organized [5] or when the state is effectively involved, only two sources are secure: public spending and donor funding.

With regard to public expenditure, the state budget is low, often well below Abuja's commitments (15%) [6]. In 2013, for example, the Congolese state allocated only 4.3% of its budget to health, while all projections for spending in 2020 are below 3%. Worse still, this state contribution has only decreased from 2013 to date.

It just so happens that a large part of the financing of the health system relies heavily on donor funding. And in order to cover all needs, donors will theoretically have to continually increase their contribution in proportion to the decrease in the state budget.

But is such a hypothesis sustainable? Logically, the answer is negative, since donors cannot set themselves up as substitutes for failing health systems. Indeed, the study of the financing mechanism supported by the World Bank Group shows that "the health sector in the DRC suffers from several ills: low budget allocation; excessive household expenditure; dependence on external financing; available resources are poorly spent; budget execution is weak; governance problems; and the decentralization process is partly theoretical." [7] The same study shows that a decrease in external financing is observed from 2017, just as the projections predict that the deficit financing observed since 2019 will have to continue until 2030.

2.2 Attempt to address the funding gap for the management of sickle cell disease

In the specific case of the management of sickle cell disease, are there other ways of compensating for this financial situation?

The first way already present in the field is that of the actions of charitable associations. The contribution of several nongovernmental organizations involved in the management of specific pathologies such as sickle cell disease is very significant and constitutes a major support, especially for the most deprived populations. The action is perceptible not only in the DR Congo but also in other countries of sub-Saharan Africa [8]. But these efforts remain insignificant compared to the magnitude of the disease, and a country's health policy cannot be based on impulses that are difficult to predict.

The second way is the frequent use of donated second-hand equipment to reduce the costs they (the equipment) represent in the health-care chain. This resource can make a great contribution if best practices for donors and donors' applicants are rigorously observed [9]. Unfortunately, very often this is not the case. Many donations still arrive in Africa without observing the prerequisites, which very often makes them either ineffective or unusable. On the other hand, recourse to donations of second-hand equipment should remain ad hoc, without becoming structural.

The third way is that of optimizing the use of the means available to approach the objectives set. At the international level, donors have understood the challenge of structured and well-executed health financing. This obliges the partners to accompany for decades the countries receiving aid through specific national programs in order to reduce deficits and achieve the objectives.

In the DR Congo, it is through the national health development program that the government and its partners express their willingness to provide effective and realistic solutions to the health problems of the DR Congo's populations. This is generally applied for a period of 5 years, iteratively after evaluation.

The partners in the health field remain practically the same for African countries, and their health problems are very similar: the fight against epidemics, malnutrition, and hereditary diseases. This probably explains why almost all countries in sub-Saharan Africa each develop a national health development plan, with virtually the same content except for a few differences. Examples include the DR Congo, Mali, Côte d'Ivoire, Burkina Faso, Benin, and Kenya. Therefore the methods applied by the partners for health support to the different countries will be very similar.

In the national health development plans drawn up in many sub-Saharan African countries since 2000 to date, the improvement of infrastructures and the strengthening of the capacities of the medical technical platforms, including the expression of needs, acquisition, and maintenance of the systems acquired, are among the issues addressed. These topics involve a lot of money that will have to be put to good use; otherwise they can be a source of conscious or unconscious waste of scarce resources.

In the case of the DR Congo, a reflection carried out on the medical technical platform shows that the objectives assigned to medical infrastructure and equipment through national programs are never achieved and the situation is getting more complicated every year. And yet, after evaluation, the same programs continue with the same objectives and use practically the same methods [10]. In order to minimize procurement costs, the WHO proposes a strategic procurement approach to achieve universal health coverage [11]. The illustration below is more explicit.

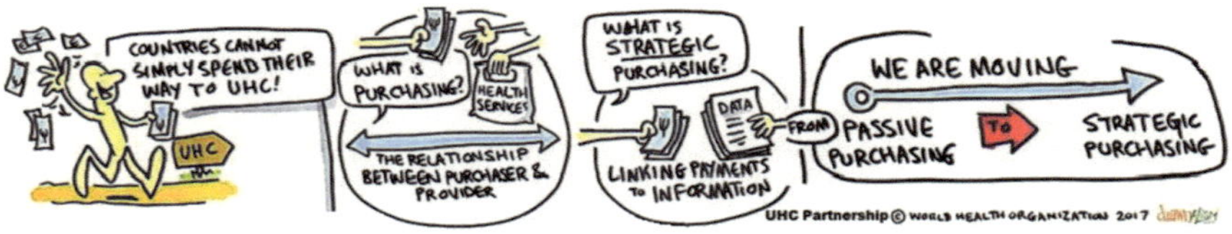
COUNTRIES CANNOT SIMPLY SPEND THEIR WAY TO UHC!
UHC
WHAT IS PURCHASING?
HEALTH SERVICES
THE RELATIONSHIP BETWEEN PURCHASER & PROVIDER
WHAT IS STRATEGIC PURCHASING?
DATA
LINKING PAYMENTS TO INFORMATION
WE ARE MOVING
FROM
PASSIVE PURCHASING
TO
STRATEGIC PURCHASING
UHC Partnership © WORLD HEALTH ORGANIZATION 2017

This diagram raises fundamental questions that need to be answered if we are to succeed in our efforts. Indeed, countries cannot simply spend their money on universal health coverage. They must master purchasing, define the relationships between suppliers and buyers, define a purchasing strategy on the basis of useful data before disbursement, and finally move from passive purchasing to strategic purchasing.

The fourth path, a corollary to the third, consists of mobilizing and structuring human skills, each in its own sector, to boost the strategic purchasing process. Since the problem of strategic purchasing concerns all sectors, what can the biomedical engineer's contribution be as far as it is concerned?

From this point of view, the biomedical engineer can play an important role as a technical interface between the hospital, suppliers, and industry to make the right choices, as he is considered responsible for the research and development, architecture, selection, management, and safe use of all types of medical devices including single-use, reusable, prosthetic, implantable, and bionic devices, among others [12].

For several decades, a developed country like France has been efficiently involving biomedical engineers in the medical equipment procurement process [13]. It organizes hospital purchasing, where biomedical engineers play a leading role in the purchasing function that has developed in companies over the last 30 years or so [14]. Better still, it is developing a purchasing policy that, among other things, brings together the skills of biomedical engineers to offer end customer equipment negotiated at attractive prices through group purchasing [15].

But in the Democratic Republic of the Congo in particular and in sub-Saharan Africa in general, the biomedical engineering component does not seem to be sufficiently integrated at its best in the administrative and technical response mechanisms for improving health care. This aspect of things can only lead to a waste of funds when the actors at this stage do not master the equipment.

3. Situation of medical equipment dedicated to the analysis of hemoglobinopathies

In the field there are currently different types of electrophoresis equipment. However, to date, it is difficult to determine their number, origins, and brands, given the country's size, diverse supply methods, and ineffective control mechanisms. Nevertheless, some facilities stand out from the others in terms of their number, mainly for historical and geographical, economic, and commercial reasons.

Historically and geographically, sickle cell disease was first discovered in black populations in Africa and in the Arabian Peninsula; to date it remains more frequent in these geographical areas. Initially, this disease, which later turned out to be hereditary, did not directly affect the Indo-European populations.

However, due to massive immigration, countries with well-organized prevention programs are now faced with the problems of uninformed couples of allochthonous origin, as well as variations in specific population characteristics, which is rare among indigenous populations [16].

In the early 1970s, screening tests were launched in the United States, and the American population of African origin was indeed very affected. In 1981, an experimental neonatal screening program began in the French Antilles and metropolitan France. It is set up by the Association Française pour le Dépistage et la Prévention du Handicap (AFDPHE). It was only in 2000 that neonatal screening for sickle cell disease was, this time, extended in whole France [17].

As a result of the above, electrophoresis systems are initially more equipped with routine programs dedicated to serum protein analysis; programs for the analysis of hemoglobinopathies will gradually come into operation. Indeed, the implementation of new programs involves significant costs that the manufacturer cannot incur without a guaranteed return on investment.

Since the greatest need for sickle cell disease management is in Africa, countries with strong historical ties to the continent will find it easier to sell their technologies to this potential market. Among them we will mention the most prominent firms such as HELENA, TITAN, BECKMAN SEBIA, and BIORAD.

In financial terms, the choice of equipment for routine needs will focus more on technical solutions that offer good results at lower cost. From this point of view, for the analysis of hemoglobinopathies, there is an established correlation between agarose gel electrophoresis on the one hand and capillary electrophoresis on the other [18]. On the other hand, high-performance liquid chromatography (HPLC) and capillary techniques are complementary and can be used routinely, knowing that capillary diagrams are easier to read and interpret than those obtained in HPLC. Even better, the development of the capillary technique for the characterization of hemoglobin variants suggested that it would become the first method of choice for screening in many clinical laboratories [19].

This trend is confirmed with regular innovations from certain manufacturers, and this is the case of SEBIA, which has added to its range for the screening of hemoglobinopathies [20]. In addition, the capillary technique is more sensitive than the HPLC technique for the detection of certain variants such as hemoglobin New York [21].

On the commercial level, thanks to their historical links with Africa, the first companies are more easily organized and set up local representations of their firms to facilitate the sale of their products. Among the first to obtain country-level representation are HELENA and BECKMAN.

But for almost two decades, we have been observing the rise of the SEBIA company, which offers different models of equipment according to the needs and which regularly innovates its products. Today, this firm, now a world leader in the field of electrophoresis, is among those with a large number of distributors in Africa.

Apart from the abovementioned brands, it is worth noting a slow penetration of products of Asian origin in the field. However, while the financial offer is attractive, distribution is still struggling to be structured in terms of regularity, reliability, and operation.

In the present case of the management of sickle cell disease and in order to make his contribution relevant and effective, the biomedical engineer must make an inventory of the existing situation in the field, evaluate the technologies in the state of the art, and propose material solutions that present a better compromise between technical and technological contributions and optimization of the financial aspect.

4. Analysis of onboard techniques on electrophoresis systems

The following theories are drawn mainly from the book *Appliances and Methods in Biochemistry and Molecular Biology*, whose pedagogical approach seems clearer.

4.1 General principles of electrophoresis

Electrophoresis has established itself over time as the method of choice for the qualification and quantification of different fractions in the management of hemoglobinopathy. It involves methods often embedded in laboratory materials. We review below the most common methods in electrophoresis of hemoglobin.

4.1.1 Definitions

Electrophoresis is a physical method of separating molecules based on their difference in mobility, under the effect of an electric field. Zone electrophoresis, carried out on a solid support, is used to essentially separate the ionizable biological macromolecules, that is to say proteins, nucleic acids, and certain polyosides and proteoglycans.

Liquid vein electrophoresis, currently capillary electrophoresis, is also applied to small molecules, organic or mineral, and not necessarily ionizable. In the most common case, the movement of the molecule depends on several intrinsic (due to the molecule itself) and extrinsic parameters, in particular linked to migration buffers which play the role of solvent [22].

4.1.2 Zone electrophoresis

This is the electrophoresis whose migration medium is stabilized by a real or sometimes virtual porous support as in the density gradient. In the case of a porous substrate, it is soaked with a buffer solution that both ensures conductivity and stabilizes the pH at the desired value. The molecules separate according to their different mobility in the system (they appear as migration zones) and will be visualized in a second time ("revelations"); we can even isolate them from the support for the preparatory purpose.

Zone electrophoresis is mainly applied to the separation of macromolecules.

4.1.2.1 Characteristics

These electrophoreses are often characterized by strong electroosmotic currents and sometimes intense Joule effect. The most common electroosmotic current is the electroendosmosis current, especially in polyosidic supports used at pH alkaline: the walls are negatively ionized as the macromolecules to be separated; positive buffer charges are attracted to the cathode and create a current that is in the opposite direction of electrophoretic migration.

Another electroosmosis phenomenon is related to the structure of the support, which can be assimilated to a capillary network; the friction forces are greater on the edges of the support, and the center moves faster, distorting the migration band. Finally, the Joule effect heats the substrate and therefore evaporates the solvent; this is gradually replaced by the liquid of the vessels which rises in the support by capillary action, opposite both ends of the support, and annulling in the middle [23].

4.1.2.2 Supports

The supports must be chemically inert (low adsorbent) and homogeneous (regular microporous structure), have good mechanical resistance (handling), and possibly allow densitometric reading [24].

4.1.2.2.1 Paper

Paper is a natural cellulose; it is no longer used much because it is not homogeneous. Paper electrophoresis provides a strong electroendosmosis current and is a source of parasitic adsorptions (added chromatography), resulting in poor resolution; the Joule effect is important with heating, evaporation, and even electrolysis of the buffer. At high pressure (1000–3000 V), paper electrophoresis is mainly used to separate peptides and amino acids.

4.1.2.2.2 Cellulose acetate

Cellulose acetate is much more homogeneous than paper; this support allows densitometric reading, but the electroendosmosis current remains high. The applications of cellulose acetate are mainly found in medical biology, allowing a quantitative densitometric reading of the protein fractions rather roughly separated (plasma and urinary proteins, lipoproteins, and hemoglobins), or finer (isoenzymes), applying the potential gradients of the order of 30 V cm^{-1}. Resolution is poor, and reproducibility is average.

However, at alkaline pH (typically pH 8.6), Hb A2, Hb C, Hb E, and Hb O migrate to the same area, and Hb S, Hb D, and Hb G migrate at the same rate. In the case of suspicions of such hemoglobin abnormalities, an additional technique should therefore be considered [25].

4.1.2.2.3 Starch gel (cross-linked starch)

Starch gel is a polyoside; electrophoresis on this gel allows the separation of complex or heterogeneous oligomeric protein associations. Starch gel is little used because it is opaque, fragile, and not very reproducible.

4.1.2.2.4 Agarose gel

Agarose is desulfonated agar (purified agar); removal of sulfonates greatly limits the flow of electroendosmosis; agarose gels between 0.5 and 2% are not very viscous. They make it possible to carry out native electrophoresis as with the previous supports, that is, without denaturation of the macromolecules. Potential gradients up to 50 V cm^{-1} are usable for protein separation; agarose gel is gradually replacing cellulose acetate in most biomedical applications because agarose improves resolution and remains colorless, allowing a good densitometric reading. The agarose gel is also very homogeneous, thus ensuring good reproducibility, and is well adapted to zymographic reading [23].

The distinction between the different variants Hb A2, Hb C, Hb E, and Hb O, as well as Hb S, Hb D, and Hb G, is most often made by electrophoresis on agarose gel at acidic pH (pH 6.0), which allows to separate Hb C, from Hb E and Hb O, as well as Hb S, from Hb D and Hb G. On the other hand, Hb E and Hb O, as well as Hb D and G, still cannot be differentiated by combining these two electrophoretic methods (cellulose acetate, agarose gel). In addition, these techniques have the disadvantage of consuming time and labor.

In addition, they lack precision for the quantification of hemoglobin in low concentrations, such as Hb A2, and for the detection of fast-migrating variants, such as Hb H or Hb Bart's. It is even now accepted that the quantification of variants by densitometry lacks precision and that these two electrophoresis techniques must be used for qualitative purposes. They are therefore most often used today in combination with another method, mainly high-performance liquid chromatography, which has a much higher accuracy.

A 1999 study by the College of American Pathologists showed a coefficient of variation (CV) of 33.6% for the quantification of Hb A2 at a concentration of 2.41% by densitometry from electrophoretic gels. By HPLC, the CV was 4.3% for Hb A2 at a concentration of 3.47%. Thus, the combination of these electrophoresis techniques with HPLC allows the identification and quantification of hemoglobin, the latter being performed by HPLC only [26].

4.1.2.2.5 Polyacrylamide

It is a polymer of acrylamide and N,N′-methylene-bisacrylamide (Bis), the acrylamide gel polymerization being obtained in the presence of a catalyst (ammonium persulfate) and a cross-linking agent (N,N,N′,N′-tetramethyl-ethylene-diamine [TEMED]). The porosity of gels can be very precise; it depends on the relative concentrations of acrylamide and Bis.

The polymer obtained is very hydrophilic although insoluble in water and easy to mold even under small thicknesses (<1 mm); it is thermostable, not fragile, transparent, and inert chemically. There is almost no electroendosmosis flow and no macromolecules are absorbed. The resolutive power is generally superior to that of polyosidic gels using gradients of similar potential. The main disadvantage is that the acrylamide in solution is neurotoxic but also that the resulting porosities are very poorly adapted to very large molecules [27].

4.1.2.3 Zone electrophoresis methods

4.1.2.3.1 Native electrophoresis (without denaturation)

It is made on paper, starch, cellulose acetate, agarose gel, and sometimes polyacrylamide whenever we do not want to touch the tertiary and quaternary structures of macromolecules, thus their biological activities. This method without denaturation is a priori applicable to all types of macromolecules, both in vertical and horizontal tanks [27].

4.1.2.3.2 Isoelectrofocusing

Isoelectrofocusing, carried out on agarose gel or polyacrylamide gel, separates hemoglobin in a pH gradient according to their isoelectric point. To do this, ampholytes are introduced into the gel in order to create a continuous pH gradient under the effect of an electric field. The different hemoglobins contained in the sample to be analyzed will migrate to the region where the pH is equal to their isoelectric pH. At this position, the net load is zero, and the hemoglobin ceases to migrate and focuses into a narrow band.

This technique, capable of separating hemoglobin variants with isoelectric points different from 0.02 pH units, has excellent resolution and is very useful for detecting abnormal hemoglobin in the newborn. In fact, it allows a good separation of hemoglobins F, A, and S. Moreover, the electrical isofocusing is perfectly adapted to the analysis of large series. On the other hand, the main limitations of this method are a long and complex implementation. Therefore, its use is almost reserved for neonatal screening of hemoglobinopathies [28, 29].

4.1.3 Liquid vein electrophoresis

4.1.3.1 Characteristics

Typically, capillary electrophoresis is performed in a fused silica capillary coated with a polyamide layer of 20–200 μm of internal diameter and 20–200 cm of length. The capillary, placed in a thermostatization system, is filled with a buffer solution and plunges into two tanks containing the same solution. Each tank is connected to an electrode connected to a current generator. A large potential difference (several thousand volts) is applied to the terminals of each capillary to separate the molecules on the basis of their charge/mass ratio [30].

The use of a capillary has a double advantage: increases the sensitivity of the detection since a reading window in the capillary allows an absorbance reading with a very small optical path and increases the resolution by applying the potential difference of more than 10,000 V since it is easy to regulate the capillary in temperature [31].

4.1.3.2 Support

In this method, the buffer solution in contact with the two tanks of the system constitutes the support. Since liquid has no specific form, the buffer uses the capillary as a solid support, contributing also to electroendosmosis current production.

4.1.3.3 Liquid vein electrophoresis methods

There are several methods used in capillary electrophoresis including capillary zone electrophoresis (CZE), capillary gel electrophoresis (CGE), and micellar electrokinetic chromatography (MECC) [32]. In this study, we will limit ourselves to capillary zone electrophoresis which is the most exploited for hemoglobinopathy.

This method can be performed on a single-fused silica capillary in which an electroosmotic flux develops. It causes the negative molecules to the cathode where the detection is carried out, the injection being anodic.

The electroosmotic flux depends on the temperature, the ionic force, and the concentration of organic solvent.

4.2 Facilities

We will limit ourselves here to the most common routine techniques for the analysis of hemoglobinopathies in the Democratic Republic of the Congo in particular and in sub-Saharan Africa in general. They are often affected by accessibility during acquisition, ease of commissioning, operation, maintenance and supply, and cost.

On one side, our analysis is based globally on equipment meeting international standards such as ISO, FDA, and CE certification. Field experience shows that such equipment can operate for about 7 years, if the manufacturer's operating recommendations are followed.

On the other hand, high-performance liquid chromatography has been developed to allow both the detection and confirmation of hemoglobinopathy in newborns with high sensitivity and specificity. In fact, its good sensitivity to the major variants involved in pathology and its speed of completion (about 3 min per sample), allowing the analysis of a large number of samples, have made HPLC a particularly suitable method for screening for hemoglobin abnormalities [33].

However, we will not discuss this technique in this study because, since its performance is comparable to that of the HPLC method, capillary electrophoresis quickly became the method of choice, just like HPLC, for the study of hemoglobinopathy. In addition, it is of economic interest: although the material cost is comparable to that of the HPLC, the expenditures on reagents are much lower. Indeed, the price of a capillary is much lower than that of a chromatography column, and the volumes of buffer used are much lower, about 1000 times less [34].

4.2.1 Manual systems

4.2.1.1 Offer

Manual systems for native electrophoresis (on cellulose acetate and agarose gel) or isoelectrofocusing offer the best acquisition possibility both in terms of cost and operational constraints. Their limits both in the separation and in the identification of hemoglobin variants will be used for the routine forms to be specified by the customer (identification of the electrophoretic profile, identification of specific variants).

The coupling of these methods to the reading system (densitometers) makes it possible to quantify the separate variants. And from this point of view, agarose gel electrophoresis offers better performance than cellulose acetate. On the other hand, the reagents are in the form of combs which often require a minimum of seven samples. Such a constraint requires, for economic reasons, to launch the samples in series of seven, which requires a consequent sizing and proper holding wire.

4.2.1.2 Facilities

For native electrophoresis the system is usually composed of a current generator and a migration tank. For isoelectrofocusing, the system consists of a stabilized supply, an isoelectrofocusing, unit, and a circulating cryostat.

The devices typically contain conventional electronic parts and boards, used in the manufacture of power generators. These components are often not complex, and do not require advanced technical repair. In addition, it has been found that when equipment actually meets ISO, FDA, or CE marking standards, it works well and lasts for a long time.

4.2.1.3 Use

These systems can be used in very small laboratories, without large volume flow of samples, for the screening of hemoglobinopathies, by planning a periodic operation. Indeed, the pre-analytical phase requires a lot of sample preparation time and immobilizes the staff for quite a long time. They can also be used in medium laboratories as a backup system.

The isoelectrofocusing system will be more targeted for newborn screening because it allows for a good separation of the Hb F, Hb A, and Hb S fractions, which assumes that the system is usually installed near a maternity ward.

4.2.2 Semiautomatic systems

4.2.2.1 Offer

Semiautomatic systems for native electrophoresis on cellulose acetate or agarose gel offer the possibility of processing large series of samples. Although the cost of the system is still high for a large number of health facilities, the manual routine is clearly improved. Semiautomatic systems (on cellulose acetate or agarose gel) are embedded on compact systems generally comprising a migration and coloring modules, which considerably reduce user handling.

The reading system, often equipped with advanced post-processing software, can be incorporated or remote. Nevertheless, the results obtained show the same limits as in the case of manual methods because the operating principles of the migration and coloring units taken separately are the same as those of the manual system.

4.2.2.2 Facilities

The semiautomatic system is generally composed of a compact unit comprising a thermoregulated migration module connected to a current generator and a fluidic module for coloring migrated gels. Technologically, an intelligent electronic unit manages the high voltage of the migration module, the fluidics of the coloring module, and the application programs for the two modules.

Generally, devices typically contain conventional electronic parts and boards. The process control is often ensured by position and temperature sensors. As their complexity is not great, maintenance can be easily carried out by a duly trained biomedical technician.

4.2.2.3 Use

These systems can equip medium-sized laboratories by planning either periodic operation or continuous operation, depending on the flow of samples. They are fairly widespread in the private laboratories which can obtain them and some public hospital laboratories often on behalf of specific programs. User maintenance monitoring must be ensured to guarantee proper functioning, and periodic annual maintenance must be carried out, insured in accordance with the manufacturer's recommendations.

4.2.3 Automatic techniques

4.2.3.1 Offer

Automatic techniques (only capillary zone electrophoresis) are the best offer, both in terms of flexibility of use and technical performance. Prices are still very high for many customers in Africa. Nevertheless, a good expression of needs and an adequate exploitation planning can allow a return on investment in an acceptable time.

4.2.3.2 Facilities

These techniques are carried out on compact systems, generally comprising capillaries at the ends plunging into reservoirs of buffer solution, themselves connected to the current generator. The apparatus also includes a detection system, most often a UV–visible spectrophotometer, linked to the wavelength of specific absorption of hemoglobin at 415 nm.

Migration support	Advantages	Disadvantages	Systems	Materials	Maintenance level	Constraints	Average cost (€)
Paper	- Native electrophoresis - Separation of amino acids and peptides	- High electroendosmosis current - Significant Joule effect - Bad resolution - Poor homogeneity - Parasite adsorptions	Manual	- Current generator	- Low	Good grounding	
				- Migration tank	- Free	Free	7000
				- Densitometer	- Low	Free	
Cellulose acetate	- Native electrophoresis - More homogeneous than paper - Separation of plasma and urine proteins, lipoproteins, hemoglobin, and isoenzymes	- High electroendosmosis currents - Poor resolution - Medium reproducibility - The hemoglobins A2, C, E, and O migrate in the same zone - The hemoglobins S, D, and G migrate at the same rate - Long implementation	Manual	- Current generator	- Low	Good grounding	
				- Migration tank	- Free	Free	7000
				- Densitometer	- Low	Free	
			Semiautomatic	- Compact staining and migration module and densitometer (integrated or no)	- Medium - Medium	- Steady voltage - Good grounding - Air-conditioned room - Inverter	15,000
Agarose gel	-Native electrophoresis - Nonnative electrophoresis - Limited electroendosmosis flow - Improved resolution - Very homogeneous - Separation of Hb C from Hb E and Hb O - Separation of Hb S from Hb D and Hb G	- No separation between HB E and Hb O - No separation between Hb D and Hb G - Inaccurate for the quantification of hemoglobin with low concentration (Hb A2) and for the detection of variants with fast migration (Hb H and Hb Bart's) - Long Implementation	Manual	- Current generator	-Low	Good grounding	
				- Migration tank	-Free	Free	7000
				- Densitometer	- Low	Free	
			Semiautomatic	- Compact staining and migration module and densitometer (integrated or no)	- Medium - Medium	- Steady stable - Good grounding - Air-conditioned room - Inverter	15,000

DOI: http://dx.doi.org/10.5772/intechopen.92546

Migration support	Advantages	Disadvantages	Systems	Materials	Maintenance level	Constraints	Average cost (€)
			Semiautomatic	-Isoelectrofocusing module	- Medium	- Steady voltage - Good grounding - Air-conditioned room - Inverter	150,000
				-Circulation cryostat	- Medium	- Steady voltage - Good grounding - Air-conditioned room - Inverter	
Liquid vein (capillaries)	- Fast - Precise quantification of hemoglobin fractions - Flexible (small and large series)	-High water quality -Demanding environment	Automatic	- Compact migration and detection module	- High	- Steady voltage - Good grounding - Air-conditioned room - Inverter - Water quality	30,000

Table 1.
Summary table of different devices.

More sophisticated technology includes a capillary thermoregulation system, a control system comprising various sensors that manage optics, robotics, pneumatics, and detection, and a set of intelligent electronic cards capable of communicating with each other. Unlike previous methods, this method allows both to launch samples in an emergency without restriction and to process large series of samples.

In view of the complexity of its technology, management requires competent personnel who are regularly trained by the manufacturer. Water quality and user maintenance of equipment are of paramount importance to ensure the quality of results. This assumes that the supplier provides user training for the best care.

4.2.3.3 Use

Thanks to their flexibility in the work organization, these automated systems can equip laboratories with small volumes of samples, as well as those which process large volumes. Indeed, there are small and large models of automata to cover all these needs. Because of their high prices, these automata are acquired in public hospitals on the basis of research projects and specific programs. Private clinics acquire them for routine because of their performance. However they do have a few requirements that must be observed: the operating environment must be less dusty, the quality of electricity flawless, the quality of pure water, and regular maintenance.

We present in **Table 1** a summary of different devices that we have reviewed.

5. Discussion on the choice to be made for equipment acquisition

For better use of data in **Table 1**, it will be broken down below with two subsidiaries: **Tables 2** and **3**.

The information contained in **Table 2** will highlight the performance of the equipment according to different migration or embedded media available, while those in **Table 3** will compare the systems sold compared to hardware, installation constraints, execution time, and cost.

A cursory reading shows that the most efficient migration support remains one of the capillary methods (liquid vein): this support brings in itself the best return for the resolution, reproducibility, discrimination, and quantification, while the parasitic effects are almost nonexistent. But medical needs and health goals differ from one level to another and do not require in all cases the acquisition of such technology.

For routine screening for sickle cell disease, for example, the performance of migration on cellulose acetate amply suffices needs. This assumes that the precise separation variants like Hb A2, Hb C, Hb E, and Hb O are not a need first. On the other hand, as part of the requirements to cover, the effective separation of Hb S and Hb C variant is needed, and migration on agarose gel will best meet this requirement.

If, during treatment, abnormal forms of hemoglobin are associated, then the choice of medium will be directed towards agarose gel for a qualitative indication or the liquid vein for a quantitative indication of Hb A2. Indeed, abnormally low Hb A and abnormally high Hb A2 correlate with the presence of some abnormal forms of hemoglobin (alpha or beta thalassemia, etc.).

If precise separation and precise quantification of the variants Hb A2, Hb C, Hb E, and Hb O are required, then the liquid vein (capillary) support should be readily chosen.

Depending on work previously defined criteria, this table can guide the choice of performance basis based migration media.

But the only performance criteria are not sufficient to make a choice of appropriate materials. It will also take into account industrial supply in terms of existing

Performances	Migration support			
	Paper	Cellulose acetate	Agarose gel	Liquid vein
Nonnative electrophoresis			✓	✓
Native electrophoresis	✓	✓	✓	✓
Separation of amino acids and peptides	✓	✓	✓	✓
Homogeneity	✓ (poor)	✓ (medium)	✓ (good)	✓
Separation of plasma and urine proteins, lipoproteins, hemoglobin, and isoenzymes	—	✓	✓	✓
Resolution	✓ (bad)	✓ (poor)	✓	✓
Separation of Hb A2 from Hb C, Hb E, and Hb O	—	x (migrate in the same area)	✓	✓
Separation of Hb C from Hb E and Hb O	—	x	✓	✓
Separation of Hb S and Hb from Hb D and G	—	x (migrate at the same rate)	✓	✓
Separation of Hb S and Hb O	—	x	x	✓
Separation of Hb D and Hb G	—	x	x	✓
Rapidity	Low	Good	Good	Fast
Quantification of hemoglobin with low concentration (Hb A2)	—	x	x	✓
Detection of fast-migrating variants (Hb H, Hb Bart's)	—	x	x	✓
Precise quantification of hemoglobin fractions	—	x	x	✓
Flexible (small and wide series)	—	x	x	✓
Electroendosmosis current	Very high	High	High	High
Joule effect	✓	—	—	—
Pest adsorption	✓	x	x	x
Reproducibility	—	✓ (medium)	✓	✓
Water quality	Normal	Normal	Normal	High
Demanding environment	Normal	Normal	Normal	High

Table 2.
Performance comparison based on migration support.

systems, the materials that make up, their costs, and maintenance requirements. Below we provide a table that can guide us in assessing the choices to be made.

The line "migration support" is added in order to link **Tables 2** and **3**.

The analysis of the table shows that as the system moves from manual to fully automated, the necessary hardware is gradually being integrated into a compact module. From this point of view, this development provides an appreciable response to the ergonomic problems that are becoming very frequent in laboratories.

On the other hand, we observe that the installation constraints are more demanding when the analysis module becomes more compact. Indeed, in addition to the quality of the electrical ground line and voltage which greatly affect the operation of systems provided, the environment requires better temperature control (air conditioning), for example, besides the requirements of the water quality.

	Systems		
	Manual	**Semiautomatic**	**Automatic**
Migration support	-Paper -Cellulose acetate -Agarose gel	Cellulose acetate -Agarose gel	-Vein liquid (capillaries)
Equipment	-Power generator -Tank migration -Densitometer	-Module staining and migration -Densitometer (integrated or not)	-Module compact migration and detection
Installation constraints	-Quality ground line -Quality voltage	-Quality ground line -Quality voltage -Quality air conditioning	-Quality ground line -Quality voltage -Quality air conditioning -Quality of water
Execution time	Très long	Long	Court
Acquisition cost (en €)	7000	15,000	3000
Maintenance level	Bas	Moyen	Haut

Table 3.
Comparison of systems in terms of hardware, installation constraints, acquisition cost, and maintenance level.

The time required to perform the analyses is a very important parameter in the choice of equipment. On the one hand, it allows better management of the patient queue, and on the other hand, it ensures the management of reagents and consumables with a limited life. When the volume of samples to be treated in a routine manner is small, manual systems are suitable for both patient satisfaction and reactive management. If the volume of samples to be processed requires more than 1 day of work, the semiautomated system should be considered to resolve the queue. Finally, if the volume of samples increases further, the fully automated system will better meet expectations.

The management of reagents in the laboratory depends heavily on two important parameters that should be noted: this is the expiry date and the stability time after opening of the reagent. The expiry date indicated on the label is usually the date after which the manufacturer no longer guarantees the validity of the results, while the stability time after opening of the reagent indicates the period after which the manufacturer no longer guarantees its reliability after the first use.

Since the stability time is shorter than the expiry date itself, it will be necessary to ensure that each open reagent is consumed before that time. For example, the use of a reagent that has a stability time of 60 days and can analyze 1000 samples in a laboratory that receives only 10 samples per day is a waste. The use of this reagent before maturity requires an average daily rate of 20 samples, considering that the laboratory operates 6 days a week. Ten samples/day instead of 20 samples/day will theoretically cause the damage of half the reagent.

The level of maintenance, and in turn cost, follows the same trend: more compact system is provided and the higher level of maintenance.

Since the cost of acquiring systems increases with the complexity of the technology, it is important to ask good questions, find good answers, and make good choices based on real needs, to achieve savings. As an example, is it necessary to acquire a semiautomatic agarose gel system when, taking into account the medical needs and the volume of samples to be treated, the manual system on agarose gel support gives us satisfaction? Affirmative answer incurs an additional a non-justified expenditure of 8000€. Worse still, such equipment oversizing compromises a substantial depreciation because it will be under-utilized.

6. Conclusion

The management of any pathology implies the appropriate choice of techniques and technologies. Indeed, beyond the medical needs that are priority, a control equipment acquisition cost is one of the major parameters providing effective support to strategies put in place.

Very often in sub-Saharan countries, the aspect of the consequent acquisition of the necessary technology is not always thorough, and this can lead a poor quality of reported results, the inaccessible test cost for the poorest people, and the delicate operation of projects being implemented.

The choice of equipment performed after an objective needs analysis enables to optimize the process of acquiring, to ensure the quality of reported results, and to provide more accessible costs to target populations generally poor.

According to WHO recommendations, technology assessment, device evaluation, needs planning, selection and acquisition, installation, commissioning, and finally monitoring should be part of a successful acquisition procedure [35].

Such an approach should involve all stakeholders, namely, doctors, managers, biomedical engineers, and users.

In the case of sickle cell anemia, the inventory of installed park shows that beside manual methods, diagnostic techniques most common in the Democratic Republic of the Congo and even in sub-Saharan Africa are phenotypic techniques. These include *the electrophoresis at different pH, the isoelectrofocusing, the capillary electrophoresis, and the high-pressure liquid chromatography.* The first three mentioned are most used for their reliability, flexibility, ease of installation, and maintenance.

The prices of the equipment listed in the table remain indicative. We have taken into account only good-quality equipment commonly used in the DR Congo and by extension in other countries of sub-Saharan Africa.

For low-income countries, the costs of such facilities are still high overall. Indeed, the increase in health expenditure, which represents 10% of the world's gross domestic product (GDP), is faster than the growth of the world economy. According to a new World Health Organization report on global health spending, it is increasing rapidly, particularly in low- and middle-income countries, where spending is increasing at an average of 6% per year, compared to 4% in high-income countries.

Health expenditure is assumed by governments, by individuals who pay for their own care (out-of-pocket payments), and by other entities such as voluntary health insurance schemes, employer-sponsored schemes, and nongovernmental organizations. On average, 51% of a country's health expenditure is assumed by general government and more than 35% by individuals in the form of direct expenditure. One of the consequences of this situation is that every year 100 million people are plunged into extreme poverty [36].

For the countries concerned, the acquisition of these health technologies requires new upstream procurement strategies to meet acquisition and operating costs. And from this point of view, some developed countries such as France are now developing group procurement procedures in public hospitals.

According to a recent study conducted in the Democratic Republic of the Congo on an investment in capillary electrophoresis equipment for a project on sickle cell disease, this can contribute to improve quality and low cost of tests, if a complete analysis of needs is carried out upstream.

In this study, for an equipment activity extending over a period of 7 years, the cost of acquisition and maintenance cost represent, respectively, 11.4% and 5.0% of the total life cycle cost.

But when the activity of the same equipment is done over a period of 2 years, the cost of acquisition and maintenance cost represent, respectively, 31.0% and 3.9% of the total life cycle cost.

Added to this, for the same annual rate, the minimum unit test cost is € 3.9 for a 7-year activity cycle, whereas it costs € 5 if the activity cycle is reduced to 2 years [37].

Therefore, it should be noted that when operating conditions remain the same, amortization of equipment carried on shorter lead times significantly increases the cost of the test at the expense of patients.

Even though this example only concerns electrophoresis capillary equipment, extrapolating conclusions on agarose gel equipment is possible for the following reasons: installation, operation, and maintenance are less demanding than for capillary technology.

While sub-Saharan Africa is the most affected region in the world for sickle cell disease, research and care are relatively slow.

At its 60th session held in Malabo from 30 August to 3 September 2010, the WHO was already raising the option of a strategy for its African region. Nine years after the effects are hardly noticeable.

The management improvement of this pathology solicits several challenges, including the one concerning the technical platform necessary for diagnosis. The costs of acquiring and operating equipment often require significant fundraising, which is often lacking. The missing financial means are often one of the first obstacles to the launching of the relevant programs.

The study mentioned above proves that it is possible to optimize the available resources, however modest they may be, in order to obtain good and lasting results.

In the case of biomedical equipment, it is sufficient to involve the right people to achieve the expected results. Policymakers in sub-Saharan African countries must therefore integrate the skills of biomedical engineers into the design and start-up of medical projects so that they, in turn, contribute effectively to improve the quality of medical care populations.

Author details

Vincent Mulunda-a-Mulunda[1]*, Pierre Kouam[2] and Taty Oke Ingwen[3]

1 Institut Supérieur de Techniques Appliquées (ISTA), Kinshasa, Democratic Republic of Congo

2 Groupe Hospitalier Nord Essonne, Lonjumeau, France

3 Wagenia Sarl, Kinshasa, Democratic Republic of Congo

*Address all correspondence to: vp_amulunda@yahoo.fr

References

[1] Tshilolo L, Aïssi LM. Guide pratique de diagnostic précoce et de prise en charge de la drépanocytose en RD Congo. CEFA; 2009. p. 7

[2] Available from: http://apps.who.int/gb/archive/pdf_files/WHA59/A59_9-fr.pdf

[3] Available from: http://www.santemondiale.org/2013/02/20/le-financement-des-systemes-de-sante-dans-les-pays-a-faible-revenus-reflexions-inspirees-de-la-situation-de-la-rdc/

[4] Available from: https://www.cabri-sbo.org/uploads/files/Documents/seminar_paper_2015_cabri_value_for_money_health _french_1.1cabri_challenges_in_financing_health_sectors_in_africa_french.pdf

[5] Stasse S et al. Improving financial access to health care in the Kisantu district in the Democratic Republic of Congo: Acting upon complexity. DOI: 10.3402/gha.v8.25480

[6] Available from: https://www.nationalplanningcycles.org/sites/default/files/planning_cycle_repository/democratic_republic_of_congo/pnds_2016-2020_version_finale_29_avril_2016.pdf

[7] Available from: https://www.globalfinancingfacility.org/sites/gff_new/files/documents/Etude-espace-budgetaire-secteur-sante-rdc-CSU.pdf

[8] Available from: https://www.fondationpierrefabre.org/fr/programmes-en-cours/lutte-contre-la-drepanocytose/

[9] Medical Devices Donation: Consideration for Solicitation and Provision. Geneva: WHO; 2011. p. 10

[10] Mulunda-a-Mulunda V, Kouam P. Réflexion sur le plateau technique médical en République Démocratique du Congo. Irbm News. 2019;**40**(4):162-174

[11] Available from: https://www.who.int/health_financing/events/strategic-purchasing-meeting-2017-report-fr.pdf?ua=1

[12] Human Resources for Medical Devices, The Role of Biomedical Engineers. Geneva: World Health Organization; 2017. p. 20. Available from: https://www.who.int/medical_devices/publications/hr_med_dev_bio-engineers/en/

[13] Broun G. Biomedical engineers in public hospitals: Observations and hypotheses. ITBM-RBM News. 2006; **27**(4):384

[14] Decouvelaere M. Hospital procurement organization: Opportunities and perspectives for biomedical and hospital engineering. IRBM News. 2013;**34**(5–6):114

[15] Available from: http://ageps.aphp.fr

[16] Giordano PC. Carrier Screening and Prevention of Hemoglobinopathies by Capillary Electrophoresis. Lisses: Sebia Laboratories; 2007. p. 7

[17] Available from: http://www.apipd.fr/wp-content/uploads/2015/05/historique-drepanocytose-new-logo.pdf

[18] Chen FA, Liu C-M, Hsieh Y-Z, Sternberg JC. Capillary electrophoresis, a new clinical tool. Clinical Chemistry. 1991;**37**(1):14-19

[19] Keren DF. Comparison of sebia capillarys capillary electrophoresis with the primus high-pressure liquid chromatography in the evaluation of hemoglobinopathies. American Journal of Clinical Pathology. 2008;**130**: 824-883

[20] Vesseron S et al. Euromedlab: Etat de l'art en biologie médicale. IRBM News. 2019:5

[21] Li Y-Q, Huang H-P, Chen Z-Z, Zhao L, Liang L, Qin G-F, et al. Comparison of capillary electrophoresis and high performance liquid chromatography for detection and quantification of hemoglobin. Clinical Chemistry and Laboratory Medicine. 2016;**54**(1):91-95

[22] Hainque B et al. Appareils et méthodes en Biochimie et Biologie Moléculaire. Paris: Flammarion; 2008. p. 274

[23] Hainque B et al. Appareils et méthodes en Biochimie et Biologie Moléculaire. Paris: Flammarion; 2008. p. 276

[24] Hainque B et al. Appareils et méthodes en Biochimie et Biologie Moléculaire. Paris: Flammarion; 2008. pp. 276-277

[25] Guerard V. Mise en place de l'électrophorèse capillaire MINICAP® (Sebia) pour le diagnostic des hémoglobinopathies au CHU de Nancy. In: Sciences Pharmaceutiques. 2014; ffhal-01733413ff. p. 22

[26] Guerard V. Mise en place de l'électrophorèse capillaire MINICAP® (Sebia) pour le diagnostic des hémoglobinopathies au CHU de Nancy. In: Sciences Pharmaceutiques. 2014; ffhal-01733413ff. pp. 22-23

[27] Hainque B et al. Appareils et méthodes en Biochimie et Biologie Moléculaire. Paris: Flammarion; 2008. p. 277

[28] Tshilolo L, Aïssi LM. Guide pratique de diagnostic précoce et de prise en charge de la drépanocytose en RD Congo. Pafoved; 2014. p. 24

[29] Guerard V. Mise en place de l'électrophorèse capillaire MINICAP® (Sebia) pour le diagnostic des hémoglobinopathies au CHU de Nancy. In: Sciences Pharmaceutiques. 2014; ffhal-01733413ff. p. 24

[30] Guerard V. Mise en place de l'électrophorèse capillaire MINICAP® (Sebia) pour le diagnostic des hémoglobinopathies au CHU de Nancy. In: Sciences Pharmaceutiques. 2014; ffhal-01733413ff. p. 32

[31] Hainque B et al. Appareils et méthodes en Biochimie et Biologie Moléculaire. Paris: Flammarion; 2008. p. 285

[32] Hainque B et al. Appareils et méthodes en Biochimie et Biologie Moléculaire. Paris: Flammarion; 2008. p. 286

[33] Guerard V. Mise en place de l'électrophorèse capillaire MINICAP® (Sebia) pour le diagnostic des hémoglobinopathies au CHU de Nancy. In: Sciences Pharmaceutiques. 2014; ffhal-01733413ff. p. 25

[34] Guerard V. Mise en place de l'électrophorèse capillaire MINICAP® (Sebia) pour le diagnostic des hémoglobinopathies au CHU de Nancy. In: Sciences Pharmaceutiques. 2014; ffhal-01733413ff. p. 34

[35] WHO Library. Procurement Process: A Practical Guide. Geneva; 2012. p. 7

[36] WHO. Press Release. 20 February 2019. Available from: https://www.who.int/fr/news-room/detail/20-02-2019-countries-are-spending-more-on-health-but-people-are-still-paying-too-much-out-of-their-own-pockets

[37] Mulunda-a-Mulunda V et al. Pérennisation des investissements en équipements biomédicaux dans les projets scientifiques. IRBM News. 2018; **39**(4–5):80-89

Chapter 10

Accuracy of Blood Group Typing in the Management and Prevention of Alloimmunization

Emilia Sippert, Evgeniya Volkova and Maria Rios

Abstract

Blood transfusion is an effective therapeutic approach for several hematological conditions including sickle cell disease (SCD), thalassaemia, myelodysplastic syndrome (MDS), and autoimmune hemolytic anemia. It is also often indicated for transplantation and for patients receiving medical treatments for cancer. However, transfusion treatment can lead to the red blood cell (RBC) alloimmunization when an incompatible antigen is inadvertently present in the transfused blood. Alloantibodies can cause RBC destruction and many other complications defeating the purpose of the treatment. The risk of development of multiple alloantibodies increases with the frequency of transfusions in transfusion-dependent patients and can be mitigated by transfusing blood type negative for multiple antigens to prevent hemolysis. This chapter discusses the transfusion's risk of RBC alloimmunization as an adverse event; consequences of alloimmunization in patients' care; approaches to prevent and/or mitigate alloimmunization and enhance transfusion efficacy; application of RBC genotyping to supplement serology for preventing alloimmunization. The currently available techniques for RBC genotyping and the importance of reference reagents for determining the genotyping accuracy will also be discussed.

Keywords: blood transfusion, RBC alloimmunization, blood groups, blood group genotyping, reference materials

1. Introduction

Blood transfusion saves lives in trauma situations and serves as a unique therapeutic treatment of various hematologic disorders where patients require lifelong regular transfusions to survive. However, in contrast to therapeutic drugs, blood cannot be manufactured and tested for quality control of purity, potency, and efficacy. Instead, each donation is a unique batch, most often single use, for which all characterization and quality assessment need to be performed individually even if several units are used in a single treatment. Since blood is a biological product, safety assessment must be done at multiple levels, including donor screening, blood collection, testing for infectious agents, blood cell typing and labeling. Checkpoints and quality control are also required at the time of transfusion to avoid human error and to guarantee that the right blood goes to the right person. Each step has its own characteristics and challenges. Screening involves the review of donor history that allows assessment for safety; requirements that need to be followed for blood collection to assure proper timing, storage, and processing so that the quality of the product is not compromised; testing for infectious agents ensures a second layer of screening for pathogens that could be transmitted to the patient with an infected blood unit; testing for blood cell typing helps to avoid improper usage of the product since non-compatible blood can produce serious consequences and even fatalities; lastly, the transfusion process itself requires strict checkpoints to prevent the use of an incompatible unit in a given patient.

The scope of this chapter focuses on blood group typing and approaches to achieve better management and prevention of alloimmunization. We will provide an overview on the following topics: blood transfusion and risk of RBC alloimmunization; approaches for prevention of alloimmunization and improvement of transfusion therapy; serology and molecular typing methods and their use for RBC matching; current technologies for RBC genotyping; and standards for red cell antigens typing including scope, importance, and description of reference reagents available for use.

2. Blood transfusion and risk of RBC alloimmunization

RBC transfusion is used for therapeutic treatment of various hematologic disorders including SCD, thalassaemia, MDS, autoimmune hemolytic anemia, and others. Management of patients may require lifelong regular transfusions for treatment of symptomatic anemia and prevention of disease complications. Although transfusion safety and donor-patient matching have improved over the years, RBC alloimmunization, transmission of infections, and iron overload are still a concern [1].

RBC alloimmunization is a serious adverse event of transfusions and can cause further clinical problems in the patients including worsening of anemia, development of autoantibodies, acute or delayed hemolytic transfusion reactions (DHTR), bystander hemolysis, organ failure, and cause serious complications during pregnancies. Frequent transfusions can lead to the production of multiple alloantibodies, which is often associated with autoantibodies requiring extensive serological workups and additional transfusions for proper treatment, increasing time and resources to find compatible RBC units [2].

Antibodies against ABO blood group antigens are naturally produced, IgM class, and are capable of rapid induction of intravascular destruction of RBCs by complement-mediated mechanism. Clinical outcome of a patient transfused with incompatible ABO blood can vary from no adverse effects to permanent organ damage and death depending on the volume of ABO-incompatible RBC transfused. As for non-ABO blood groups, clinically significant antibodies against non-ABO antigens are from IgG class and rarely activate complement. Instead, they cause DHTR or hemolytic disease of fetus and newborn (HDFN) by extravascular destruction of RBCs marked with IgG [3]. DHTR has been ranked as second or third most commonly reported cause of fatal transfusion reactions secondary to non-ABO antibodies in many countries including the United States [4–8]. However, experts believe that DHTR has been under-recognized or under-reported to biovigilance agencies and FDA, possibly because the reactions can be obscured by underlying disease (liver disease, massive trauma, and SCD), lack of knowledge among clinicians regarding the reactions, or lack of knowledge regarding the mechanism of reporting [7].

Reported RBC alloimmunization rates have considerable variations depending on the population and disease studied [9]. The rates are estimated between 1 and 3% in patients that receive episodic transfusions, while for patients who receive chronic blood transfusions like patients with SCD and MDS, rates vary between 8 and 76% [9–12]. Although the most commonly observed alloantibodies of clinical relevance are against antigens belonging to RH (D, C, c, E, e), KEL (K, k, Js^a, Kp^a), JK (Jk^a, Jk^b), FY (Fy^a, Fy^b), and MNS (M, S, s) blood group systems [9], alloantibodies against Rh variants [13–15] and other rare blood group phenotypes have also been implicated in shortened survival of transfused RBCs by causing DHTR [13, 16] or HDFN [17]. In addition, some antibodies only have occasional reports of being clinically significant, that is, anti-Yt^a, -Ge, and -N or have no clinical significance unless reactive at 37°C, that is, anti-Le^a, -Le^b, -M, -N, -P1, -Lu^b, -A1, and -Bg [18].

The development of RBC antibodies is influenced by many factors including recipient's gender, age, and underlying disease. The diversity of the blood group antigen expression among the donor and patient populations contribute substantially to the high alloimmunization rates [15]. Other factors that might be associated with alloimmunization risk have been actively explored in seeking novel strategies for prevention of alloimmunization [19]. Studies in both animal models and SCD patients have reported that inflammation is associated with higher likelihood of alloimmunization and it is suggested that the extent of the alloimmune response is higher when RBCs are transfused in the presence of an inflammatory signal [19–23]. Several studies have suggested that genetic variation in immune-related genes such as *TNFA*, *IL1B*, *CTL4*, *CD81*, *TRIM21*, *TLR1/TANK*, *MALT1* [24–28], and human leukocyte antigens (HLA) [24, 29] might be associated with susceptibility to or protection from alloimmunization. Importance of unit's age and blood product modifications like leukoreduction or irradiation has also been investigated but their impact remains unclear.

3. Prevention of alloimmunization and improvement of transfusion therapy

Prevention of alloimmunization is desirable for any blood transfusion; however, for patients not previously transfused or only having episodic blood transfusions, matching for all clinically significant antigens is not of great concern, but can result in alloimmunization against non-matched antigens. For patients previously transfused, particularly transfusion-dependent patients, the alloimmunization risk is higher and management of alloimmunized patients is of greater concern. Their alloimmunization status, including antigens of low clinical significance, is a critical part of their clinical history that may enable health care providers to take measures to prevent further alloimmunization.

As of May 2019, the International Society of Blood Transfusion (ISBT) recognizes 36 blood group systems. Of the 360 identified antigens, 322 have been assigned to a specific blood group system. These antigens have variable immunogenicity and not all blood group antigens are involved with the production of clinically significant antibodies after blood transfusion or pregnancy. Ideally, every blood transfusion should be compatible for the most clinically significant antigens in the RH (D, C, E, c, e), KEL (K), FY (Fy^a, Fy^b), JK (Jk^a, Jk^b), and the MNS (S, s) systems to prevent alloimmunization; however, the standard pre-transfusion cross-matching is only performed for ABO blood group and the Rh(D) antigen; ABO matching is performed to avoid acute hemolytic transfusion reactions caused by natural IgM antibodies against ABO antigens, and Rh(D) matching is performed because of the high immunogenicity of the Rh(D), which is implicated in DHTR and HDFN.

Currently, recommendations for partial and extended donor unit/patient matching are limited to specific groups including [1] patients on long-term transfusion protocol (i.e. SCD, MSD, thalassaemia, and aplastic anemia), [2] patients who have developed alloantibodies, and [3] patients with warm autoimmune hemolytic anemia.

Verification of compatibility for Rh (D, E, C, c, e) and K, which are the most frequent antigens involved in alloimmunization, is considered partial matching. Extended matching should include at least RH (D, C, E, c, e), KEL (K), FY (Fy^a, Fy^b), JK (Jk^a, Jk^b), MNS (S, s) and, if available, additional antigens.

3.1 Serology typing

Knowledge of the role of blood groups with their antigens and variants in alloimmunization was pivotal for the development of transfusion practices and medical interventions that require blood transfusion such as trauma, hematological diseases (e.g. SCD, MDS, thalassaemia, and aplastic anemia) and later for transplantation and cancer treatment.

Serology has been considered the gold standard technique for blood group typing for a long time. Serological methods detect the antigen expressed on the red cell using specific antibodies and can be carried out manually or by automated platforms. Typing of blood group antigens using this method is easy, fast, reliable, and accurate for most of the antigens. However, serology has limitations, some of which cannot be overcome when it is used as a standalone testing platform (**Table 1**). Scarcity of serological reagents for some blood group systems for which there is no monoclonal antibody available is a major limitation. In addition, human serum samples from different donors vary in reactivity, which is an issue when a nearly exhausted batch of reagent needs to be replaced. This is especially problematic when an alloantibody for that antigen is suspected to be causing adverse events after transfusion. In those circumstances, molecular methods can be used as an alternative or as a complementary test for identification of genes associated with the blood group antigens expression and prediction of antigenic profile (see **Table 1**).

3.2 Molecular typing

The identification of genes that encode proteins carrying blood group antigens and the molecular polymorphisms that result in distinct antigenicity of these proteins is possible using molecular typing methods, which facilitate blood typing

Serology limitation	**Genotyping application**
No available antisera, weak or limited antisera (i.e. Do^a, Do^b, Js^a, Js^b, Kp^a, Kp^b, V and VS)	Blood group typing can be easily performed by single PCR and/or high throughput platform
Mixed field caused by the presence of donor's RBCs in patient's sample (i.e. patients with recent blood transfusions) Presence of interfering antibodies (i.e. autoantibodies, multiple antibodies, antibodies against high prevalence antigens)	Genotyping is performed with extracted DNA from nucleated cells (e.g. leukocytes, epithelial). The presence of donor's RBCs or interfering antibodies in patient's sample does not interfere with the results
Presence of variant antigens (i.e. hybrid RH types, FY silencing mutations, MNS hybrids)	Detection of genes and molecular mechanisms associated with variant antigen expression
Detection of blood type of fetus at risk of HDFN without invasive procedure	Detection of blood type and zygosity on DNA extracted from maternal plasma
Mass screening for antigen-negative and rare RBC phenotypes	Use of high throughput platforms for donor screening allows mass scale typing and creation of databases

Table 1.
Benefits of genotyping over serology.

resolution in complex cases and overcome limitations of serological techniques when dealing with alloimmunized and multitransfused patients. In addition, molecular techniques have allowed identification of genes encoding clinically relevant antigens for which serological reagents are not available (see **Table 1**). In those instances, genotyping is critical to resolve clinical challenges.

Blood group genotyping is performed to predict blood group antigens by identifying specific polymorphisms associated with the expression of an antigen. Most variations in the blood group antigens are linked to point mutations, but for some, other molecular mechanisms are responsible, such as deletion or insertion of a gene, an exon or a nucleotide sequence (i.e. ABO, RH, and DO blood group systems), sequence duplication, (i.e. RHD gene and GE blood group system), nonsense mutation (i.e. RHD gene), and hybrid genes (i.e. RH, MNS, ABO, and CH/RG blood group systems) [30].

In contrast to serology, molecular tests are performed on DNA obtained from nucleated cells and are not affected by the presence of donor's red cells in patient's sample, which is a common occurrence in samples of patients with recent/multiple blood transfusions. Thus, RBC genotyping can resolve blood group typing discrepancies in multitransfused patients presenting with mixed field reactions, alloantibodies, or autoantibodies (**Table 1**). Also, blood group genotyping can substantially help patients who were not previously phenotyped and need regular transfusions by facilitating management of these patients and preventing alloimmunization [31].

Studies comparing serology and genotyping in multitransfused population such as patients with thalassaemia and SCD have shown that genotyping is superior to serology for resolving discrepancies [31–35]. Use of genotyped matched units has been shown to decrease alloimmunization rates [36], increase hemoglobin levels and in vivo RBC survival, and diminish frequency of transfusions [37–39].

3.3 Sickle cell disease

SCD is the most common congenital red blood cell disorder affecting millions of people worldwide with high mortality and morbidity rates [40]. It is considered a major public health issue by the WHO. Characterized by an abnormal synthesis of hemoglobin, this genetic trait is most common among people of African ancestry. Abnormal hemoglobin carried in red cells causes these cells to sickle (thus the name SCD), which as early symptoms produces swelling of the hands and feet, anemia, fatigue, and jaundice. Long-term effects of the disease include serious damage in spleen, brain, eyes, lungs, liver, heart, kidneys, bones, and/or skin that can accumulate over a person's lifetime. Patients can survive beyond their 50s, and most fatalities are not associated with chronic organ failure but occur due to an acute episode of one of the SCD complications. SCD can be cured by bone marrow transplantation, but only a few patients get transplant.

Blood transfusion therapy is part of treatment for SCD patients and it is mainly indicated for prevention of stroke and vaso-occlusive crisis. However, transfusion benefits are limited upon development of alloantibodies, a common adverse event of transfusion. The high incidence of RBC alloimmunization in SCD is multifactorial, but lack of blood group compatibility between donor and recipient is a key factor. This is more evident in countries where donors' and patients' ethnicities significantly diverge, that is, in North America, where blood donors are mostly Caucasians while SCD patients are predominantly of African descent; thus, SCD patients are frequently exposed to foreign antigens and, consequently, have higher risk of developing multiple alloantibodies.

Transfusion protocols for management of SCD and prevention of alloimmunization vary among the hospitals and transfusion services. In many centers that provide care to SCD patients, transfusions are phenotypically matched for RH

(D, C/c, E/e) and K [41], while others provide extended matching including RH (D, C, c, E, e), KEL (K, k), FY (Fy^a, Fy^b), JK (Jk^a, Jk^b), and MNS (S, s) in addition to the standard ABO and Rh(D). Less frequently, extended matching is performed by genotyping [36]. However, a wide range of institutions do not request phenotypically matched RBC units until the patient has produced an alloantibody [42].

It has been reported that antibodies against Rh antigens are the most frequently identified antibodies in multitransfused SCD patients despite transfusion from Rh phenotype matched donors [15]. The main reason for that is the high frequency of Rh variants in people of African descent. It has been reported that 90% of SCD patients and donors of African ancestry have at least one variant *RHD* or *RHCE* allele [15, 43]. The term "variant" is used when *RHD* and/or *RHCE* genes are carrying genetic alterations that may affect the RhD and RhCe protein expression. Variant alleles can encode weak and/or altered antigens and serological methods are limited in which variant Rh antigens can be identified and might not be reliable [44, 45].

The prophylactic RBC matching performed by serology typing, before exposure to RBC transfusions, can decrease transfusion complications in SCD patients substantially, but does not eliminate the occurrence of alloimmunization against Rh variants and other non-matched antigens that can cause DHTR [41]. Currently available molecular typing methods can predict several blood group antigens allowing a more precise RBC matching and can support transfusion decision-making. *RHD* and *RHCE* genotype matching particularly benefits SCD patients carrying Rh variants. For instance, SCD patients presenting D+ or e+ phenotype can make alloantibodies to these antigens despite receiving Rh phenotyped matching RBCs. The molecular analysis in such individuals may identify polymorphisms in *RH* genes responsible for the phenotypic alteration, confirming the alloimmune status of the antibody. In such cases, provision of *RH* genotype matched units or units negative for the specific antigen would be recommended, because the antibodies produced may be clinically relevant [13, 15].

An additional benefit of blood group genotyping on transfusion management of SCD patients is the capability of identifying silence mutations like −67T>C in the ACKR1 gene (Duffy gene). Patients carrying the mutation can receive Fy(b+) units, because the mutation only abolishes expression of Fy(b) on red cells but not in other tissues. The detection of this mutation avoids unnecessary use of Fy(b−) and increases the chances to find compatible units available even for highly restrictive matching.

Extended genotyping including Dombrock: Do^a, Do^b, Jo^a, Hy; Kell: Kp^a, Kp^b, Js^a, Js^b; Rh: V, VS; Colton: Co^a, Co^b; Cartwright: Yt^a, Yt^b; Lutheran: Lu^a, Lu^b; Diego: Di^a, Di^b; and Scianna: Sc1, Sc2 may help prevent development of clinically significant antibodies that can be potentially life-threatening.

3.4 Thalassaemia

Thalassaemia is an inherited blood disorder associated with a mutation in one of the genes involved in hemoglobin production resulting in abnormal form or an inadequate amount of hemoglobin. RBCs carrying abnormal hemoglobin do not function properly and are destroyed in large numbers leading to anemia. People with thalassaemia may have mild or severe anemia depending on the type of thalassaemia. Severe anemia requires regular blood transfusions to maintain the hemoglobin and RBCs levels, and to suppress the ineffective erythropoiesis but can lead to alloimmunization.

The prevalence of alloimmunization in patients with thalassaemia varies among geographical locations and may be related to the heterogeneity of population, transfusion exposure frequency, patients age, antigen matching policy, recipient related factors, and other factors [46]. The most common alloantibodies reported in these patients are against RH (primarily anti-E and anti-C) and K, followed by antigens of the FY, JK, MNS, and other blood group systems. Development of autoantibodies is also commonly observed in these patients. A policy for RH and KEL matching been introduced worldwide and its effectiveness has been demonstrated by the decreasing rates of alloantibody and autoantibody formation [46–48].

The *Thalassaemia International Federation* guidelines for transfusion-dependent thalassaemia published in 2014 recommends that all patients should receive prophylactic ABO, RH (D, C, c, E, e), and KEL (K) matched transfusions identified either with serology or genotyping. In addition, it is indicated that antigen typing should be performed using molecular rather than serologic testing if the patient had received transfusions previously [49]. However, surveys have reported that there is still a lack of adherence to recommendations and a large variation in transfusion practices for thalassaemia and SCD patients among the health care systems [42]. Some of the challenges for transfusion centers include difficulty in obtaining a reliable antibody and transfusion history and the lack of standards regarding procedures for phenotyping and transfusion matching [42].

Molecular typing has been introduced in several centers to confirm extended blood group profiles obtained through serological methods, however, it is not routine yet [31, 32, 42]. This approach is particularly important for thalassaemia patients because these patients are transfusion-dependent and, in many circumstances, might have received transfusions at hospitals with different transfusion matching policies, therefore the phenotyping might not be reliable.

3.5 Rare type blood donor selection

Alloimmunized patients require transfusion of RBCs that are negative for a particular antigen. Historically, serology methods, which are labor-intensive and time-consuming, have been used to screen for antigen-negative units. However, the standard practice is likely to change with the high-throughput platforms for blood group genotyping being approved by regulatory bodies and becoming more widely used. High-throughput platforms allow identification of a higher number of antigens compared with serology, increasing the availability of blood characterized for clinically relevant antigens.

The implementation of RBC mass scale genotyping for donor screening has started in blood centers, especially in large collecting facilities [50–53]. The successful establishment of a blood group genotype database has already been accomplished aiming to fulfill antigen-negative requests, especially for SCD patients receiving regular transfusions, and to create an inventory of frozen red cell units with rare blood types [51]. The refereed database comprises 43,066 non-Caucasian blood donors genotyped for 32 single nucleotide polymorphisms, related to the expression of 42 blood group antigens. The report showed that within 4 years of starting RBC genotyping, the blood group antigen database generated on blood donors was fivefold larger than that obtained by serology methods over 30 years. In addition, most antigen-negative units requests to that center were met using exclusively the genotyping database.

Strategies for finding units to fulfill transfusion requests for SCD patients have included RBC genotyping of non-Caucasian blood donors and donors with altered Rh antigen expression [54, 55]. The genotyping selection of donors with a genetic background similar to that of SCD patients' increases the chances of finding compatible blood for these patients, including RH-genotype matching. However, the low percentage of blood donors with African ethnic background combined with the cost of genotyping are limiting factors for widespread use of extended RBC genotyping matching strategy.

4. Molecular testing: current technologies

Polymerase chain reaction (PCR) and further advancements in molecular methods such as DNA sequencing and recombinant DNA technology allowed elucidation of the molecular basis of most of the blood group antigens and subsequent use of molecular techniques employed for blood group genotyping initially as in-house assays or laboratory developed tests (LDT) and later as commercially available assays.

While molecular basis for many of the blood group systems is relatively straightforward, with two antithetical alleles differing by a single nucleotide polymorphism (SNP) and responsible for one of the two possible phenotypes, some blood group systems are very complex. RH blood group system has over 50 antigens described

Name/manufacturer	Principle	Number of polymorphisms/antigens identified
Immucor PreciseType HEA Molecular BeadChip Test#,$ [56] BioArray Solutions	Multiplex PCR followed by hybridization of amplified DNA to probes attached to spectrally distinguishable beads and elongation	24 polymorphisms associated with 38 antigens plus phenotypic variants and Hemoglobin S
BioArray RHCE and RHD BeadChip$ [57] BioArray Solutions	Multiplex PCR followed by hybridization of amplified DNA to probes attached to spectrally distinguishable beads and elongation	35+ *RHCE* variants; 80+ *RHD* variants
ID CORE XT#,$ [58] Progenika Biopharma	Multiplex biotinylating PCR followed by hybridization to probes on color-coded microspheres	29 polymorphisms associated with 37 antigens and phenotypic variants
ID RHD XT$ [59] Progenika Biopharma	Multiplex biotinylating PCR followed by hybridization to probes coupled to color-coded microspheres	6 *RHD* variants and HPA-1
Hemo ID DQS Panel$ [60, 61] Agena Bioscience	Multiplex end-point PCR and single base primer extension	101 antigens associated with 16 systems, and 23 platelet and neutrophil antigens, in modules
HIFI Blood 96$ [62] AXO Science	Automated multiplex PCR and microarray-based assay	15 polymorphisms associated with 24 antigens
RBC-FluoGene vERYfy eXtend$ [63] inno-train diagnostik GMBH	Automated TaqMan-based assay	70 antigens and phenotypic variants associated with 12 systems
RBC-ReadyGene$ [64] inno-train diagnostik GMBH	PCR-SSP-based assay	16 modules encompassing antigens and variant phenotypes within 13 systems
TaqMan genotyping on OpenArray [65, 66] BioTrove	Nanofluidic TaqMan assays performed in OpenArray plates	16, 32 or 64 assays (custom designed)
Pre-designed TaqMan assays Thermo Fisher Scientific	Real-time allelic discrimination PCR	Polymorphisms associated with 8 systems

#*FDA approved.*
$*CE mark certification.*

Table 2.
Commercial solutions available for blood group genotyping.

Name	Principle	Number of polymorphisms/ antigens identified
Multiplex PCR-single-strand conformation polymorphism (SSCP) analysis [67]	Denaturation of PCR product followed by fragment analysis in polyacrylamide gel	9 polymorphisms associated with 1 blood group
PCR-RFLP [68–74]	Amplification of target sequence followed by enzyme digestion (PCR-RFLP)	Varies
PCR-SSP [75–77]	Amplification of single alleles using allele-specific primers	Singleplex or multiplex
Multiplex-PCR [78, 79]	Amplification with multiple primers followed by gel electrophoresis	Polymorphisms associated with 6 exons of *RHD*
Quantitative multiplex PCR of short fluorescent fragments (QMPSF) [80]	Amplification of multiple targets using both specific and universal-FAM-labeled primers detected by electrophoresis	10 exons of both *RHD* and *RHCE*
Denaturing high-performance liquid chromatography (DHPLC) analysis [81]	Amplification followed by enrichment with a known sample and DHPLC analysis	Entire *RHD* gene
Multiplex ligation-dependent probe amplification (MLPA) [82]	MLPA probes hybridized to DNA target sequence followed by fragment amplification and detection	48 alleles encoding blood group antigens and 112 variant alleles of 18 blood groups
GenomeLab SNPStream [83]	Multiplex PCR followed by single-nucleotide extension and hybridization to complementary oligonucleotides	12 polymorphisms associated with 6 blood groups and platelet antigens
High-resolution melting analysis [84, 85]	PCR with gene-specific primers and probes followed by melting curve analysis	Various—customized
Single nucleotide primer extension minisequencing assay (SNaPshot) [86]	Multiplex PCR followed by SNaPshot reaction and fragment analysis	Various—customized
Microsphere-based array [87]	Multiplex PCR followed by hybridization to probes coupled to fluorescent microspheres	8 polymorphisms associated with 6 blood groups
Multiplex PCR and DNA microarray hybridization [88]	Chimeric primers (specific-universal tag) are used along with fluorescent-label universal primers followed by products hybridization to a DNA array	Gene fragments of 19 different RBC and platelets antigen systems
Sanger sequencing [89]	Classical DNA sequencing of single fragment using dye terminators	Various—customized
Next generation sequencing (NGS) [90]	Sequencing of entire genome or specific regions. Millions of small fragments of DNA are simultaneously sequenced	Various—customized

Table 3.
Other techniques developed for blood group genotyping.

to date, more than 500 alleles, and 2 highly homologous genes that, in addition to SNPs, insertions, and deletions, may have hybrid configurations. Other systems with more than 50 alleles currently identified include MNS, Diego, and Kell. Genotyping strategies are often based on a SNP altering a restriction site or punctuating otherwise perfectly matched sequence for primers or probe annealing site. These approaches may be suboptimal for designing genotyping assays of complex systems and fail to reveal rare variants. Next generation sequencing (NGS) is the only method that can reliably detect the exact genetic composition of the site making it possible to predict the phenotype.

Genotyping methodologies vary widely and include labor-intensive techniques that are best suited to test individual samples for limited number of polymorphisms (i.e. PCR-RFLP and PCR-SSP), high-throughput commercial kits that are relatively easy to use (i.e. real-time PCR and arrays), and methods that require specialized equipment to differentiate between alleles in multiple blood group systems at once (i.e. NGS). Most of assays described to date rely on enzyme-mediated DNA amplification at some point in their workflow and on sequence-specific primers or probes (**Tables 2** and **3**).

At the time of this writing, several platforms have been commercialized, but only two commercial assays have been approved by the US FDA. Immucor PreciseType by BioArray Solutions was approved in May 2014 and ID CORE XT manufactured by Progenika Biopharma was approved in October 2018. Due to less stringent requirements to obtain the European Conformity (CE mark), this certification has been granted to most of the commercial devices described here (see **Table 2**). Commercial assays not approved by the FDA can be labeled and utilized for research or investigational use only. Some commercial platforms (such as OpenArray or GenomeLab SNPStream) are used to run LDT assays to increase the throughput (**Table 3**).

5. Molecular testing: standards for RBC antigens

The use of molecular typing for characterization of blood group genes has been steadily increasing in the last few decades due to the transfusion benefits for the patients, technological advances in molecular techniques, and expanding availability of mass-scale genotyping. While blood group genotyping is becoming increasingly used, typing errors have been documented indicating the need for quality control.

International Workshops on Molecular Blood Group Genotyping have reported discrepancies between laboratories studying the same samples indicating that there is room for improvement [91, 92]. As a genotyping test may only be done once in a person's lifetime, errors can have serious consequences. A major challenge in performing routine RBC genotyping is controlling for process variability of molecular assays that arises due to scarcity of reference materials. This limitation has been circumvented by using clinical specimen leftovers from previous testing, which lack proper characterization. Reference materials are critical for the development and manufacture of testing kits, for test calibration and for monitoring of assay performance.

Recommendations on which targets and recommended controls to use for prediction of RBC antigens have been published by international societies offering proficiency test programs such as INSTAND [93], The Consortium for Blood Group Genes (CBGG) [94], College of American Pathologists (CAP), and International Society of Blood Transfusion (ISBT) [91, 92] and also by The American Association of Blood Banks (AABB) [95] whose focus is on creating guidelines for AABB accreditation aiming to certify laboratories that perform molecular testing for red cell, platelet, and neutrophil antigens.

Molecular testing laboratories participate in accreditation programs to validate their activities. In the US, the requirements for AABB accreditation are described in the 4th edition of standards for molecular testing for red cell, platelet, and neutrophil antigens (updated in October 2018) [95]. According to the document, "laboratories shall use appropriate reference DNA to validate and control the reported test" and further, "the reference DNA needs to contain the target polymorphisms reported by the laboratory". The same publication lists the blood group alleles within 17 blood group systems that should be included in the reference DNA materials by the lab seeking to meet the minimum requirements for accreditation.

Various preparations have been used as controls to monitor performance of blood group genotyping assays, including synthetic DNA (such as PCR products, plasmid-cloned PCR products) and genetic material from human samples col¬lected and characterized for that purpose following standard guidelines [96]. PCR products and plasmid-cloned PCR products are simple and easy to produce and use as controls for SNPs, but they lack the genomic complexity of human sample and do not represent the clinical analyte (genomic DNA); moreover, the synthetic material can be a source of contamination for the laboratory if not carefully handled and well diluted. Although well-characterized human specimens are the best representation of clinical samples, they are of limited source and the replenishment may not come from the same donor. The alternative to overcome source limitation is to transform human cells into immortalized cell lines and use those for characterization and formulation of reference reagents. This approach has been successfully used to produce reference DNA using B-lymphoblastoid cell lines (B-LCLs), which are an appropriate representation of the genetic material of the donor [97].

B-LCLs can be generated by Epstein Barr Virus (EBV) infection of peripheral mononuclear cells from genetically characterized donors carrying specific blood group antigens and variants. The infection leads to proliferation and subsequent cell immortalization, providing an unlimited source of donor's genomic DNA. Once the B-LCLs are established, master and working cell banks are maintained in liquid nitrogen to ensure long-term survival of the cell line and continuous supply of the DNA. To produce the DNA reagent, B-LCLs from the working cell banks are expanded for bulk DNA extraction and subsequent DNA lyophilization. Tests on the lyophilized reagents are performed for assessment of their stability under accelerated degradation conditions and under normal conditions over longer periods of time as long-term stability. The material must be validated via collaborative studies with laboratories that routinely perform molecular blood typing.

The first DNA reference reagents for blood group genotyping developed using B-LCLs were produced in 2013 by the National Institute for Biological Standards and Control (NIBSC) and serve as World Health Organization (WHO) International Reference Reagents (IRR) for common blood group alleles found in ancestral Caucasians and Black African populations. The panel includes four DNA samples covering the most clinically important homozygous and heterozygous genotypes within RH, FY, KEL, JK, DO, and MNS blood group systems (**Table 4**). The material was validated in an international collaborative study by PCR-ASP or PCR-SSP, PCR-RFLP, Multiplex SSP assays, real-time PCR, Immucor Beadchip array, Progenika BLOODchip array, Luminex array, and 5′ Nuclease assay [98].

Additional cell lines were produced by CBER-FDA for use as source of genomic DNA for development of reference reagents to expand the number of red cell blood group polymorphisms represented in the first WHO IRR from 2013 for blood group genotyping. The CBER reference panel consists of 18 members, covering genotypes associated with 40 polymorphisms within 17 blood group systems, including alleles present in the existing WHO IRR-2013 except for *RHD*ψ* (**Table 4**). The CBER panel was also characterized and validated for additional genotypes belonging to systems already included in the WHO IRR-2013 (RH, KEL, FY, JK, DO, and MNS) (**Table 4**), and for additional systems only represented in CBER panel (ABO, LU, DI, YT, SC, CO, LW, CR, KN, IN, and OK) (**Table 5**) [89].

Participants in the international collaborative study to validate the CBER panel used traditional molecular techniques and additional genotyping techniques not available at the time of the first WHO IRR production. The most common methods

Blood group system	WHO IRR [98]	CBER RR [89]
Rh	*RHD* positive (zygosity not determined)	*RHD*01/RHD*01* (*RHD* homozygous)
		*RHD*01/RHD*01N.01* (*RHD* hemizygous)
	*RHD*01 N.01/RHD*01 N.01*	*RHD*01 N.01/RHD*01N.01* (homozygous *RHD* deletion)
	*RHD*01 N.01/RHD*ψ*	
	*RHCE*C/RHCE*c*	*RHCE*C/RHCE*c* (307T/C; 109 bp intron 2 ins present)
	*RHCE*C/RHCE*C*	*RHCE*C/RHCE*C* (307T/T; 109 bp intron 2 ins present)
	*RHCE*c/RHCE*c*	*RHCE*c/RHCE*c* (307C/C; 109 bp intron 2 ins absent)
	*RHCE*E/RHCE*e*	*RHCE*E/RHCE*e* (676C/G)
	*RHCE*e/RHCE*e*	*RHCE*e/RHCE*e* (676G/G)
		Additional polymorphisms:
		***RHCE* c. 122A>G (genotypes A/A; A/G)**
		***RHCE* c. 106G>A (genotype G/G)**
		***RHCE* c. 733C>G (genotype G/C; G/G; C/C)**
		***RHCE* c. 1006G>T (genotype G/G)**
Kell	*KEL*01/KEL*02*	*KEL*01/KEL*02* (578T/C)
	*KEL*01/KEL*01*	*KEL*01/KEL*01* (578T/T)
	*KEL*02/KEL*02*	*KEL*02/KEL*02* (578C/C)
		Additional polymorphisms:
		***KEL* c. 841C>T (genotypes C/C; C/T; T/T)**
		***KEL* c. 1790T>C (genotypes T/T; C/T; C/C)**
Duffy	*FY*01/FY*02*	*FY*01/FY*02* (125G/A)
		*FY*01/FY*01*(125G/G)
	*FY*02/FY*02*	*FY*02/FY*02* (125A/A)
	*FY*02N.01/FY*02N.01*	*FY*02N.01/FY*02N.01* (–67T/T)
		*FY*01/FY*02N.01* (–67T/C)
		Additional polymorphisms:
		***FY* c. 265C>T (genotypes C/C; C/T)**
Kidd	*JK*01/JK*02*	*JK*01/JK*02* (838G/A)
	*JK*01/JK*01*	*JK *01/JK*01* (838A/A)
	*JK*02/JK*02*	*JK *02/JK*02* (838G/G)
Dombrock		*DO*01/DO*02* (793A/G)
		*DO*01/DO*01* (793A/A)
	*DO*02/DO*02*	*DO*02/DO*02* (793G/G)
		Additional polymorphisms:
		***DO* c. 323G>T (genotypes G/G; G/T)**
		***DO* c. 350C>T (genotype C/C; C/T; T/T)**

Blood group system	WHO IRR [98]	CBER RR [89]
MNS	*GYPA*M/GYPA*M*	*GYPA*M/GYPA*M* (59C/C)
	*GYPA*M/GYPA*N*	*GYPA*M/GYPA*N* (59C/T)
	*GYPA*N/GYPA*N*	*GYPA*N/GYPA*N* (59 T/T)
		*GYPB*S/GYPB*S* (143 T/T)
	*GYPB*S/GYPB*s*	*GYPB*S/GYPB*s* (143C/T)
	*GYPB*s/GYPB*s*	*GYPB*s/GYPB*s* (143C/C)
		Additional polymorphisms:
		***GYPB* c. 230C>T (genotype C/C)**
		***GYPB* c. 270+5G>T (genotype G/G)**

Notes: Additional polymorphisms and genotypes included in the CBER panel are in bold; in parentheses are genotypes represented in the CBER panel members; descriptions of the polymorphism positions/genotypes are not available for WHO panel. For additional details see references [89, 98].

Table 4.
Alleles or genotypes included in the WHO IRR and CBER RR for the overlapping blood group systems.

Blood group system	Gene	Polymorphism	Genotypes included
ABO	*ABO*	c.1061delC	CC; C/delC
		c.526C>G	C/C; G/C
		c.703G>A	G/G; G/A
		c.796C>A	C/C; C/A
		c.803G>C	G/G; G/C
		c.261delG	G/G; G/delG, delG/delG
Lutheran	*BCAM*	c.230G>A	A/A; G/A; G/G
Diego	*SLC4A1*	c.2561C>T	C/T; C/C
Cartwright	*ACHE*	c.1057C>A	C/C; C/A; A/A
Scianna	*ERMAP*	c.169G>A	G/G; G/A
Colton	*AQP1*	c.134C>T	C/C; C/T; T/T
Landsteiner-Wiener	*ICAM4*	c.299A>G	A/A; A/G
Cromer	*CD55*	c.679G>C	G/G; G/C
Knops	*CR1*	c.4681G>A	G/G; G/A
		c.4768A>G	A/A; A/G
		c.4801A>G	A/A; A/G; G/G
Indian	*CD44*	c.137G>C	G/G
OK	*BSG*	c.274G>A	G/G

For additional details, see reference [89].

Table 5.
Genotypes from additional blood group systems covered by the CBER panel members.

used by the collaborators were PCR-SSP, either single- or multiplex, the HEA (human erythrocyte antigen), RHD, and RHCE BeadChip arrays from Immucor, Sanger sequencing, PCR-RFLP, and real-time PCR based assays. Less common methods included ID-CORE XT and BLOODchip REFERENCE by Progenika, MALDI-TOF-based assays such as Hemo ID from Agena Bioscience, NGS, RBC-Ready Gene and

RBC-FluoGene by Inno-train Diagnostik GmbH, droplet digital PCR, HI-FI Blood by AXO Science, SNaPshot, and high-resolution melting analysis (HRMA) [89].

6. Conclusions

Alloimmunization remains a major risk for transfusion-dependent patients for whom transfusion is critical for survival. The transfusion management of patients who have already been alloimmunized is still a challenge when rare blood types are involved, but for new patients there is a hope that genotyping will help minimize exposure, except for those very rare alleles which are hard to find. One approach to overcome this limitation is to create a database for rare and very rare RBC alleles where donor selection is based on genotyping and the donor pool is constantly enhanced and updated. The use of RBC genotyping for both rare donor selection and patient care is path forward in transfusion therapy and transfusion safety. The development of new assays and high throughput platforms will enable mass-scale genotyping at lower cost and rapid pace to select rare and very rare donors. The development and availability of reference reagents will allow better quality control in assay development and evaluation of performance and proficiency of testing by specialized laboratories making patient care easier and safer to provide.

Conflict of interest

The authors have no conflict of interest.

Disclaimer

The content of this chapter represents the authors' opinion and does not represent FDA judgment; therefore, it does not bind or obligate the FDA.

Author details

Emilia Sippert, Evgeniya Volkova and Maria Rios*
Office of Blood Research and Review (OBRR), Center for Biologics Evaluation and Research (CBER), U.S. Food and Drug Administration (FDA), Silver Spring, MD, USA

*Address all correspondence to: maria.rios@fda.hhs.gov

References

[1] Liu C, Grossman BJ. Red blood cell transfusion for hematologic disorders. Hematology American Society of Hematology Education Program. 2015;**2015**:454-461

[2] Brand A. Immunological complications of blood transfusions. La Presse Médicale. 2016;**45**(7-8 Pt 2):e313-e324

[3] Flegel WA. Pathogenesis and mechanisms of antibody-mediated hemolysis. Transfusion. 2015;**55** (Suppl 2):S47-S58

[4] Keller-Stanislawski B, Lohmann A, Gunay S, Heiden M, Funk MB. The German Haemovigilance system—Reports of serious adverse transfusion reactions between 1997 and 2007. Transfusion Medicine. 2009;**19**(6):340-349

[5] Robillard P, Nawej KI, Jochem K. The Quebec hemovigilance system: Description and results from the first two years. Transfusion and Apheresis Science. 2004;**31**(2):111-122

[6] Stainsby D, Jones H, Asher D, Atterbury C, Boncinelli A, Brant L, et al. Serious hazards of transfusion: A decade of hemovigilance in the UK. Transfusion Medicine Reviews. 2006;**20**(4):273-282

[7] Flegel WA, Johnson ST, Keller MA, Klapper EB, Khuu HM, Moulds JM, et al. Molecular immunohaematology round table discussions at the AABB Annual Meeting, Boston 2012. Blood Transfusion. 2014;**12**(2):280-286

[8] U.S. Food and Drug Administration. Fatalities Reported to FDA Following Blood Collection and Transfusion: Annual Summary for Fiscal Year [internet]. 2011. Available from: https://www.fda.gov/downloads/BiologicsBloodVaccines/SafetyAvailability/ReportaProblem/TransfusionDonationFatalities. [Accessed: 07/07/2019]

[9] Karafin MS, Westlake M, Hauser RG, Tormey CA, Norris PJ, Roubinian NH, et al. Risk factors for red blood cell alloimmunization in the recipient epidemiology and donor evaluation study (REDS-III) database. British Journal Haematology. 2018;**181**(5):672-681

[10] Chou ST, Fasano RM. Management of patients with sickle cell disease using transfusion therapy: Guidelines and complications. Hematology/Oncology Clinics of North America. 2016;**30**(3):591-608

[11] Singhal D, Kutyna MM, Chhetri R, Wee LYA, Hague S, Nath L, et al. Red cell alloimmunization is associated with development of autoantibodies and increased red cell transfusion requirements in myelodysplastic syndrome. Haematologica. 2017;**102**(12):2021-2029

[12] Guelsin GA, Rodrigues C, Visentainer JE, De Melo Campos P, Traina F, Gilli SC, et al. Molecular matching for Rh and K reduces red blood cell alloimmunisation in patients with myelodysplastic syndrome. Blood Transfusion. 2015;**13**(1):53-58

[13] Sippert E, Fujita CR, Machado D, Guelsin G, Gaspardi AC, Pellegrino J Jr, et al. Variant RH alleles and Rh immunisation in patients with sickle cell disease. Blood Transfusion. 2015;**13**(1):72-77

[14] Moores P. Rh18 and hrS blood groups and antibodies. Vox Sanguinis. 1994;**66**(3):225-230

[15] Chou ST, Jackson T, Vege S, Smith-Whitley K, Friedman DF, Westhoff CM. High prevalence of red

blood cell alloimmunization in sickle cell disease despite transfusion from Rh-matched minority donors. Blood. 2013;**122**(6):1062-1071

[16] Cooling L, Dake LR, Haverty D, Mullis N, Ellis S, Shayman J, et al. A hemolytic anti-LKE associated with a rare LKE-negative, "weak P" red blood cell phenotype: Alloanti-LKE and alloanti-P recognize galactosylgloboside and monosialogalactosylgloboside (LKE) antigens. Transfusion. 2015;**55**(1):115-128

[17] Mattaloni SM, Arnoni C, Cespedes R, Nonaka C, Trucco Boggione C, Lujan Brajovich ME, et al. Clinical significance of an alloantibody against the Kell blood group glycoprotein. Transfusion Medicine and Hemotherapy. 2017;**44**(1):53-57

[18] Poole J, Daniels G. Blood group antibodies and their significance in transfusion medicine. Transfusion Medicine Reviews. 2007;**21**(1):58-71

[19] Hendrickson JE, Tormey CA. Understanding red blood cell alloimmunization triggers. Hematology American Society of Hematology Education Program. 2016;**2016**(1):446-451

[20] Hendrickson JE, Chadwick TE, Roback JD, Hillyer CD, Zimring JC. Inflammation enhances consumption and presentation of transfused RBC antigens by dendritic cells. Blood. 2007;**110**(7):2736-2743

[21] Ryder AB, Zimring JC, Hendrickson JE. Factors influencing RBC alloimmunization: Lessons learned from murine models. Transfusion Medicine and Hemotherapy. 2014;**41**(6):406-419

[22] Yazdanbakhsh K, Ware RE, Noizat-Pirenne F. Red blood cell alloimmunization in sickle cell disease: Pathophysiology, risk factors, and transfusion management. Blood. 2012;**120**(3):528-537

[23] Zimring JC, Hendrickson JE. The role of inflammation in alloimmunization to antigens on transfused red blood cells. Current Opinion in Hematology. 2008;**15**(6):631-635

[24] Sippert EA, Visentainer JE, Alves HV, Rodrigues C, Gilli SC, Addas-Carvalho M, et al. Red blood cell alloimmunization in patients with sickle cell disease: Correlation with HLA and cytokine gene polymorphisms. Transfusion. 2017;**57**(2):379-389

[25] Oliveira VB, Dezan MR, Gomes FCA, Menosi Gualandro SF, Krieger JE, Pereira AC, et al. -318C/T polymorphism of the CTLA-4 gene is an independent risk factor for RBC alloimmunization among sickle cell disease patients. International Journal of Immunogenetics. 2017;**44**(5):219-224

[26] Tatari-Calderone Z, Minniti CP, Kratovil T, Stojakovic M, Vollmer A, Barjaktarevic I, et al. rs660 polymorphism in Ro52 (SSA1; TRIM21) is a marker for age-dependent tolerance induction and efficiency of alloimmunization in sickle cell disease. Molecular Immunology. 2009;**47**(1):64-70

[27] Tatari-Calderone Z, Tamouza R, Le Bouder GP, Dewan R, Luban NL, Lasserre J, et al. The association of CD81 polymorphisms with alloimmunization in sickle cell disease. Clinical & Developmental Immunology. 2013;**2013**:937846

[28] Meinderts SM, Gerritsma JJ, Sins JWR, de Boer M, van Leeuwen K, Biemond BJ, et al. Identification of genetic biomarkers for alloimmunization in sickle cell disease. British Journal Haematology. 2019;**186**(6):887-899

[29] Schonewille H, Doxiadis II, Levering WH, Roelen DL, Claas FH, Brand A. HLA-DRB1 associations

in individuals with single and multiple clinically relevant red blood cell antibodies. Transfusion. 2014;**54**(8):1971-1980

[30] International Society of Blood Transfusion (ISBT). Red Cell Immunogenetics and Blood Group Terminology [Internet]. 2019. Available from: http://www.isbtweb.org/working-parties/red-cell-immunogenetics-and-blood-group-terminology/ [Accessed: 08/06/2019]

[31] Shah A, Patel P, Patel K, Patel B, Jariwala K, Sharma P, et al. Comparison of serology and molecular detection of common red cell antigens in multitransfused thalassemia major and sickle cell disease patients. Transfusion and Apheresis Science. 2019. [Internet]. Available from: https://www.sciencedirect.com/science/article/pii/S1473050219301302?via%3Dihub [Accessed: 11/05/2019]

[32] Castilho L, Rios M, Pellegrino J Jr, Saad STO, Costa FF. Blood group genotyping facilitates transfusion of beta-thalassemia patients. Journal of Clinical Laboratory Analysis. 2002;**16**(5):216-220

[33] Guelsin GA, Sell AM, Castilho L, Masaki VL, Melo FC, Hashimoto MN, et al. Benefits of blood group genotyping in multi-transfused patients from the south of Brazil. Journal of Clinical Laboratory Analysis. 2010;**24**(5):311-316

[34] Bakanay SM, Ozturk A, Ileri T, Ince E, Yavasoglu S, Akar N, et al. Blood group genotyping in multi-transfused patients. Transfusion and Apheresis Science. 2013;**48**(2):257-261

[35] Kulkarni S, Choudhary B, Gogri H, Patil S, Manglani M, Sharma R, et al. Molecular genotyping of clinically important blood group antigens in patients with thalassaemia. The Indian Journal of Medical Research. 2018;**148**(6):713-720

[36] Castilho L, Dinardo CL. Optimized antigen-matched in sickle cell disease patients: Chances and challenges in molecular times—The Brazilian way. Transfusion Medicine and Hemotherapy. 2018;**45**(4):258-262

[37] Legler TJ, Eber SW, Lakomek M, Lynen R, Maas JH, Pekrun A, et al. Application of RHD and RHCE genotyping for correct blood group determination in chronically transfused patients. Transfusion. 1999;**39**(8):852-855

[38] Castilho L, Rios M, Bianco C, Pellegrino J Jr, Alberto FL, Saad ST, et al. DNA-based typing of blood groups for the management of multiply-transfused sickle cell disease patients. Transfusion. 2002;**42**(2):232-238

[39] da Costa DC, Pellegrino J Jr, Guelsin GA, Ribeiro KA, Gilli SC, Castilho L. Molecular matching of red blood cells is superior to serological matching in sickle cell disease patients. Revista Brasileira de Hematologia e Hemoterapia. 2013;**35**(1):35-38

[40] Kato GJ, Piel FB, Reid CD, Gaston MH, Ohene-Frempong K, Krishnamurti L, et al. Sickle cell disease. Nature Reviews Disease Primers. 2018;**4**:18010

[41] Vichinsky EP, Luban NL, Wright E, Olivieri N, Driscoll C, Pegelow CH, et al. Prospective RBC phenotype matching in a stroke-prevention trial in sickle cell anemia: A multicenter transfusion trial. Transfusion. 2001;**41**(9):1086-1092

[42] Fasano RM, Branscomb J, Lane PA, Josephson CD, Snyder AB, Eckman JR.Transfusion service knowledge and immunohaematological practices related to sickle cell disease and thalassemia. Transfusion Medicine. 2019;**29**(3):185-192

[43] Reid ME, Halter Hipsky C, Hue-Roye K, Hoppe C. Genomic analyses of RH alleles to improve transfusion therapy in patients with sickle cell disease. Blood Cells Molecules and Diseases. 2014;**52**(4):195-202

[44] Wagner FF, Ladewig B, Flegel WA. The RHCE allele ceRT: D epitope 6 expression does not require D-specific amino acids. Transfusion. 2003;**43**(9):1248-1254

[45] Raud L, Ferec C, Fichou Y. From genetic variability to phenotypic expression of blood group systems. Transfusion Clinique et Biologique. 2017;**24**(4):472-475

[46] Singer ST, Wu V, Mignacca R, Kuypers FA, Morel P, Vichinsky EP. Alloimmunization and erythrocyte autoimmunization in transfusion-dependent thalassemia patients of predominantly Asian descent. Blood. 2000;**96**(10):3369-3373

[47] Seferi I, Xhetani M, Face M, Burazeri G, Nastas E, Vyshka G. Frequency and specificity of red cell antibodies in thalassemia patients in Albania. International Journal of Laboratory Hematology. 2015;**37**(4):569-574

[48] Gupta R, Singh DK, Singh B, Rusia U. Alloimmunization to red cells in thalassemics: Emerging problem and future strategies. Transfusion and Apheresis. 2011;**45**(2):167-170

[49] Trompeter SC. A. Blood transfusion. In: Cappellini MD, Cohen A, Porter J, Taher A, Viprakasit V, editors. Guidelines for the Management of Transfusion Dependent Thalassaemia (TDT) [Internet]. 3rd ed. Nicosia (CY): Thalassaemia, International Federation N; 2014. Available from: https://www.ncbi.nlm.nih.gov/books/NBK269382/. pp. 28-41. [Accessed: 8/21/2019]

[50] Portegys J, Rink G, Bloos P, Scharberg EA, Kluter H, Bugert P. Towards a regional registry of extended typed blood donors: Molecular typing for blood group, platelet and granulocyte antigens. Transfusion Medicine and Hemotherapy. 2018;**45**(5):331-340

[51] Flegel WA, Gottschall JL, Denomme GA. Integration of red cell genotyping into the blood supply chain: A population-based study. The Lancet Haematology. 2015;**2**(7):e282-e289

[52] St-Louis M, Perreault J, Lavoie J, Emond J, St-Laurent J, Long A, et al. Genotyping of 21,000 blood donors in Quebec and RHD analysis. Transfusion Clinique et Biologique. 2010;**17**(4):242-248

[53] Perreault J, Lavoie J, Painchaud P, Cote M, Constanzo-Yanez J, Cote R, et al. Set-up and routine use of a database of 10,555 genotyped blood donors to facilitate the screening of compatible blood components for alloimmunized patients. Vox Sanguinis. 2009;**97**(1):61-68

[54] Gaspardi AC, Sippert EA, De Macedo MD, Pellegrino J Jr, Costa FF, Castilho L. Clinically relevant RHD-CE genotypes in patients with sickle cell disease and in African Brazilian donors. Blood Transfusion. 2016;**14**(5):449-454

[55] Prisco Arnoni C, Guilhem Muniz J, de Paula Vendrame TA, de Medeiros Person R, Roche Moreira Latini F, Castilho L. RHCE variants inherited with altered RHD alleles in Brazilian blood donors. Transfusion Medicine. 2016;**26**(4):285-290

[56] Paccapelo C, Truglio F, Antonietta Villa M, Revelli N, Marconi M. HEA BeadChip technology in immunohematology. Immunohematology. 2015;**31**(2):81-90

[57] Bioarray RHCE and RHD Beadchip [Internet]. Available from: http://www.immucor.com/en-us/Products/Documents/BioArray_RH_SalesSheet.pdf [Accessed: 08/28/2019]

[58] Goldman M, Nuria N, Castilho LM. An overview of the Progenika ID CORE XT: An automated genotyping platform based on a fluidic microarray system. Immunohematology. 2015;**31**(2):62-68

[59] Molano A, Apraiz I, Espana P, Azkarate M, Vesga MA, Rubia M, et al. Performance evaluation study of ID RHD XT, a new genotyping assay for the detection of high-prevalence RhD negative and weak D types. Vox Sanguinis. 2018;**113**(7):694-700

[60] HEMO ID Blood Group Genotypig Panel User Guide. Agena Bioscience [Internet]. 2015. Available from: http://agenabio.com/wp-content/uploads/2015/05/51-20004R2.0-Hemo-ID-Flyer_WEB.pdf [Accessed: 8/21/2019]

[61] McBean RS, Hyland CA, Flower RL. Blood group genotyping: The power and limitations of the Hemo ID panel and MassARRAY platform. Immunohematology. 2015;**31**(2):75-80

[62] Boccoz SA, Le Goff GC, Mandon CA, Corgier BP, Blum LJ, Marquette CA. Development and validation of a fully automated platform for extended blood group genotyping. The Journal of Molecular Diagnostics. 2016;**18**(1):144-152

[63] inno-train Diagnostic GMGH. RBC-FluoGene vERYfy eXtend [Internet] 2019. Available from: https://www.inno-train.de/fileadmin/user_upload/Produktflyer/englisch/Flyer_RBC-Fluogene_vERYfy_eXtend_QMS0418.pdf [Accessed: 8/25/2019]

[64] inno-train Diagnostic GMBH. RBC-Ready Gene [Internet]. 2019. Available from: https://www.inno-train.de/en/products/rbc-typing/rbc-ssp-pcr/ [Accessed: 8/25/2019]

[65] Hopp K, Weber K, Bellissimo D, Johnson ST, Pietz B. High-throughput red blood cell antigen genotyping using a nanofluidic real-time polymerase chain reaction platform. Transfusion. 2010;**50**(1):40-46

[66] Denomme GA, Schanen MJ. Mass-scale donor red cell genotyping using real-time array technology. Immunohematology. 2015;**31**(2):69-74

[67] Yip SP. Single-tube multiplex PCR-SSCP analysis distinguishes 7 common ABO alleles and readily identifies new alleles. Blood. 2000;**95**(4):1487-1492

[68] Hummel S, Schmidt D, Kahle M, Herrmann B. AB0 blood group genotyping of ancient DNA by PCR-RFLP. International Journal of Legal Medicine. 2002;**116**(6):327-333

[69] Mifsud NA, Haddad AP, Condon JA, Sparrow RL. ABO genotyping by polymerase chain reaction-restriction fragment length polymorphism. Immunohematology. 1996;**12**(4):143-148

[70] Rios M, Cash K, Strupp A, Uehlinger J, Reid M. DNA from urine sediment or buccal cells can be used for blood group molecular genotyping. Immunohematology. 1999;**15**(2):61-65

[71] Nishihara S, Narimatsu H, Iwasaki H, Yazawa S, Akamatsu S, Ando T, et al. Molecular genetic analysis of the human Lewis histo-blood group system. The Journal of Biological Chemistry. 1994;**269**(46):29271-29278

[72] Male DA, Phillips P, Turner DR. Improved polymerase chain reaction-based glycophorin-A M/N blood group allelotyping. Vox Sanguinis. 2002;**83**(2):170-171

[73] Rios M, Hue-Roye K, Lee AH, Chiofolo JT, Miller JL, Reid ME. DNA analysis for the Dombrock polymorphism. Transfusion. 2001;**41**(9):1143-1146

[74] Reid ME, Rios M, Powell VI, Charles-Pierre D, Malavade V. DNA from blood samples can be used to genotype patients who have recently received a transfusion. Transfusion. 2000;**40**(1):48-53

[75] Shao CP, Zhao CJ, Wu CL, Xu H, Wang XD, Wu XY, et al. Rh-matched transfusion through molecular typing for beta-thalassemia patients is required and feasible in Chinese. Transfusion Medicine and Hemotherapy. 2018;**45**(4):252-257

[76] Gassner C, Schmarda A, Kilga-Nogler S, Jenny-Feldkircher B, Rainer E, Muller TH, et al. RHD/CE typing by polymerase chain reaction using sequence-specific primers. Transfusion. 1997;**37**(10):1020-1026

[77] Rink G, Scharberg EA, Bugert P. PCR with sequence-specific primers for typing of diallelic blood groups. Methods in Molecular Biology. 2015;**1310**:71-81

[78] Maaskant-van Wijk PA, Faas BH, de Ruijter JA, Overbeeke MA, von dem Borne AE, van Rhenen DJ, et al. Genotyping of RHD by multiplex polymerase chain reaction analysis of six RHD-specific exons. Transfusion. 1998;**38**(11-12):1015-1021

[79] Intharanut K, Bejrachandra S, Nathalang S, Leetrakool N, Nathalang O. Red cell genotyping by multiplex PCR identifies antigen-matched blood units for transfusion-dependent Thai patients. Transfusion Medicine and Hemotherapy. 2017;**44**(5):358-364

[80] Fichou Y, Le Marechal C, Bryckaert L, Dupont I, Jamet D, Chen JM, et al. A convenient qualitative and quantitative method to investigate RHD-RHCE hybrid genes. Transfusion. 2013;**53**(11 Suppl 2):2974-2982

[81] Le Marechal C, Guerry C, Benech C, Burlot L, Cavelier B, Porra V, et al. Identification of 12 novel RHD alleles in western France by denaturing high-performance liquid chromatography analysis. Transfusion. 2007;**47**(5):858-863

[82] Haer-Wigman L, Ji Y, Loden M, de Haas M, van der Schoot CE, Veldhuisen B. Comprehensive genotyping for 18 blood group systems using a multiplex ligation-dependent probe amplification assay shows a high degree of accuracy. Transfusion. 2013;**53**(11 Suppl 2):2899-2909

[83] Denomme GA, Van Oene M. High-throughput multiplex single-nucleotide polymorphism analysis for red cell and platelet antigen genotypes. Transfusion. 2005;**45**(5):660-666

[84] Polin H, Danzer M, Proll J, Hofer K, Heilinger U, Zopf A, et al. Introduction of a real-time-based blood-group genotyping approach. Vox Sanguinis. 2008;**95**(2):125-130

[85] Tanaka M, Takahahi J, Hirayama F, Tani Y. High-resolution melting analysis for genotyping Duffy, Kidd and Diego blood group antigens. Legal Medicine. 2011;**13**(1):1-6

[86] Latini FR, Castilho LM. An overview of the use of SNaPshot for predicting blood group antigens. Immunohematology. 2015;**31**(2):53-57

[87] Drago F, Karpasitou K, Spinardi L, Crespiatico L, Scalamogna M, Poli F. A microsphere-based suspension array for blood group molecular typing: An update. Transfusion Medicine Hemotherapy. 2010;**37**(6):336-338

[88] Beiboer SH, Wieringa-Jelsma T, Maaskant-Van Wijk PA, van der

Schoot CE, van Zwieten R, Roos D, et al. Rapid genotyping of blood group antigens by multiplex polymerase chain reaction and DNA microarray hybridization. Transfusion. 2005;**45**(5):667-679

[89] Volkova E, Sippert E, Liu M, Mercado T, Denomme GA, Illoh O, et al. Validated reference panel from renewable source of genomic DNA available for standardization of blood group genotyping. The Journal of Molecular Diagnostics. 2019;**21**(3):525-537

[90] Fichou Y, Mariez M, Le Marechal C, Ferec C. The experience of extended blood group genotyping by next-generation sequencing (NGS): Investigation of patients with sickle-cell disease. Vox Sanguinis. 2016;**111**(4):418-424

[91] Daniels G, van der Schoot CE, Gassner C, Olsson ML. Report of the third international workshop on molecular blood group genotyping. Vox Sanguinis. 2009;**96**(4):337-343

[92] Daniels G, van der Schoot CE, Olsson ML. Report of the fourth international workshop on molecular blood group genotyping. Vox Sanguinis. 2011;**101**(4):327-332

[93] Flegel WA, Chiosea I, Sachs UJ, Bein G. External quality assessment in molecular immunohematology: The INSTAND proficiency test program. Transfusion. 2013;**53**(11 Suppl 2): 2850-2858

[94] Denomme GA, Westhoff CM, Castilho LM, St-Louis M, Castro V, Reid ME. Consortium for blood group genes (CBGG): 2009 report. Immunohematology. 2010;**26**(2):47-50

[95] American Association of Blood Banks (AABB). Standards for Molecular Testing For Red Cell, Platelet, and Neutrophil Antigens. 4th Edition ed: AABB; 2018 October 1. 2018

[96] World Health Organization (WHO) Expert Committee on Biological Standardization. WHO Technical Report Series. Recomendations for the preparation, characterization and establishment of international and other biological reference standards (revised 2004). 2004; Fifty-fifth report, Series No 932. 137 p

[97] Londin ER, Keller MA, D'Andrea MR, Delgrosso K, Ertel A, Surrey S, et al. Whole-exome sequencing of DNA from peripheral blood mononuclear cells (PBMC) and EBV-transformed lymphocytes from the same donor. BMC Genomics. 2011;**12**:464

[98] Boyle J, Thorpe SJ, Hawkins JR, Lockie C, Fox B, Matejtschuk P, et al. International reference reagents to standardise blood group genotyping: Evaluation of candidate preparations in an international collaborative study. Vox Sanguinis. 2013;**104**(2):144-152